AF556721

Arthroscopy:
Diagnostic and Surgical Practice

Arthroscopy: Diagnostic and Surgical Practice

S. Ward Casscells, M.D.

Associate Clinical Professor of Orthopedics
Thomas Jefferson University Medical School
Philadelphia, Pennsylvania
Attending Chief of Orthopedics
Wilmington Medical Center
Wilmington, Delaware

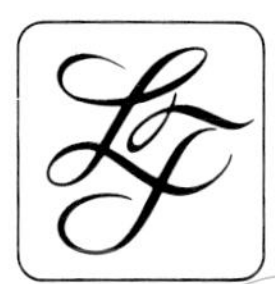

Lea & Febiger 1984 Philadelphia

Lea & Febiger
600 South Washington Square
Philadelphia, Pa. 19106
U.S.A.

Library of Congress Cataloging in Publication Data

Main entry under title:

Arthroscopy, diagnostic and surgical practice.

Includes bibliographies and index.
1. Knee—Examination. 2. Arthroscopy. 3. Knee—Surgery. 4. Joints—Examination. I. Casscells, S. Ward.
[DNLM: 1. Knee joint—Surgery. WE 870 A7866]
RD561.A77 1984 671'.582 83-11289
ISBN 0-8121-0888-4

Printed in the United States of America

Print Number: 3 2 1

To my sons who honor me by pursuing careers in medicine and to my wife and daughters who are tolerant and understanding of my neglect while laboring over the preparation of this book.

Foreword

"Ah, but a man's reach should exceed his grasp," said the poet Robert Browning. This seems to be the credo of most arthroscopists, who are still reaching, still exploring, and still seeking the better way to treat knee pathology. At times it appears that technique triumphs over reason; however, as arthroscopic surgery clearly is less traumatic, less costly, and often more effective than traditional knee surgery, mankind will undoubtedly benefit.

This text is a compendium of knowledge and skill that will not be surpassed for years to come. It truly is a state-of-the-art publication. Dr. Casscells and his co-authors were the original lone voices in the wilderness during the early years. Now diagnostic and operative arthroscopic procedures are routine in most centers. All these men have played a significant role in elevating arthroscopy from an interesting academic toy to a dynamic working tool.

History will probably confirm that the advent of arthroscopy is as great a contribution to orthopaedics as the techniques of internal fixation and total joint replacement. Although we have grasped much in the past few years, we are still reaching.

Toronto, Canada R.W. Jackson, M.D., M.S., F.R.C.S. (C)

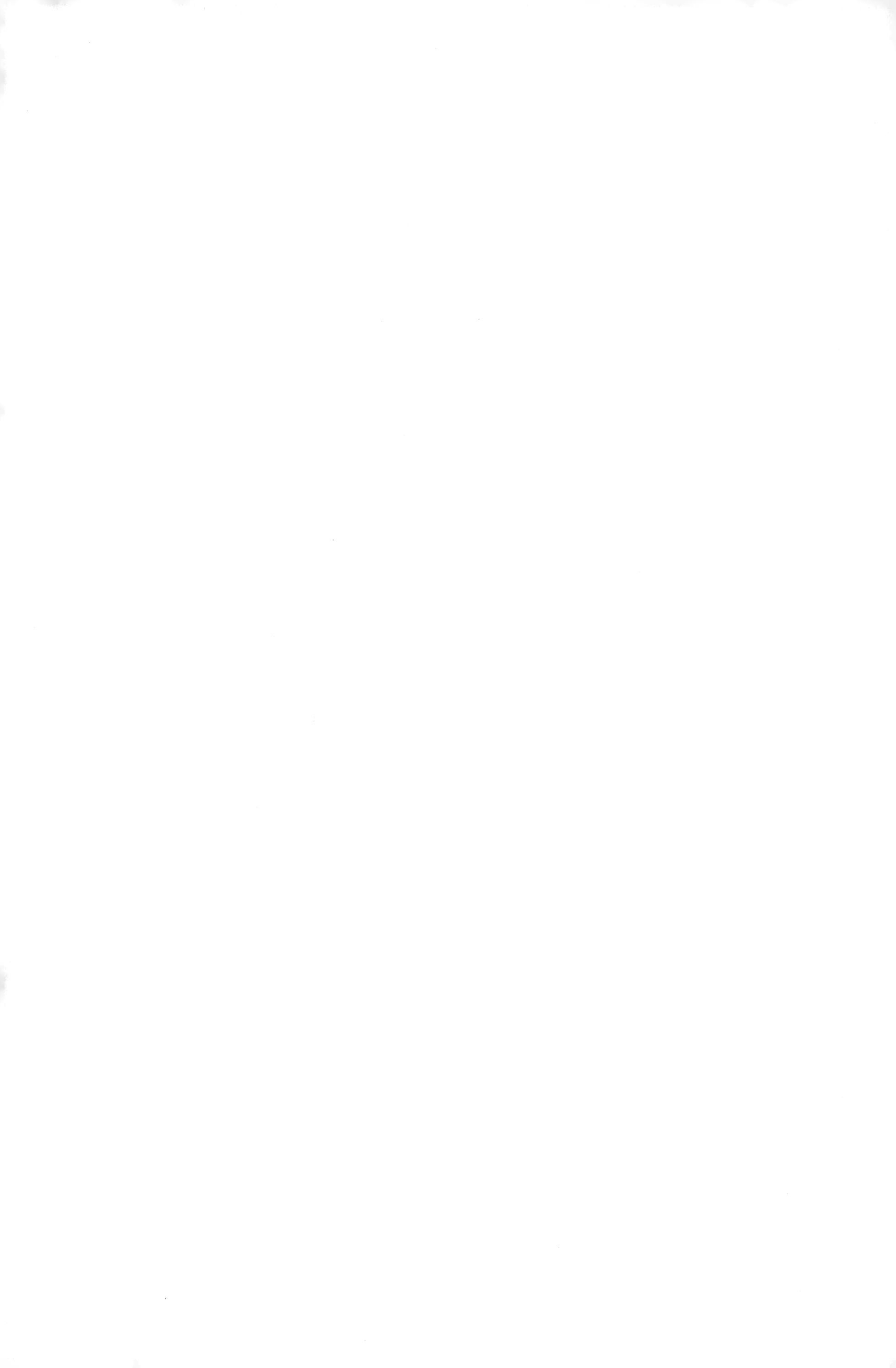

Preface

Probably, no area in the wide world of orthopedics has stimulated so much interest in the past few years as arthroscopy. This interest is evidenced by the plethora of courses given throughout the country during the past six years, virtually all of them oversubscribed. Many surgeons have taken more than one course because they have felt the need for more knowledge and more experience, having learned how difficult it is to put into practice what one has learned in only one of these courses. It is hoped that this book by experts will help to fulfill this need.

There has been such an explosion in this field of knowledge in recent years that subspecialties have been created within a subspecialty. As an example, only a few arthroscopists have had wide experience in treating osteochondritis dissecans arthroscopically. It is becoming increasingly obvious that no one orthopedist has acquired the experience to write knowledgeably on all aspects of diagnostic and surgical arthroscopy. The contributing authors to this volume are pioneers in the field, each of whose experience runs to several thousand cases, and they are writing on subjects in which they have the greatest knowledge and experience.

Arthroscopy has not yet found its proper place in the world of orthopedics. Espoused by many enthusiastically, it is still rejected by some, including not a few in academic circles who still feel that it is superfluous. This opinion will also change, if it has not already.

I hope that this book will help to establish arthroscopy in its proper place, used widely but not abused. As Dr. George Silver of Yale has so aptly stated, "medical technology is a good servant but a bad master." These wise words should be kept in mind by all who must decide when and if an arthroscopic evaluation of a joint is indicated.

Wilmington, Del. S. Ward Casscells, M.D.

Acknowledgment

I wish to acknowledge the invaluable help of the photographic department of the Wilmington Medical Center in the preparation of many of the illustrations.

S.W.C.

Contributors

Alan L. Bass, M.D., F.R.C.P (Edin.), F.R.C.P. (C.)
Clinical Professor of Medicine Emeritus
McMaster University
Hamilton, Ontario
Regional Director of Rehabilitation
City of Victoria, British Columbia, Canada

Robert W. Carson, M.D.
Clinical Associate Professor of Orthopaedic Surgery
University of Utah
Active Staff Surgeon
Holy Cross Hospital
Salt Lake City, Utah

S. Ward Casscells, M.D.
Associate Clinical Professor of Orthopedics
Thomas Jefferson University Medical School
Philadelphia, Pennsylvania
Attending Chief of Orthopedics
Wilmington Medical Center
Wilmington, Delaware

Lawrence Crane, M.D.
Clinical Assistant Professor of Orthopaedics
University of Vermont College of Medicine
Burlington, Vermont
Chief of Orthopaedics Emeritus
Maine Medical Center
Portland, Maine

Kenneth E. DeHaven, M.D.
Professor of Orthopaedics
Head, Section of Athletic Medicine
University of Rochester School of Medicine
Senior Surgeon
Strong Memorial Hospital
Chief of Orthopaedics
Monroe Community Hospital
Rochester, New York

James M. Glick, M.D.
Associate Professor of Orthopaedic Surgery
University of California Medical Center
Assistant Chief of Orthopaedic Surgery
Mount Zion Hospital and Medical Center
Team Physician
San Francisco State University
San Francisco, California

James F. Guhl, M.D.
Clinical Instructor of Orthopedic Surgery
Medical College of Wisconsin
Chief of Orthopedics
St. Francis Hospital
Milwaukee, Wisconsin

Michael Harty, M.D., F.R.C.S.
Emeritus Professor of Anatomy and Orthopaedic Surgery
University of Pennsylvania School of Medicine
Philadelphia, Pennsylvania

Robert W. Jackson, M.D., F.R.C.S.(C.)
Professor of Surgery
University of Toronto
Chief of Orthopaedic Surgery
Toronto Western Hospital
Toronto, Ontario, Canada

John J. Joyce III, M.D.
Clinical Professor of Orthopaedic Surgery
University of Pennsylvania School of Medicine
Senior Orthopedic Surgeon
Germantown Hospital
Philadelphia, Pennsylvania

Ralph T. Lidge, M.D.
Clinical Associate Professor of Orthopaedic Surgery
Abraham Lincoln School of Medicine
University of Illinois at the Medical Center
Chicago, Illinois

John B. McGinty, M.D.
Clinical Professor of Orthopaedic Surgery
Tufts University School of Medicine
Boston, Massachusetts
Chief of Orthopedic Surgery
Newton-Wellesley Hospital
Newton, Massachusetts

Vincent K. McInerney, M.D.
Director of Orthopaedic Education
Director of Sports Medicine/Human Performance Center
St. Joseph's Hospital and Medical Center
Paterson, New Jersey

Robert W. Metcalf, M.D.
Professor of Orthopedic Surgery
University of Utah School of Medicine
Salt Lake City, Utah

Nils Y. Oretorp, M.D.
Chief of Orthopedic Surgery
Central Hospital
Jönköping, Sweden

Dinesh Patel, M.D.
Clinical Instructor of Orthopaedic Surgery
Harvard Medical School
Assistant Orthopaedic Surgeon, Massachusetts General Hospital
Chief of Arthroscopic Surgery Unit
Massachusetts General Hospital
Boston, Massachusetts

George T. Shybut, M.D.
Associate in Orthopaedic Surgery
Northwestern University Medical School
Co-Director of Center for Sports Medicine
Northwestern University
Associate in Orthopaedics
Northwestern Memorial Hospital
Chicago, Illinois

John E. Tetzlaff, M.D.
Formerly, Resident in Orthopaedic Surgery
Hospital of the University of Pennsylvania
Philadelphia, Pennsylvania

Bertram Zarins, M.D.
Assistant Clinical Professor of Orthopaedic Surgery
Harvard Medical School
Chief of Sports Medicine Unit
Massachusetts General Hospital
Boston, Massachusetts

Contents

PART I: DIAGNOSTIC ARTHROSCOPY

PART II: ARTHROSCOPIC SURGERY

Part I

DIAGNOSTIC ARTHROSCOPY

Diagnostic arthroscopy and, perhaps even more important, arthroscopic surgery constitute what is probably the outstanding achievement in orthopedic surgery in the past decade. Almost universally accepted now, arthroscopy is indispensable to those who specialize in the care of athletes and is relied upon more and more by general orthopedists because its diagnostic accuracy in experienced hands is at least 20% greater than that of clinical diagnostic techniques.[1-4] Perhaps no other advance in orthopedic surgery was so long delayed. The articles by Burman, Finkelstein, and Mayer in the early 1930s provoked no surge of interest in the orthopedic world,[5] and even the authors themselves abandoned their early efforts. Although lack of sophisticated arthroscopes may have been in part responsible, the available scopes enabled these clinicians to make an outstanding, if unappreciated, contribution to orthopedic surgery. The same indifference greeted the early efforts of Takagi and his successor, Watanabe,[6] who developed the first practical arthroscope in 1960. Their efforts, however, did not come to the attention of orthopedic surgeons in other parts of the world until some years later. Although rheumatologists were among the early users of the arthroscope in the late 1960s,[7,8] orthopedic surgeons are primarily responsible for its development and progress.

Papers on the subject appeared in the *Journal of Bone and Joint Surgery* in 1971 by Casscells[1] and in 1972 by Jackson and Dandy,[2] and these were followed in 1973 by the first course in arthroscopy, organized by Joyce and Harty at the University of Pennsylvania.

The International Arthroscopy Association was founded in Philadelphia in 1974, and in 1975 the first course was given, under the sponsorship of the American Academy of Orthopaedic Surgeons in Boston, with McGinty as course chairman. This course was followed by many others throughout the country, and the trend continues. Despite the location of the first course at the University of Pennsylvania, arthroscopy, both diagnostic and surgical, grew up largely outside the confines of academia, and most of the pioneers in the field were physicians in private practice, an indication that all orthopedic surgeons are in a position to make a contribution to our specialty.

As with so many technical advances in surgery, problems pose questions to which we have inconclusive answers. In arthroscopy, some of the problems stem from the difficulty inherent in diagnostic and surgical arthroscopy as a skill, both to learn and to teach. Until as late as 5 years ago, there was a paucity of interest in arthroscopy, and the voices crying in the wilderness who advocated its use were lonely indeed. It has recently become evident, however, that many orthopedic surgeons wish to learn both diagnostic and surgical arthroscopy. As a direct result, the demand for courses on this subject has risen, perhaps because no orthopedic procedure requires so much experience for the learner to become proficient. Those with the greatest experience in this field now realize that many surgeons are unable to acquire the needed hand-eye skills, partly because the volume of cases needed to obtain the necessary experience is larger than encountered in many orthopedic practices. Those who contemplate arthroscopy would be wise to review the amount of clinical material available to them. Younger surgeons, whose minds are perhaps more receptive to new ideas and techniques, seem to learn more quickly.

In 1975, arthroscopy was underused, and needless arthrotomies were performed. The pendulum is now swinging rapidly in the other direction. The current tendency in arthroscopy is toward overuse. Some surgeons seem to be unable to distinguish between patients who are good candidates for arthroscopy and those who are not, and the trend is toward arthroscopy in patients in whom little likelihood exists of finding any treatable disorder. As has been pointed out,[9] the yield in any diagnostic test may be too low to justify the cost. In the case of arthroscopy, the cost is considerable. Walter Alvarez has said that "the average patient demands tests, plenty of them." This statement now applies to arthroscopy because, as a result of national publicity in lay publications, patients want the procedure to be performed on their own knees and are often unwilling to be treated by anyone who is not familiar with arthroscopy.

In this book, technique is discussed, but more important, it is related to the underlying disorder suspected, to the need for such a test, and to the benefits to the patient from such a test. That arthroscopy does not appeal to all who practice general orthopedics is fortunate, considering the learning difficulties. Many orthopedic surgeons, however, still wish to acquire the necessary expertise and perform arthroscopic examinations on patients in whom the likelihood of finding articular disease is remote. Just as the pendulum in arthroscopy has swung from underuse to overuse, so will it find its proper place between these extremes. I hope that this book helps those who read it to distinguish between patients who should be treated arthroscopically and those who should not.

REFERENCES

1. Casscells, S.W.: Arthroscopy of the knee joint: a review of 150 cases. J. Bone Joint Surg. (Am.), *53*:287, 1971.
2. Jackson, R.W., and Dandy, D.: The role of arthroscopy in the management of disorders of the knee: an analysis of 200 consecutive examinations. J. Bone Joint Surg. (Br.), *54*:310, 1972.
3. Poehling, G., Bassett, F., and Goldner, L.: Arthroscopy: its role in treating non-traumatic and traumatic lesions of the knee. South. Med. J., *70*:465, 1977.
4. DeHaven, K.E.: Diagnosis of internal derangement of the knee. J. Bone Joint Surg. (Am.), *57*:802, 1975.
5. Burman, N.S., Finkelstein, H., and Mayer, L.: Arthroscopy of the knee joint. J. Bone Joint Surg., *16*:255, 1934.
6. Watanabe, M., Takeda, S., and Ikeuchi, H.: Atlas of Arthroscopy. 2nd Ed. Tokyo, Igaku Shoin, 1969.
7. Robles, G.J., and Katona, G.: Arthroscopy as a Means of Diagnosis and Research; A Review of 80 Arthroscopies. Proceedings of the Fourth Pan-American Congress of Rheumatology, Mexico City, 1967. Amsterdam, Excerpta Medica, 1969.
8. Jayson, M., and Dixon, A. StJ.: Arthroscopy of the knee in rheumatic diseases. Ann. Rheum. Dis., *27*:503, 1968.
9. Casscells, S., Schoenberger, A., and Graboys, T.B.: Interpretation by physicians of clinical laboratory results. N. Engl. J. Med., *299*:999, 1978.

Chapter 1

KNEE JOINT ANATOMY

Michael Harty

Although the pathology, the biochemistry, and the biomechanics of intra-articular changes have been the subject of extensive research and publications, intra-articular anatomy has been a neglected and static feature for many years. The recent advances in the fields of arthroscopy and arthrography, however, have stimulated a renewed interest in joint anatomy and its variations. The arthroscope magnifies the viewing area from two to ten times, but this magnification in turn restricts and reduces the size of the anatomic field under inspection.

The region may be probed, photographed, and palpated, but the overall picture must be reconstructed and evaluated from individual pictures. A clear mental picture of the changes in anatomic relationships that occur during the full range of joint movement forms an indispensable adjunct to a precise diagnosis—the prerequisite to correct management.[1] The joint cavity is limited by articular cartilage and synovial membrane, which lines the fibrous capsule and may cover fat, ligaments, tendons, or muscles, all containing a rich and sensitive neurovascular plexus. The synovial membrane has recesses, pouches, and many folds or plicae that present an everchanging picture in direction, length, and tension during the full range of joint motion.[2]

Inspection and the palpation of bony landmarks provide the major orientation guidelines to joint anatomy. The flexor aspect of skeletal joints is covered by muscle masses and fat, which often contain the neurovascular bundle to the distal limb segment.[3] The more obvious bony prominences are found on the extensor and collateral aspects and are commonly covered only by skin and aponeuroses or tendons, thus allowing more accurate palpation and localization of the underlying joint anatomy. A loose articular capsule allows joint distension, which is essential for adequate arthroscopic visualization; however, separation of bone ends, also desirable, is often restricted by the reinforcing ligaments. At the knee, distraction strains on the lateral side allow 3- to 8-mm separation of the lateral condyles, but on the medial side the intact large, dense, tibial collateral ligament rarely allows more than 2 to 3 mm of separation.[4] The freely movable shoulder joint has a loose capsule that distends readily in the relaxed patient, but the normal, deeply placed hip joint is difficult to distract or to distend.

KNEE JOINT CAVITY

Situated between the longest, strongest, and most rigid lever arms in the body, the knee joint is exposed to a great number and variety of strains and stresses. It flexes from 0 to 135° and, when flexed, allows 20 to 30° of leg rotation, but it was never designed to permit abduction, adduction, or hyperextension. The patella, the femoral condyles, the tibial plateaus, and the fibular head present the palpable bony features, and the muscle masses include the quadriceps, the hamstrings, and the gastrocnemius.

In the extended knee, the sensitive infrapatellar fat pad bulges at each side of the ligamentum patellae, but it retracts during flexion into the intercondylar notch of the femur, to leave a lateral and medial triangle outlined by the femoral condyles, the tibial plateaus, and the edges of the ligamentum patellae. These triangles provide the usual sites for insertion of the arthroscope, but the menisci project about 15 mm proximal to the tibial plateaus and must be carefully considered.

The arthroscopist concentrates on the areas seen from the joint cavity, but without a working knowledge of some basic biomechanics and anatomy, visualization and interpretation of the intra-articular features and changes can be difficult and misleading.

PATELLA

The quadriceps femoris muscles converge onto the patella. Where two or more muscles with differently directed axes insert by a common tendon that plays over a movable bony surface, a sesamoid bone usually develops in the tendon, becomes incorporated in the joint capsule, and acquires an articular surface on its deep aspect.[5] The sesamoid bone provides a number of advantages: it directs the tendon pull perpendicular to the joint axis; it increases the length of the lever arm, thereby enhancing muscle power; and it ensures an adequate blood supply to a possibly compressed tendon. The knee and first metatarsophalangeal joints are typical examples of the development of such bones.

The large and powerful vastus lateralis muscle, assisted by the vastus intermedius muscle, pulls the patella proximally and laterally during the later stages of knee extension. The vastus medialis obliquus muscle (distal portion) counteracts this lateral pull. In well-developed, muscular subjects, the vastus medialis muscle reaches distally to the medial margin of the patella. The vastus medialis muscle has the most extensive direct relations to the joint cavity. It is the first muscle to show wasting in knee disorders and is the last to gain full functional recovery. In the distal thigh, the massive vastus lateralis and intermedius muscles lose their muscle fibers and become aponeurotic, thus allowing lateral release to occur in a bloodless, aponeurotic field. The medial and lateral patellar retinacula are aponeurotic prolongations of the insertion of the quadriceps muscles, but both present condensations that connect the patella to the femoral epicondyles and to the peripheral margins of the menisci, often called the patellofemoral and patellomeniscal bands.

LIGAMENTS

Many ligaments are derived from condensations of the adjoining capsule. They become taut at certain phases of joint motion, but at other phases are more relaxed. Ligaments maintain stability, direct the movements of joint surfaces on one another, and guide the surfaces into a congruent relationship for weight bearing. In the position of full passive extension, the patella is freely mobile, but the collateral ligaments and posterior capsule are tense. Knee flexion allows some relaxation of all these structures, except the tibial collateral ligament, which rarely permits much condylar separation.

The cruciate (crossed) ligaments placed in the center of the joint pass from the sides of the femoral intercondylar notch to the anterior and posterior margins of the intercondylar eminences of the tibia. They are intra-articular but extrasynovial. As these ligaments enter the intercondylar area from behind, they push the synovium anteriorly into the intercondylar space. The synovium lies directly on the anterosuperior aspect of the anterior cruciate ligament and on the upper posterosuperior aspect of the posterior cruciate ligament, outlining what the arthrographist calls the synovial or cruciate "tent." On arthroscopy, the distal three-quarters of the anterior cruciate ligament can be seen directly under the synovium. The proximal anterior aspect of the posterior cruciate ligament may be hidden by a subsynovial fat pad and possibly by Humphry's ligament. The proximal half of the superior surface of the posterior cruciate ligament, covered by the synovium, can only be visualized from the posteromedial aspect. The anterior (or lateral) cruciate ligament passes from the anterior intercondylar tibial area to the posterior margin of the lateral femoral condyle. The posterior (or medial) cruciate ligament passes to the anterior margin of the medial femoral condyle. Both cruciate ligaments contain two or three longitudinal bundles that are parallel in extension, but rotate on themselves during flexion.

In today's nomenclature, the term "intercondylar eminence" has replaced the old and honored "tibial spine." The eminence has a medial and lateral tubercle separated by a sulcus occupied by the anterior cruciate ligament in the position of full flexion. The anterior cruciate ligament does not attach to the medial or lateral tubercle; rather, it gains firm anchorage to the anterior slope of the intercondylar eminence. The cruciate ligaments control and limit anterior and posterior displacement of the proximal tibia on the distal femur.

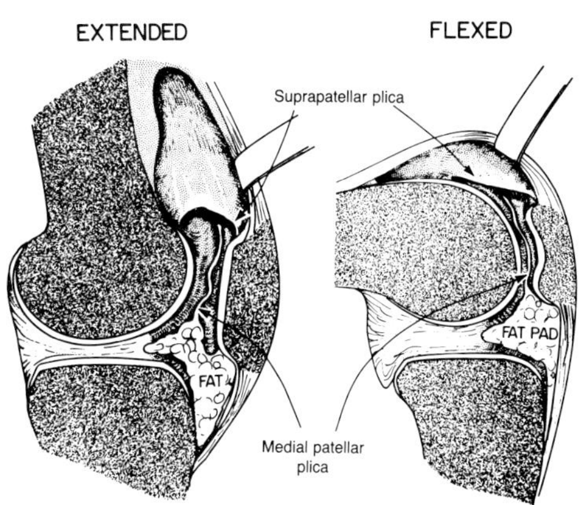

Fig. 1–1. Diagram to show the site and direction of the suprapatellar and medial patellar plicae during extension and flexion.

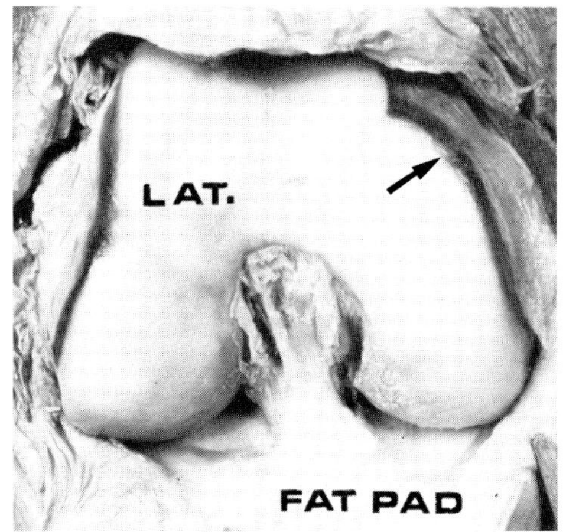

Fig. 1–2. View of distal right femur showing indentation on medial condyle and adjacent medial patellar plicae shelf (arrow) stretching distally to the fat pad.

SYNOVIAL MEMBRANE

The knee joint has the largest synovial cavity in the body. Embryologically, this joint is made up of three loculi: a medial and a lateral articular space and a suprapatellar bursa. The medial and lateral compartments are separated by the infrapatellar fold (ligamentum mucosum), which may remain as a single strand, a fenestrated partition, or rarely, as a total synovial fold. A complete suprapatellar septum persists in 8% of knees, but partial remnants of it are found in 80% of specimens. A constant wreath of synovial-covered fat surrounding the articular margins

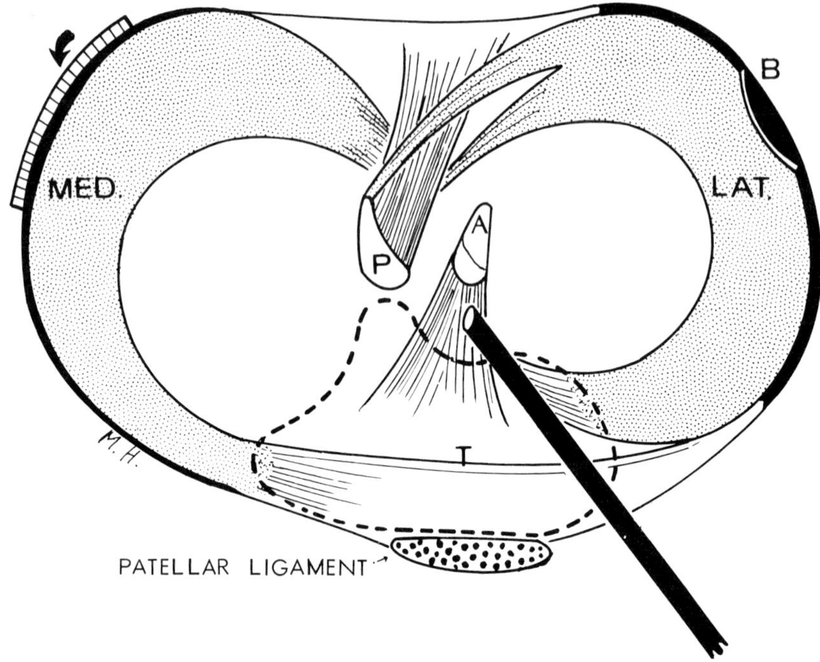

Fig. 1–3. Left knee. Diagram of menisci. The anterior (A) and the posterior (P) cruciate ligaments split the meniscofemoral ligament into anterior (Humphry) and posterior (Wrisberg) components. The area outlined by the heavy broken line is covered by the infrapatellar fat pad. The meniscal attachment to the medial ligament is indicated by the curved arrow, upper left. The popliteal bursa and tendon (B) are at the upper right. The transverse ligament (T) is below the anterior cruciate ligament. (From Harty, M., and Joyce, J.J.: Surgical anatomy and exposures of the knee joint. Am. Acad. Orthop. Surg. Instruct. Course Lect., *20*:206, 1971.)

of the patella is most obvious inferiorly as the infrapatellar fat pad. Additional folds or plicae are commonly encountered in the knee synovium. Current plica nomenclature recognizes (1) infrapatellar plica (ligamentum mucosum), (2) suprapatellar plica, and (3) medial patellar plica. The fat pad covered posteriorly by synovium fills the incongruous space between the intercondylar notch and the ligamentum patellae; it then fans and attaches to the collateral synovial walls. Like all intra-articular fat collections, this fat pad has a large concentration of sensory nerve endings and is therefore sensitive.

The suprapatellar plica, when intact (suprapatellar septum), separates the bursa from the joint cavity. In extension, it is directed horizontally and posteriorly from the superior patellar pole. During flexion, this plica is stretched over the femoral trochlea and adjacent condylar margins (Fig. 1–1). The medial patellar plica (shelf) is really a continuation of the alar fold ascending on the synovial wall to reach the medial suprapatellar area or the suprapatellar plica. When well developed, the medial patellar plica covers the underlying margin of the medial femoral condyle and may even groove that bone at the articular area demarcated between the patella and the medial meniscus (Fig. 1–2).

Like all serous membranes, the synovium is thin, smooth, glistening, and transparent, but in pathologic conditions it becomes thick, rough, dull, and opaque. These changes are more obvious in the plicae, which may be rough, thickened, frayed, or perforated. The free margin of a perforated plica is often called the chorda synovialis.

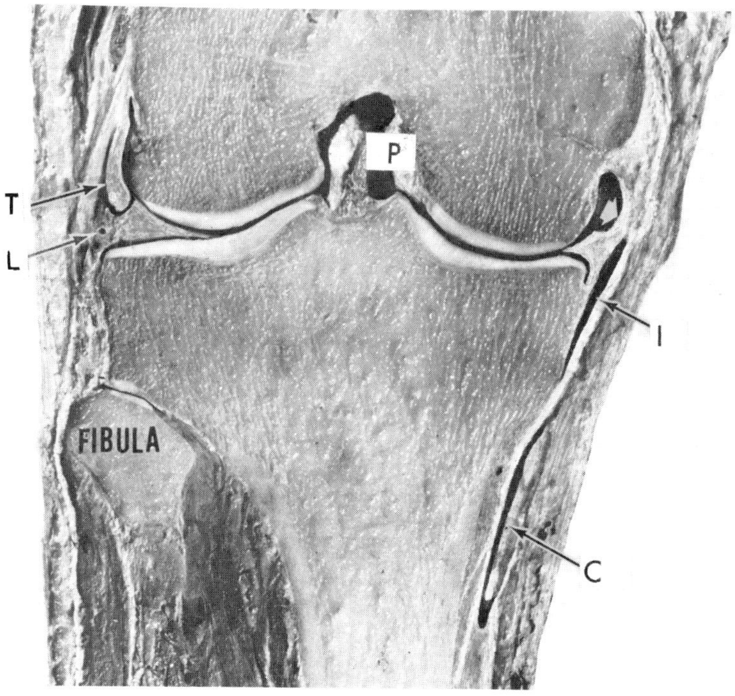

Fig. 1–4. Coronal section of left knee joint. Superficial and deep parts of the medial ligament are retracted (white arrow). P, Posterior cruciate ligament; T, tendon of popliteus muscle; A, lateral genicular artery; C, pes anserinus bursa; I, intraligamentus bursa. (From Harty, M., and Joyce, J.J.: Surgical anatomy and exposures of the knee joint. Am. Acad. Orthop. Surg. Instruct. Course Lect., *20*:206, 1971.)

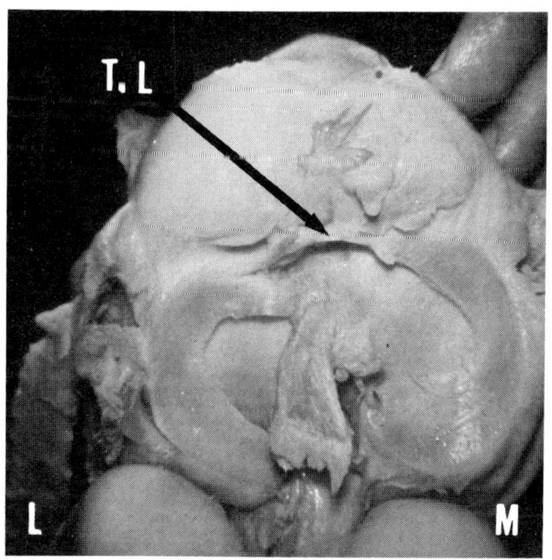

Fig. 1–5. The attachment of the anterior horn of the medial meniscus is variable. Commonly, it goes to the intercondylar area of the tibia and to the transverse ligament, but never to the anterior cruciate ligament, as does the lateral meniscus. TL, transverse ligament; L, lateral; M, medial.

MENISCI

The menisci are crescent-shaped, fibrous discs that occupy the incongruous areas between the femur and the tibia. Although often called semilunar cartilages, they are composed of tough, fibrous tissue with few cartilage cells. The ends of the menisci are tethered by fibrous horns to the intercondylar area of the tibia and are attached to the margins of the tibial plateaus by the short coronary ligaments corresponding to the meniscotibial capsule and synovium. The so-called long coronary ligaments connect the superior margins of the menisci to the chondrosynovial margins of the femur. They are concave superiorly where flexion and extension occur and are flat inferiorly where rotation takes place (Figs. 1–3 to 1–5). The menisci have a limited blood supply. Small vessels may be seen fanning outward from the anterior and posterior horns for about 10 mm, but in the central area, short vessels extend into the thick peripheral margin for only 2 to 4 mm from smaller vessels in the coronary ligaments. No vessels have been demonstrated in the thinner central regions of the menisci. The posterolateral area of the lateral meniscus is separated from the tendon of the popliteus muscle by a synovial diverticulum that may mimic a peripheral meniscal tear.

The advent of diagnostic and operative arthroscopy has again emphasized the major role that anatomy must play in reaching a correct evaluation of intra-articular structures and their variations under different functional circumstances. The arthroscope adds another avenue of exposure to the human eye, our paramount sense organ.

REFERENCES

1. Harty, M., and Joyce, J.J.: Surgical anatomy and exposures of the knee joint. Am. Acad. Orthop. Surg. Instruct. Course Lect., *20*:206, 1971.
2. Harty, M.: Synovial folds in the knee joint. Orthop. Rev., *6*:10, 91, 1977.
3. Joyce, J.J., and Harty, M.: Orthopaedic Approaches. Baltimore, Williams & Wilkins, 1961.
4. Harty, M.: Knee joint anatomy. Orthop. Rev., *5*:9, 23, 1976.
5. Walmsley, T.: Practical Anatomy. London, Longmans Green, 1938.

Chapter 2

PHOTOGRAPHY IN ARTHROSCOPY

John B. McGinty

Because arthroscopy is now an essential part of a thorough evaluation of the knee, and because arthroscopic techniques are becoming widespread in the treatment of intra-articular disorders, the need for documentation of arthroscopic procedures has arisen. To provide satisfactory documentation, proper photographic equipment and a knowedge of endoscopic photographic techniques are mandatory.

If the surgeon is primarily a diagnostic arthroscopist and prefers conventional surgical techniques for definitive management, a good photographic record will be useful when he returns to execute the surgical plan. No better way exists to approach an intra-articular lesion surgically than to know exactly what it is and where it is located. If a surgeon sees a small lesion in the knee and decides not to treat it surgically, an accurate photograph will help in assessing the knee if the patient's symptoms change. When consultation with another surgeon is required, a photographic record is of inestimable value.

The fields of arthroscopy and arthroscopic surgery are unusual in that peer review is almost impossible. When a surgeon claims to perform a particular procedure through an arthroscope, a person who has not looked through the arthroscope can hardly debate the surgeon's findings. Therefore, an accurate photographic record on film or on videotape can protect both patient and surgeon.

Liability claims have complicated the life of orthopedic surgeons, who are often called on to establish a cause-and-effect relationship between an accident and an anatomic abnormality or absence of it. Because these judgments are frequently made by nonmedical people, such as juries or workmen's compensation boards, photographic documentation of the pathologic anatomy can make the physician's role as an expert witness clearer, and one hopes that these decisions will thereby be more just.

Finally, photographic documentation is essential to arthroscopy, both with still photographs, including slides for lectures and photographs to supplement written texts, and with live video and videotape, to teach the new and difficult skills of arthroscopic surgery.

HISTORICAL BACKGROUND

The first development in endoscopic photography occurred in 1840, when Alfred Donné presented microscopic daguerreotypes to the French Academy in Paris. In 1845, Léon Foucault, a French physicist, published a microscopic atlas illustrated with copper engravings from daguerreotypes. In 1882, an effective method of photographing the larynx and nasopharynx by indirect laryngoscopy was developed by Thomas R. French of New York.

Max Nitze developed the first successful photographic endoscope in 1882 (Fig. 2–1). He used a rotating glass disc covered with a photographic emulsion that could selectively take the image from the cystoscope by movement of a prism while the operator viewed through an offset eyepiece. Nitze produced some astounding photographs in his *Cystophotographic Atlas*, published in 1894.

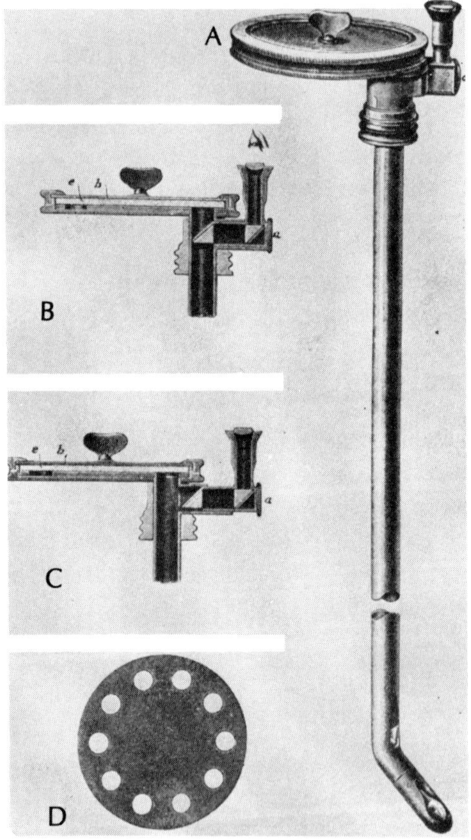

Fig. 2–1. *A,* **Photographic cystoscope developed by Nitze.** *B,* **The prism in the down position allows the image to pass to the eye of the endoscopist.** *C,* **The prism in the up position allows the image to pass to the photographic emulsion.** *D,* **Perforated disc of the camera. (From Medicine and early photography. Ciba Symp., 4, 1942. Copyright 1942, Ciba-Geigy Corporation. Reprinted with permission from Ciba Symposia by George Rosen, M.D.)**

Kenji Takagi, who developed the first arthroscope, in Tokyo in 1918, produced the first black-and-white arthroscopic photographs in 1932, followed by color photographs and moving pictures in 1936. Arthroscopic photography was further refined by Masaki Watanabe in 1957, when he developed an automated, 35-mm system coupling an Olympus half-frame with his No. 21 arthroscope. This development has progressed to reliable 35-mm photographic systems, fully automated to provide the surgeon with prints or slides for documentation and teaching.

Since the mid-1970s, television has become an integral part of arthroscopy, and particularly of arthroscopic surgery. Video cameras, first with black-and-white film and then with color, have dropped in size from four pounds to three ounces. Now most manufacturers have a video camera in their system or arthroscopic instrumentation. The ability to use a video camera directly coupled to the arthroscope allows the surgeon to operate directly from a video monitor and thereby involves the surgical team in the procedure, frees up a hand for the surgeon (Fig. 2–2), and provides an opportunity for instantaneous documentation on videotape.

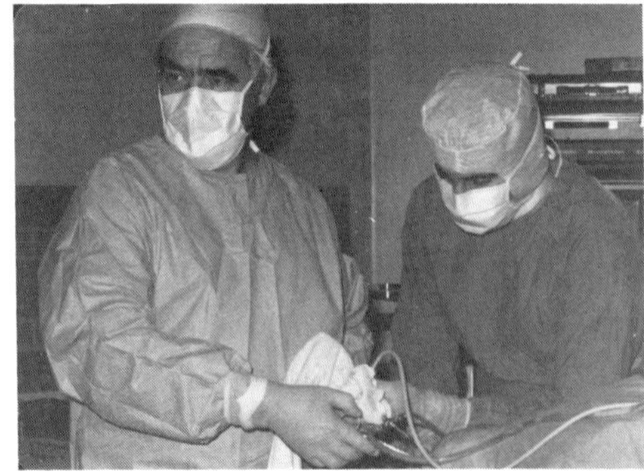

Fig. 2–2. The surgeon on the left holds the instrument with his right hand and concentrates on the monitor while the assistant on the right holds the video camera.

In the past decade in North America, we have progressed from crude diagnostic arthroscopy accomplished by looking directly into the telescope to arthroscopic knee operations aided by a magnified image on a television monitor.

OPTICAL PRINCIPLES

Every telescope has an optical point of reference called the exit pupil, at which the image is focused at its brightest point. The pupil of a camera lens is usually located behind the front element of the lens in the general location of the iris diaphragm. In the ideal arthroscopic photographic system, the camera's diaphragm and the exit pupil of the arthroscope are in the same plane. The camera's diaphragm is usually behind the exit pupil of the arthroscope, however. Therefore, the camera lens should be left wide open to allow the exit pupil of the arthroscope (usually 2 mm) to determine the diameter and therefore the brightness of the system. For example, with a 100-mm lens in the camera, the f-stop can be calibrated thus:

$$f = \text{stop} = \frac{\text{focal length of lens}}{\text{diameter of system}} = \frac{100}{2} = 50$$

The f-50 stop is a tiny aperture with the disadvantage that a small quantity of light reaches the film plane. Therefore, a large quantity of light must be delivered from the source, with high-speed film to allow a fast enough shutter speed to obtain a crisp image. On the other hand, this small aperture allows a tremendous depth of field, thereby creating essentially a fixed-focus system.

LIGHT SOURCE

Using present photographic systems in arthroscopy, electromagnetic energy from the visible spectrum is the basic element essential to recording images either chemically on film or electronically on television. The source of this energy is visible light.

Direct visual arthroscopic examination can readily be performed using a 150-watt tungsten light source. Satisfactory still photography with a 35-mm system is possible with such a light source, provided fast film (400 ASA) and a metering system are used; the surgeon can then photograph at shutter speeds of 1/8 to 1/30 second with minimal camera motion. The standard fiberoptic light sources using this type of illumination result in images of a warm color temperature. These images may also be less clear than desirable if the subject is highly absorbent of light, as is synovium, which requires a slower shutter speed and therefore a greater chance of camera motion at the time of exposure.

If high-quality photographs, such as slides for projection to large audiences or prints for publication, are desired, high-intensity light sources are advisable. In making high-quality videotapes, the color balance is the first to suffer if light intensity is insufficient. Therefore, when using television, equipment, high-intensity light sources are recommended.

Several types of high-intensity light sources are produced by arthroscopic manufacturers, all considerably more expensive than standard light sources. These may be high-intensity tungsten illumination (1000 watt), xenon arc lamps, or mercury vapor lamps. In some housings, a standard and a high intensity lamp may be interchanged by a switch.

Some manufacturers provide a strobe unit that can be fired through the fiberoptic cable. This unit must be calibrated, requiring bracketing exposures unless an automatic sensor in the camera quantitates the light delivered based on metering. This sophisticated system will probably be more readily available in the future.

In any fiberoptic system, approximately 5% of light is lost for every foot of cable it must pass through, and approximately 30% is lost at each connection. Therefore, it is best to have as little distance from the light source to the subject and as few connections as possible. Any light source has a color temperature that must be balanced with the film or the video system if acceptable color balance is to be attained in the final result. Tungsten light is usually around 3000 to 3200° Kelvin and must be balanced accordingly. High-intensity light sources, such as xenon or mercury vapor, are usually around 5000° K and require daylight film. Most video cameras have a control feature that electronically compensates for color temperature.

SUBJECT

The reflective properties of the subject to be photographed affect the amount of light that ultimately reaches the film. For example, the amount of light reflected from shiny white articular cartilage is considerably greater than that reflected from red synovium, even though the original light source is the same. This discrepancy can be compensated for by metering the light as it enters the camera and by controlling the shutter speed (explained in the next section).

CAMERA

Still Photography. Any high-quality 35-mm single-lens-reflex camera can be adapted to an arthroscope (Fig. 2–3). The camera should be aperture-preferred with a center-weighted meter capable of fully automatic, variable shutter speeds. The sequence of events is as follows:

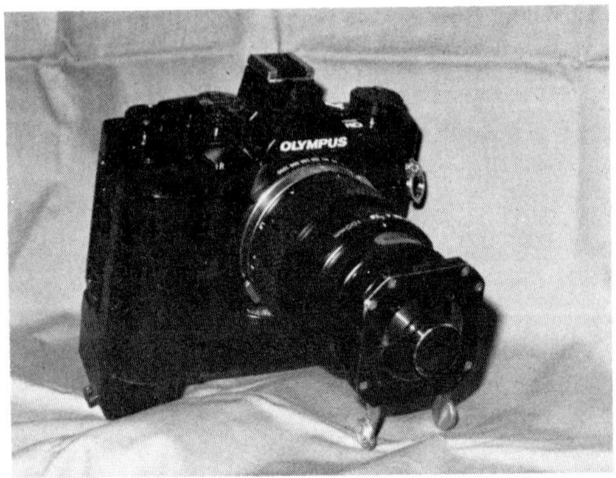

Fig. 2–3. A 35-mm camera, fully automatic (aperture-preferred) with motor drive, a 100-mm lens, and an adapter to couple the front of the lens onto an arthroscope.

1. The light from the light source enters the joint through the fiberoptic bundles around the arthroscope and is reflected from the object to be photographed.
2. The reflected light then passes through the telescope to the camera. The exit pupil of the telescope determines the diameter of the system and hence the f-stop and depth of field. Therefore, the lens should be set fully open, and the focusing mount should be set to the near point.
3. The light then passes through the camera's meter, which instantly determines the camera's shutter speed. The camera is set in the automatic mode.
4. The shutter is then tripped, and the exact amount of light is passed onto the film to record an image because the camera's automatic system selects the proper shutter speed for the film's ASA number.

Lenses. The most desirable focal length of lens is that which fills the negative with the image. The longer the focal length of the lens, the more light required to produce an acceptable image. I feel that a lens of approximately 100 mm in a 35-mm system is the best compromise. It fills about 70% of the negative. A lens greater than 100 mm requires too much light, and the result is diminished brilliance in the periphery of the image.

Having selected an appropriate camera and lens, the surgeon may then order an adapter to the telescope from the arthroscope manufacturer. It is necessary to provide the manufacturer with the diameter of the lens objective.

Accessories. Most 35-mm systems have an optional "data back" for their camera. This interchangeable back codes the film for identification. On the other hand, the surgeon can ask a nurse to photograph the patient's name and the date before each arthroscopic procedure. These data then appear sequentially when the film is developed, and one thereby avoids distracting numbers when a slide is projected.

A macrolens or a bellows with a strobe unit can be placed on the camera to photograph specimens or operative work during the same procedure.

A special back can be attached to most cameras to adapt them for Polaroid film, to obtain immediate prints in color or black and white.

A motor drive, available for most 35-mm cameras, permits the surgeon to trip the shutter and wind the film in one motion with one hand. The surgeon can wear an extra glove on one hand and take the camera once the circulating nurse has attached it to the arthroscope. Upon completing the photographic exposures with only one hand, the surgeon returns the camera to the nurse, strips off the extra glove, and is back in a sterile field (Fig. 2–4).

FILM

Generally, fast film is advisable for arthroscopic photography. If transparencies are desired, Ektachrome 400 is recommended. Kodacolor 400 is recommended for prints. The negative from Kodacolor film can be converted either to prints or to slides. Prints from an Ektachrome transparency are usually not as satisfactory and may bleach with time.

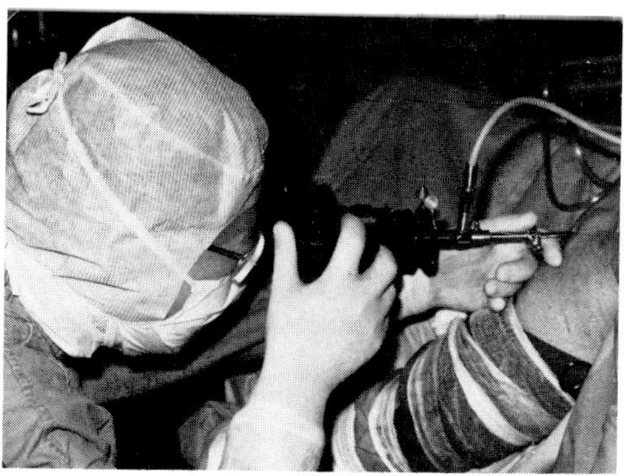

Fig. 2–4. One-hand operation of the camera on an arthroscope. The left hand is sterile and holds the arthroscope. The right hand with an extra glove controls the camera through motor drive.

The following are recommended for still photography in arthroscopy:

1. A high-quality, medium-to-large-diameter arthroscope.
2. A standard 150-watt light source.
3. A 35-mm, single-lens-reflex camera, with aperture-preferred, meter-controlled automation (preferably a center-weighted meter).
4. A lens compatible with the camera of a focal length of 100 to 110 mm and an appropriate adapter to the arthroscope; the lens should be left wide open when exposing the film.
5. Ektachrome 400 or Kodacolor 400 films.
6. A system for filing finished photographs.

I use 35-mm transparencies for documentation. They are filed chronologically and are cross-indexed alphabetically by the patient's name. Photographs of particular interest are kept in special folders filed by topic and hence are readily available for lectures or publications.

TELEVISION

Since it was first used in arthroscopy in 1974, television has become much more prevalent, particularly as an aid to teaching and performing arthroscopic surgical procedures. The photographic principles are the same as for conventional photography with film in that an object is transferred to an image, but with television, this image is visualized electronically instead of optically and is stored electromagnetically instead of chemically. The object is photographed through the arthroscope by a videocamera and is electronically registered on a monitor for instantaneous visualization. The circuit can be bypassed at any time to record the image on electromagnetic videotape.

The camera comprises a lightweight vidicon pickup tube (Fig. 2–5) connected to

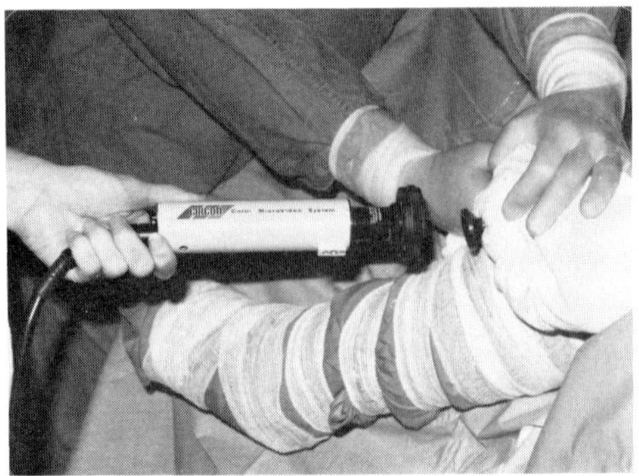

Fig. 2–5. Six-ounce vidicon tube about to be coupled to an arthroscope. Note that the stockinette is rolled back on the telescope to cover the camera to provide sterility. Commercial plastic drapes are available for this purpose.

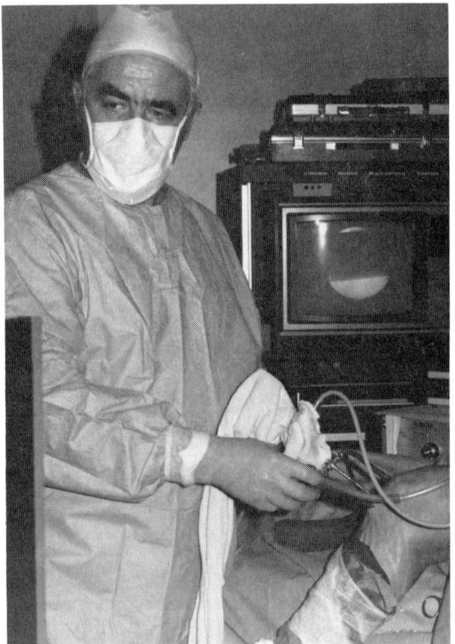

Fig. 2–6. The camera is covered with a stockinette and the surgeon is working from the monitor in the foreground.

the electronic amplifier by a 20-foot cable. The pickup tube usually weighs 6 ounces or less, a size and weight suitable for a handle on the arthroscope. With direct coupling, the tube may be handed to an assistant to allow the surgeon both hands with which to operate. The tube may also be connected to the arthroscope through a beam splitter, which passes 85% of the light to the video system and 15% to the eyepiece for the surgeon to view directly (Fig. 2–6).

A high-intensity light source is desirable for the use of television in arthroscopy. Most cameras today can automatically compensate for changing light levels and therefore provide consistently accurate pictures unless the intensity of light is too low for the camera.

The camera is electronically coupled to a video recorder, which is then connected to a video monitor. The recorder can be placed in the record mode by a foot switch, so that any sequence can be recorded by the surgeon. Although half-inch videotape is adequate for most documentation, a three-quarter-inch video cassette recorder is recommended if editing and big-screen projection are planned. Three-quarter-inch videotape, though more expensive, gives better image resolution, an increasingly important factor in second- and third-generation edited tape.

The use of television in arthroscopic surgery has resulted in a valuable tool for education. One-on-one teaching in the operating room can be performed by placing the student at the table with the telescope and a beam-splitter, and the teacher at the monitor instructing him. The system also allows students to watch the procedures, either in the operating room or on a monitor in another room or an auditorium. Edited videotapes can be shown on monitors in small conferences, or they may be shown to large audiences with the newer large-screen projectors.

Television has changed arthroscopy from a procedure in which only the surgeon could see to one in which the entire surgical team is involved. By working from a video monitor, the surgeon involves the assistant surgeon, nurses, residents, and students and makes learning the procedure a more active process.

In summary, photography in arthroscopy, both conventional and electronic, provides a method of documentation for patients' records, consultations, expert witnesses, planning future management of patients, and publication. Arthroscopic photography is useful for education, whether one on one, in small conferences, or in large lectures, as well as in solving problems arising from personal interactions.

SUGGESTED READINGS

Berci, G.: Endoscopy. New York, Appleton-Century-Crofts, 1975.

McGinty, J.B.: Closed circuit television in arthroscopy. *Rheumatology, 33*:45, 1976.

McGinty, J.B.: Photography in arthroscopy. *In* Symposium on Arthroscopy and Arthrography of the Knee. American Academy of Orthopaedic Surgeons, 1978.

Medicine and early photography. Ciba Symp., *4*, 1942.

Prescott, R.: Optical principles of endoscopy. J. Med. Primatol., *5*:133, 1976.

Chapter 3

TECHNIQUE OF DIAGNOSTIC ARTHROSCOPY

Lawrence Crane

PREPARATION FOR ARTHROSCOPY

Clinical Examination

It seems almost redundant to stress the importance of a proper clinical evaluation of the patient, who may or may not require arthroscopy. Such an evaluation is important for two reasons. First, the diagnostic accuracy of arthroscopy reported by most experienced arthroscopists is not possible without an adequate clinical examination. It is important not only to bring the results of the clinical examination to the operating room, but also to review the clinical notes just prior to the arthroscopy; it is often necessary to review the clinical picture again during the course of the arthroscopic procedure. If the clinical picture does not fit the arthroscopic findings, the surgeon should redouble his efforts to find a lesion that does explain the clinical picture. Frequently, a patient has separate lesions that are unrelated.

The second reason for a thorough clinical examination is to find other disorders in the extremity that make arthroscopy unnecessary. Most orthopedists have patients with pain referred to the knee from lesions in the femur or the hip joint. Despite this knowledge, reports exist of patients with Legg-Calvé-Perthes disease and malignant tumors of the femur who underwent arthroscopic procedures on the knee before the definitive diagnosis was made. Young patients with pain in the knee are not good candidates for arthroscopy, and the search for the cause of the knee pain should not begin with the knee. The elements of a proper medical history and physical examination are beyond the scope of this book.

Draping

Draping of the knee for arthroscopy is essentially the same as that for arthrotomy. Recently, however, several excellent arthroscopy packs have appeared on the market and include disposable paper gowns and drapes with adhesive backing to seal off any potential source of contamination such as a television camera. These drapes also have extra holes for light cords, inflow and outflow drains, and other accessories. The cost of these packages is about the same as for standard methods of draping.

Tourniquet

The difference of opinion among arthroscopists regarding the use of tourniquets is considerable. In general, most arthroscopic surgeons employ a tourniquet for performing arthroscopic surgical procedures, and many do for simple diagnostic arthroscopy. A tourniquet simplifies and speeds the procedure, but of course, certain risks exist, such as an increased incidence of thrombophlebitis. In my experience, a tourniquet is helpful for patients who are under general or spinal anesthesia in whom epinephrine is not or cannot be used. If a leg-holding device is used, venous engorgement takes place, and again, a tourniquet may be essential. If, on the other hand, epinephrine is mixed with a long-lasting anesthetic such as bupivacaine (Marcaine) a tourniquet is rarely required. In my last 200 operative cases, including meniscectomies and lateral retinacular releases, only 5 patients required inflation of the tourniquet.

Anesthesia

I find local anesthesia effective for diagnostic arthroscopy, as well as for almost all arthroscopic surgical procedures. My technique is as follows: (1) the surgical site is washed for 2 minutes in the induction room; (2) 25 ml 0.25% bupivacaine with epinephriine 1:200,000 U are injected into the skin and subcutaneous tissues of the 3 or 4 portals to be used. Another 25 ml 0.25% bupivacine with epinephrine are injected into the patient's knee joint itself. If the central patellar approach is to be used, this structure is also injected. Nothing more is necessary. The patient is then taken to the operating room, and a tourniquet is applied to the thigh. This tourniquet is inflated only if excessive bleeding is encountered.

Indications for local anesthesia are: (1) a patient who expresses this preference and who appears to be stable and cooperative; and (2) a patient who is a poor risk for general anesthesia. Contraindications are: (1) a patient who has hypertension, in which case epinephrine is contraindicated, or is allergic to local anesthesia; (2) a patient with an acutely injured knee in which one must evaluate the ligaments, best done under general anesthesia; (3) a young, heavily muscled athlete with a tight knee in which a thigh-holding brace is indicated; and (4) a nervous patient or a nervous or inexperienced arthroscopist. Although local anesthesia is my preference, I feel that it is desirable for an anesthesiologist to be available in the event of vascular collapse or a nervous or restless patient. All my patients are prepared for general anesthesia, including laboratory work, even though I infrequently require the services of a standby anesthesiologist. Of 250 patients given local anesthetics in the last year and a half, approximately 20 have required general anesthesia, usually because of the escape of saline solution into the subcutaneous tissues, which is apt to be painful.

Spinal anesthesia is rarely used because it usually requires postoperative hospital admission, and the advantages of outpatient surgery are thereby lost.

General anesthesia for arthroscopy is essentially similar to general anesthesia for any other procedure, except deep anesthesia for the relaxation of the patient is not necessary. Most patients can go home after about an hour in the recovery room.

Inflation of the Knee Joint

At least one 3000-ml bag of saline solution should be suspended 3 to 4 feet above the table to ensure maximal distension of the knee. This procedure is essential for arthroscopic viewing. A large-bore needle or cannula is attached to the tubing and is inserted into the patient's knee through a medial or superior lateral portal. If the knee fluid is at all cloudy, a constant flow of saline solution through the knee is desirable. The inflow may be through the cannula, and the outflow may be connected to the arthroscope, or the positions may be

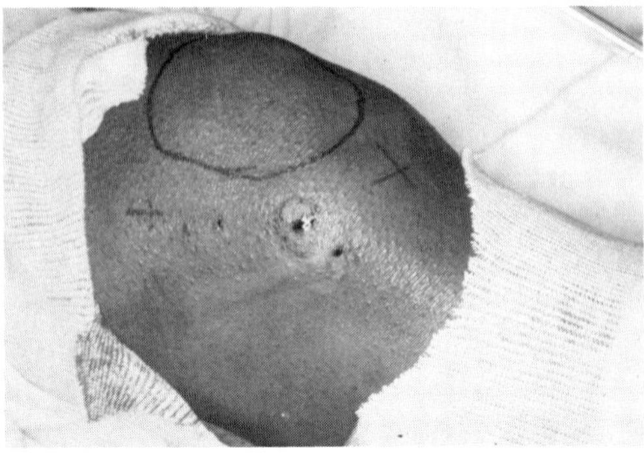

Fig. 3–1. Left knee showing portals.

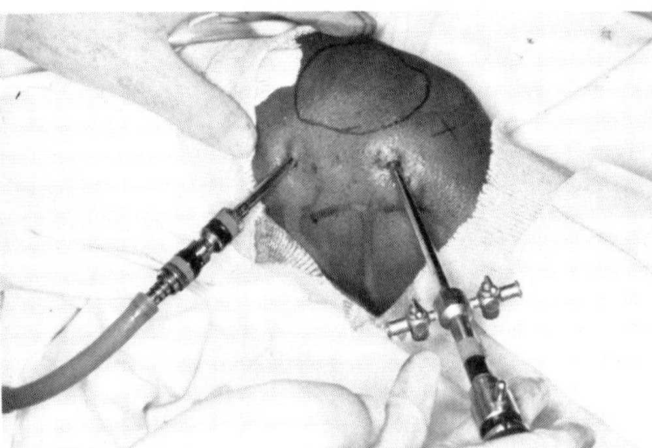

Fig. 3–2. Left knee showing an inflow in the medial suprapatellar area and the arthroscope high in the anteromedial triangle.

reversed. Some surgeons prefer to have both the inflow and the outflow connected to the arthroscope, with the outflow tubing attached to the suction equipment.

TYPE OF ARTHROSCOPE

The available arthroscopes vary in outer diameter and in the lens angle, which may be straight or angled from 10 to 70°. The most versatile arthroscope and the one preferred by most surgeons has a 4.5-mm outer diameter and a 25 or 30° lens angle.

An arthroscope with an angled lens of 30° has several advantages. By rotating the arthroscope, one can increase the field of vision and obviate the need for moving the arthroscope about the joint which can be difficult in some situations. This is true when the intercondylar notch approach is used, in which angled arthroscopes of 30 and 70° are essential for viewing the entire posterior joint. The angled arthroscopes can also be inserted at some distance from the disorder, to allow the instruments easier access to the area. The midpatellar approach of Patel is an example.

TECHNIQUE

Arthroscope Insertion

Numerous portals exist for insertion of the arthroscope (Figs. 3–1 and 3–2). For diagnostic purposes, most arthroscopists in the United States use the anterolateral triangle formed by the upper edge of the tibia, the lateral margin of the patellar tendon, and the lateral femoral condyle. A similar triangle on the medial side is also used. If the anterior two-thirds of the menisci need to be thoroughly examined, the arthroscope should be inserted higher, at the midpatellar position. In Sweden, the central approach is most often used, in which the arthroscope is inserted through the center of the patellar ligament about 1 cm distal to its lower pole. This approach permits visualization of both sides of the joint as well as the popliteal area when the arthroscope is advanced through the intercondylar notch.

Whichever portal is used, a skin incision 3 to 4 mm long is made, and the trocar is inserted through the subcutaneous tissue layer down to the synovium. A blunt obturator is then used to pass through the synovial membrane. The blunt obturator does not damage the articular surface as does the sharp trocar. When the obturator is well into the suprapatellar pouch, it is removed, and the knee is then thoroughly irrigated to ensure adequate visualization. In an acutely injured knee, which may contain fresh blood, 500 to 1000 ml saline solution may be required to flush the knee prior to insertion of the arthroscope. When the outflow of the saline solution from the arthroscopic sheath is perfectly clear, the sheath is further inserted into the suprapatellar pouch to block the outflow. This technique keeps the table dry because one rarely needs a wet table to perform diagnostic arthroscopy.

Compartmental Examination

If we think of the knee as divided into three compartments, anterior, medial, and lateral, we realize that the knee must be positioned differently to obtain the most advantageous view of each compartment. Free mobility of the knee is essential to exploring all compartments.

Anterior Compartment. The anterior compartment, which consists of the suprapatellar pouch, the patellofemoral area, and the medial and lateral gutters, is best viewed with the knee in hyperextension or extension. These positions allow maximum expansion of the patellofemoral area. If the knee is flexed 90°, the patellofemoral joint obviously cannot be seen. Some flexion, on the other hand, often helps one to evaluate the tracking of the patella. Subtle variations in the alignment of the patella may be visualized. It is important to try to get into the habit of viewing the knee the same way each time, to avoid missing an area. Most arthroscopists first view the anterior compartment, carefully observe the suprapatellar pouch, and note any abnormal plicae or loose bodies as well as the condition of the cartilage of the patella, the femoral condyles, and the synovium. In studying the tracking of the patella, it is important that the arthroscope not distort the patellofemoral relationship. To be certain, it is often helpful to insert the angled arthroscope through an anterosuperior medial or superolateral portal and to study patellar tracking from that position.

Medial Compartment. A view of the medial condyle determines the presence or absence of a medial patellar plica or shelf. As the arthroscope slides down the medial condyle while keeping the horizon in view, one must flex the knee. When the joint line is seen, placing of the knee in a valgus position permits visualization of the medial meniscus. A lateral post or a thigh holder fastened to the operating table serves as a fulcrum to help one to visualize the posteromedial compartment when the knee is placed in a valgus strain (Figs. 3–3 and 3–4). Not only should the meniscus be carefully examined and probed, but also attention should be paid to the articular surface of the femur and the tibia. It is most important to evaluate and to record the state of the articular surface.

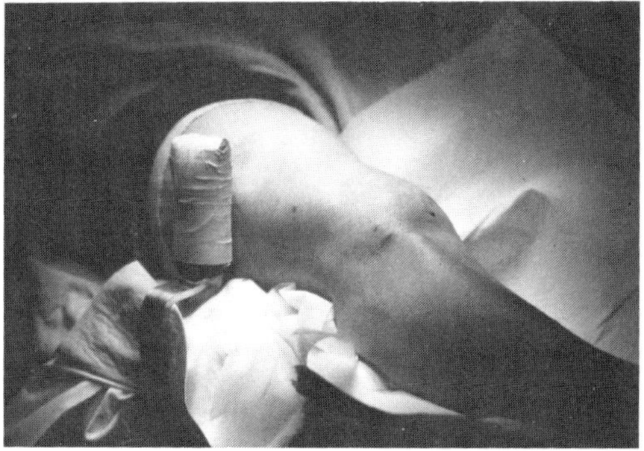

Fig. 3–3. Shoulder brace attached to the bed can act as a lever to open the medial compartment.

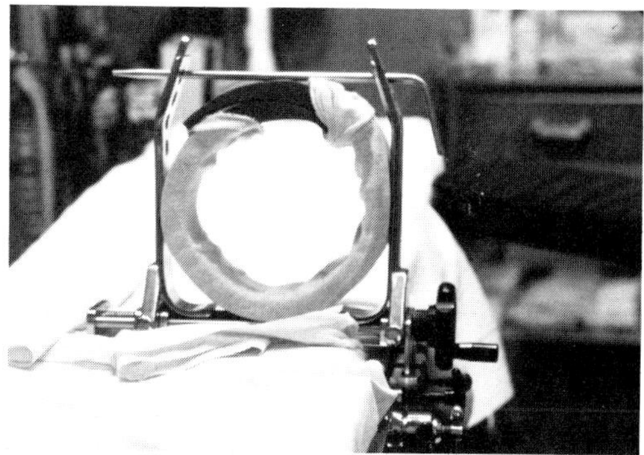

Fig. 3–4. Thigh brace.

In the event of an unusually tight medial collateral ligament, it may be difficult or impossible to view the posterior third of the meniscus adequately. In such cases, one should place the arthroscope through the intercondylar notch into the posteromedial compartment. This procedure is probably most easily accomplished by the transpatellar approach, in which one slides the sheath and blunt obturator between the cruciate ligaments and the lateral margin of the medial femoral condyle. In many patients, insertion of the arthroscope immediately adjacent to the patellar tendon permits one to enter the popliteal area. The size and configuration of the intercondylar notch vary widely, and occasionally it may be difficult or impossible to insert the arthroscope through that structure. The arthroscope should not be inserted into the sleeve until the obturator is in the posterior compartment. To do so may result in damage to the lens. To view the posterior compartment completely, a 70° angle scope is helpful.

If the arthroscope cannot be inserted through the intercondylar notch, or for some other reason one may wish to use a posteromedial approach, the surgeon should flex the patient's knee 60° to 90° and should palpate the joint line just behind the medial collateral ligament. A small incision is made at this point, and the sheath and obturator are inserted through the skin and subcutaneous tissue (see Fig. 17–2). Injecting 50 ml saline solution under pressure from the front of the knee then distends the posterior capsule and allows easier entrance of the arthroscope. When the obturator is removed from the sheath, a gush of fluid tells the surgeon that the arthroscope is properly placed. It is then possible to place a probe through the intercondylar notch, or the positions can be reversed. With a 70° arthroscope inserted through the intercondylar notch, it is simple to apply external pressure to the skin and to watch the tenting of the synovium that permits easy entrance of a probe or operating instrument.

When the arthroscope is still in the anterolateral portal, the anterior cruciate ligament should be evaluated. This examination may either be simple or difficult, depending upon the size of the anterior fat pad and the ligamentum mucosum. At times, these structures are so large that the anterior cruciate ligament is obscured. The femoral attachment of the posterior cruciate ligament is covered by a fat pad, but the tibial attachment of the posterior cruciate ligament can usually be seen when the arthroscope is introduced through the intercondylar notch.

Lateral Compartment. After viewing the medial compartment and the intercondylar notch, the arthroscope is passed into the lateral compartment. To open the joint, the knee must be placed into a varus position. One can often obtain an excellent view of the lateral meniscus with the arthroscope in the anterolateral portal, but it may be necessary to insert the arthroscope from the anteromedial portal. No one position of flexion or extension is consistently best for viewing either the medial or lateral compartment, especially the lateral compartment. In most patients, the figure 4 position opens the lateral compartment sufficiently to permit an adequate view of most of the lateral meniscus and the joint space. Again, it is important to examine the articular cartilage thoroughly. With the arthroscope inserted from an anteromedial portal, the entire lateral femoral condyle can be seen. When the arthroscope is in the anterolateral portal, the lateral gutter and popliteal tendon can be seen. Loose bodies are often found in this area. The posterolateral compartment can be viewed in a manner similar to that on the medial side, although this approach is more difficult.

At times, the patient's collateral ligaments are so tight that no position of the leg permits an adequate view of the posterior recesses of the joint. In such a case, a small, 2.7-mm arthroscope should be used. This size is probably the safest for entering the posterolateral compartment.

Central Approach

In the central approach, one flexes the patient's knee 60 to 70° and makes a 4-mm skin incision 2 cm above the tibial tubercle. Some surgeons use the lower pole of the patella as a point of reference and make the incision 1 cm distal to this point. The tibial tubercle is a more reliable landmark than the patella, which may be in an abnormally superior position. The trocar then passes through the patellar ligament if it is in the midline. Occasionally, an increase in the quadriceps angle brings the patellar tendon lateral to the midline, and then a slight adjustment has to be made. When the sharp trocar reaches the synovium, it is replaced by the blunt obturator. If the knee is extended to 20 to 30°, the obturator can slip superior to the fat pad into the patellofemoral joint with ease. This approach allows instruments to be inserted into the medial and lateral triangles for arthroscopic surgical procedures. It also permits easy passage into the posterior compartment adjacent to the anterior cruciate ligament either medially or laterally.

Handling the Arthroscope

The arthroscope should be handled firmly but delicately. It should be squeezed like a fountain pen, with the surgeon's fourth and fifth fingers braced against the skin of the patient's knee for better control. When viewing inside the knee, the surgeon must remember that the arthroscope magnifies objects and that at 1 mm from the object, the magnification is 10 times. At 1 cm distance, no magnification occurs.

Because most arthroscopes in current use have a lens angled at 25 to 30°, it is important to remember that one can rotate the arthroscope to permit a wide field of view without having to aim the instrument in another direction, which may be difficult. The arthroscope should not be kept at the same distance from the object; pistoning gives one a much more accurate picture. Scanning is also an important maneuver in arthroscopy. One should proceed from a known area, such as the patellofemoral joint, to other areas of the knee, and one should keep a known horizon in view such as the femoral condyle. If the end of the arthroscope is pushed against tissue, one will see nothing, but pistoning the arthroscope provides orientation within the joint.

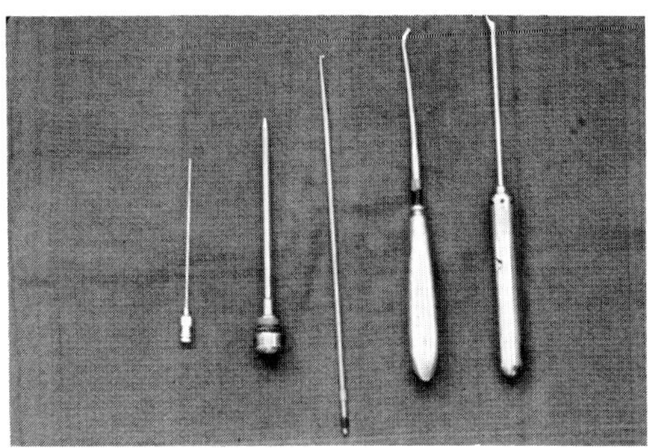

Fig. 3–5. Various types of probes.

Use of the Probe

Probes currently used in arthroscopy are blunt ended, with a tip 3 to 4 mm in length at right angles to the main body of the probe (Fig. 3–5). It is impossible to overemphasize the value of a probe. One can detect the difference between soft and hard articular cartilage, and the probe can be dropped into unseen tears in the posterior horn of a meniscus to test meniscal mobility. The probe can also be used as a retractor to remove soft tissue from in front of the arthroscope. Of course, the probe must be accurately placed within the joint, and to locate the proper point of entrance, an 18-gauge needle can be first used. After locating the joint line with a needle, one may make a small incision in the skin and capsule, to introduce the probe. Triangulating with the probe is the first step in arthroscopic surgery. No arthroscopic examination is complete unless the probe has been used to evaluate the interior of the joint (Fig. 3–6).

STERILIZATION

Some hospitals continue to require arthroscopic instruments to be either gas or steam autoclaved. Repeated steam autoclaving damages these expensive instruments. Gas autoclaving is excellent, however, and most hospitals use this procedure overnight, to have the arthroscope and an-

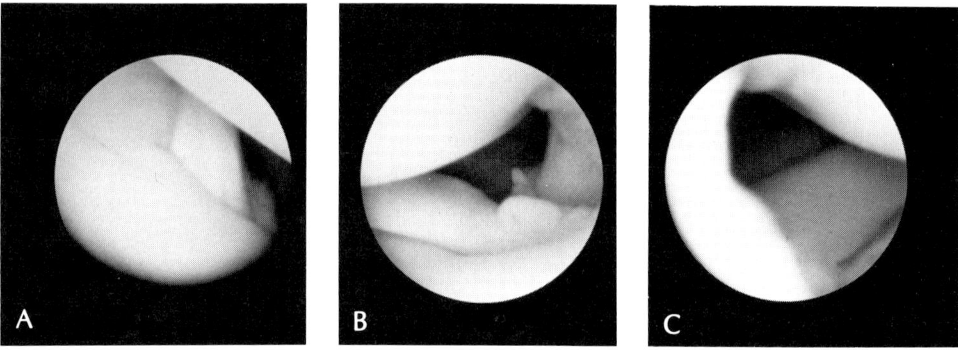

Fig. 3–6. Anatomic landmarks. ***A,*** **Popliteal sheath;** ***B,*** **medial dark hole;** ***C,*** **lateral dark hole.**

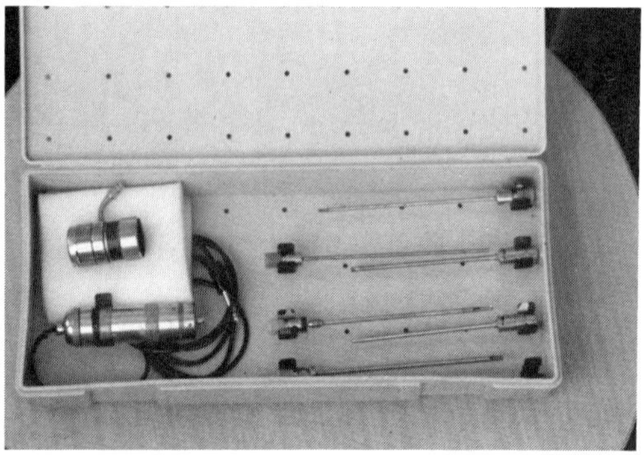

Fig. 3–7. Tray to hold instruments.

cillary instruments ready for the morning. Few hospitals have sufficient equipment to permit more than one or two arthroscopic procedures per day. As a result, almost all hospitals now place arthroscopic instruments in glutaraldehyde (Cidex) if they must be used more than once a day.

The usual technique is to place the instruments in glutaraldehyde for 12 minutes, after which time the instruments are washed with sterile saline solution. Several different containers have been designed to hold arthroscopic instruments (Fig. 3–7). I have found the fiberglass trays most effective. Once the instruments have soaked in the tray for 12 minutes, the tray is rotated 90° to allow the solution to drain from the instruments. The tray is then passed into a second container filled with a saline solution. The fiberglass tray does not damage the end of the instruments or the lenses, as does the stainless steel tray. Although a 12-minute soaking in glutaraldehyde does not kill spores, this objection to its use is without much merit because the only known infections in arthroscopy have been bacterial. Johnson has reviewed over 10,000 cases by many prominent arthroscopists using glutaraldehyde solution and has reported an infection rate of under 0.01%.[1] Certainly, this rate is far lower than that following arthrotomies, in which all the instruments have been steam autoclaved.

REFERENCE

1. Johnson, L.: Two percent glutaraldehyde: a disinfectant in arthroscopy and arthroscopic surgery. J. Bone Joint Surg. (Am.), *64*:237, 1982.

Chapter 4

LESIONS OF THE SYNOVIUM

Alan L. Bass

The illustrations in this chapter are presented to help the practitioner of arthroscopy to recognize synovial lesions. The most important point is that many variations of normal synovium exist, and until one learns to recognize these variations, it is virtually impossible to notice abnormalities. For example, a perfectly normal knee may have areas of villous hypertrophy, usually just superior to the femoral condyles and sometimes around the patella itself.

Figure 4–1 demonstrates normal synovium. It is a pale salmon pink, and the blood vessels are easily visualized, arranged in a radicular pattern best seen in the suprapatellar pouch. Figure 4–2 demonstrates hypertrophied synovial villi. This feature is commonly seen in patients with no inflammatory reaction. Figure 4–3 shows a tight fibrous plica over the medial femoral condyle. Figure 4–4 shows heavy postoperative adhesion in the suprapatellar pouch.

Figure 4–5 demonstrates acute synovitis in the intercondylar notch in a patient with a torn anterior cruciate ligament. Figure 4–6 is acute synovitis associated with tearing of the medial capsular wall in a patient with recent patellar dislocation. Figure 4–7 shows subsiding acute traumatic synovitis in a patient who had taken anti-inflammatory drugs for 5 days. Instead of tall or long synovial villi interspersed with a clear reticulation of blood vessels, one sees a generalized matte appearance with some loss of definition and some thickening and edema of the synovium itself, which appears to be heaped into gentle, undulating folds. Figure 4–8 represents a free fragment of torn synovium in a patient who had extensive synovial tearing following a fall.

Figure 4–9 shows an unusual chronic synovitis secondary to a foreign-body reaction. Two years previously, this patient had a Guepar-type total joint replacement. In this type of prosthesis, tiny metallic fragments have broken off and have caused an intense inflammatory reaction and much synovial debris.

Figure 4–10 shows calcium pyrophosphate crystals in the synovium. This patient was asymptomatic, and the crystal deposition was an incidental finding during a routine arthroscopy in a case of pseudogout. Figure 4–11 shows another patient with crystalline synovitis, in this case from gout. The villi, although having the classic appearance of chronic synovitis, appear to be more edematous and slightly glazed.

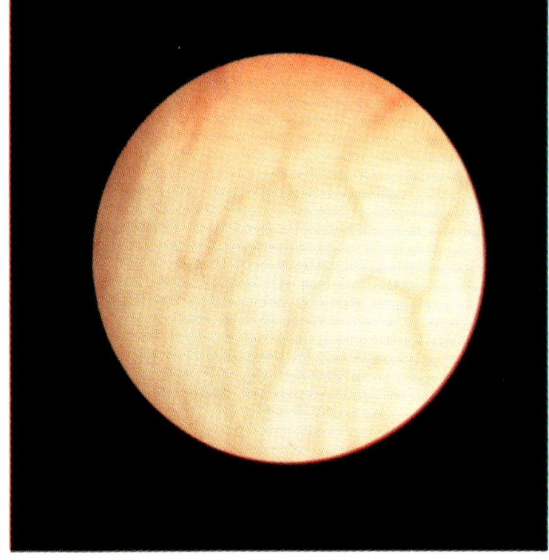

Fig. 4–1.

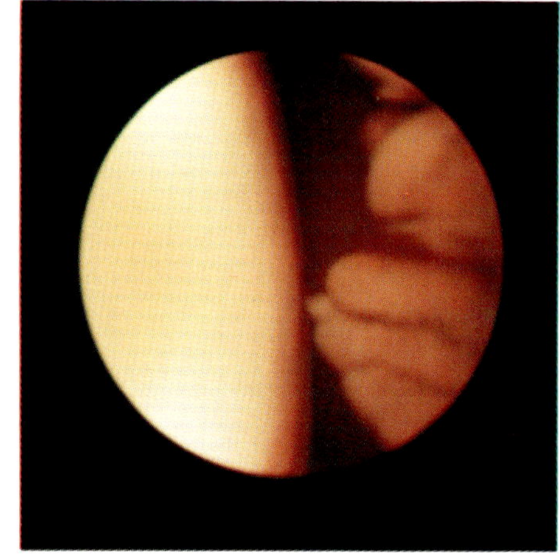

Fig. 4–2.

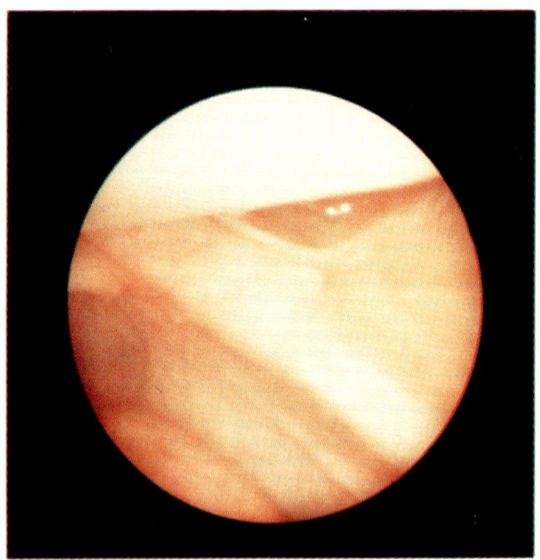

Fig. 4–3.

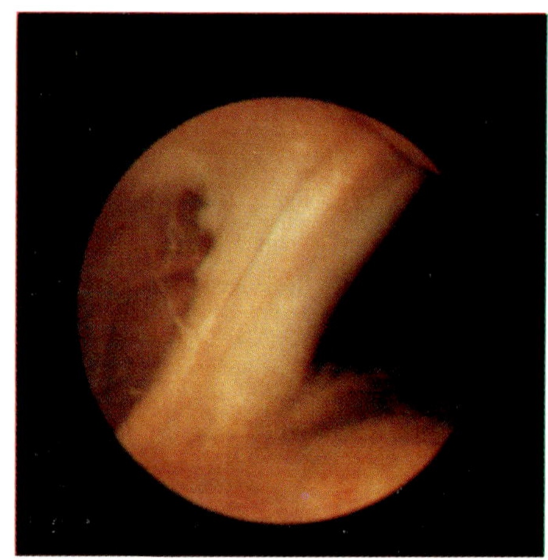

Fig. 4–4.

Fig. 4–1. Normal synovium.

Fig. 4–2. Hypertrophy of synovial villi.

Fig. 4–3. Fibrous medial plica that became trapped in flexion between the patella and the femoral condyle.

Fig. 4–4. Postoperative suprapatellar adhesion.

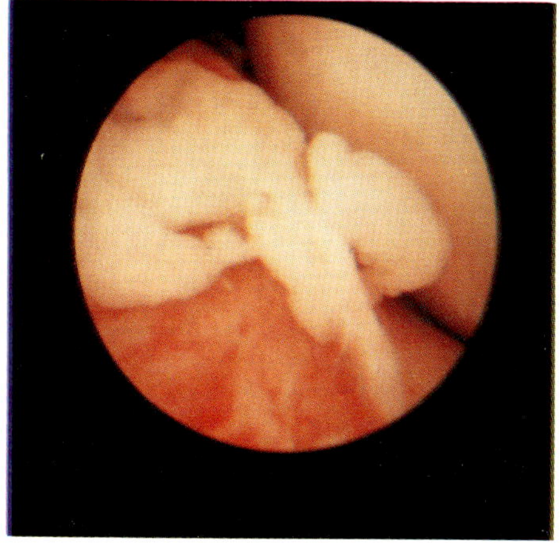

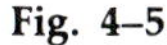

Fig. 4–5.

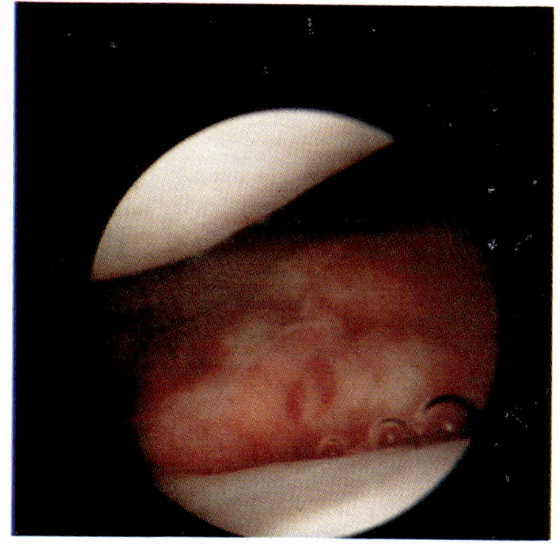

Fig. 4–6.

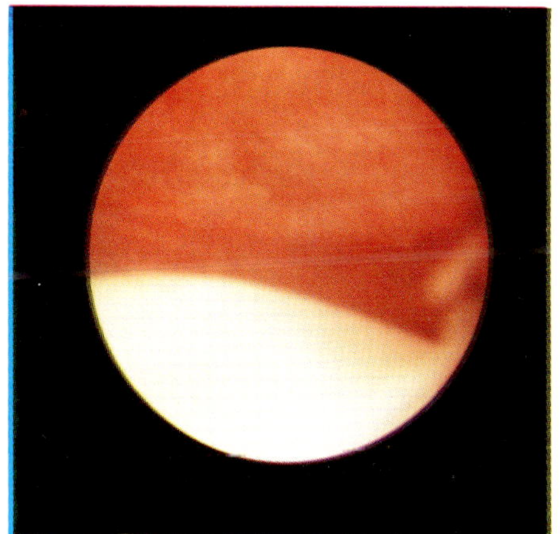

Fig. 4–7.

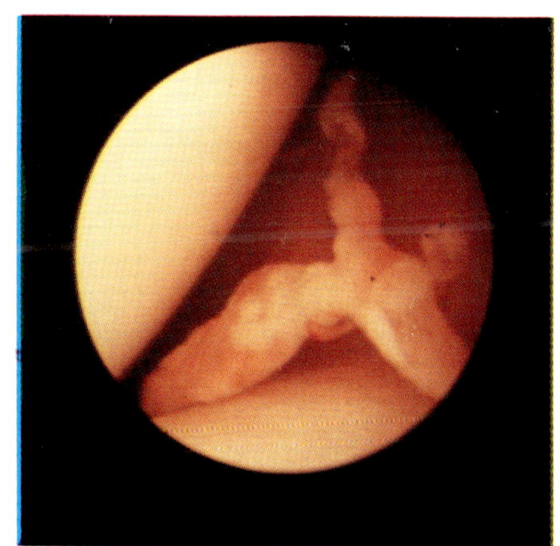

Fig. 4–8.

Fig. 4–5. Acute synovitis of the intercondylar notch in a patient with an acute rupture of the anterior cruciate ligament.

Fig. 4–6. Acute synovitis and tearing of medial capsular wall.

Fig. 4–7. Subsiding acute synovitis.

Fig. 4–8. Fragment of torn synovium loose in the joint.

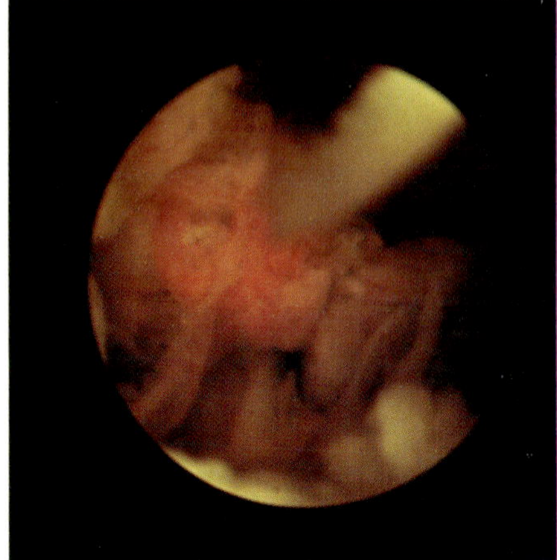
Fig. 4–9.

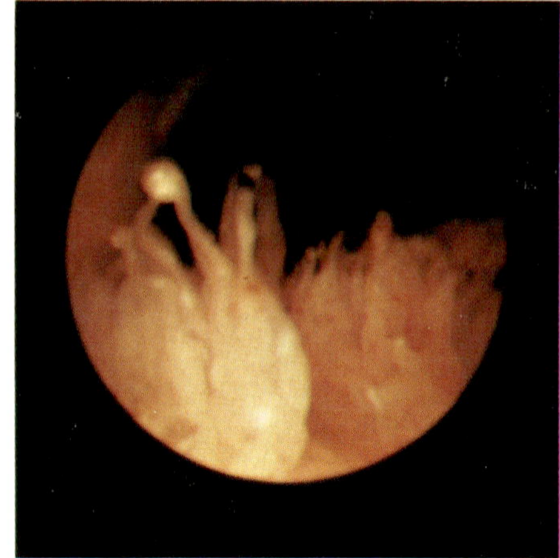
Fig. 4–10.

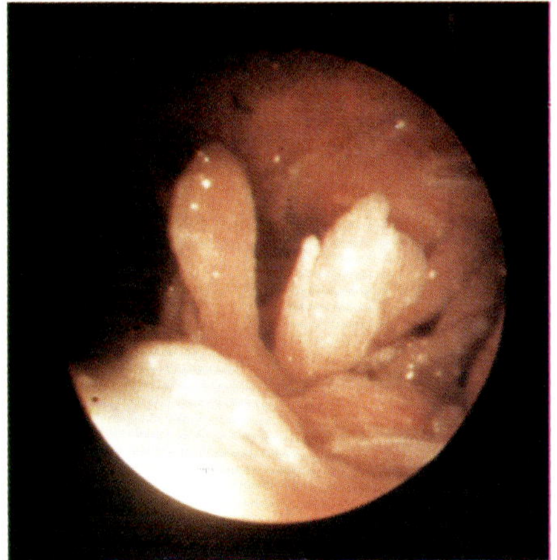
Fig. 4–11.

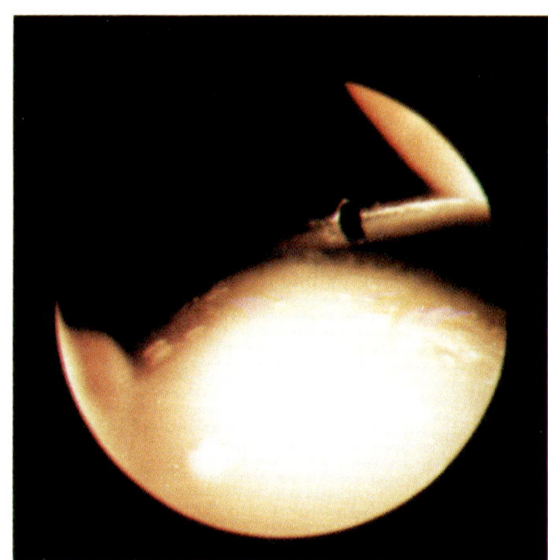
Fig. 4–12.

Fig. 4–9. Chronic synovitis due to foreign body reaction due to tiny metal fragments from a Guepar prosthesis.

Fig. 4–10. Crystalline synovitis due to pseudogout.

Fig. 4–11. Crystalline synovitis due to gout.

Fig. 4–12. Urate deposits on femoral condyle.

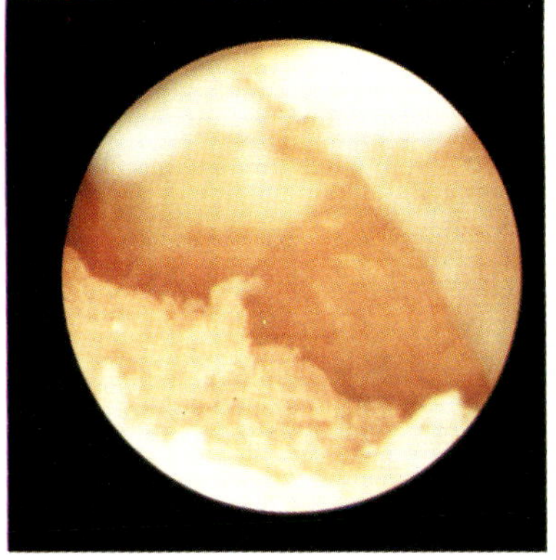

Fig. 4–13.

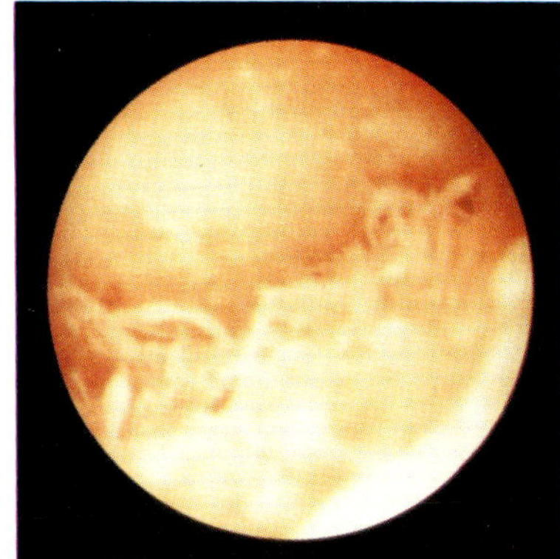

Fig. 4–14.

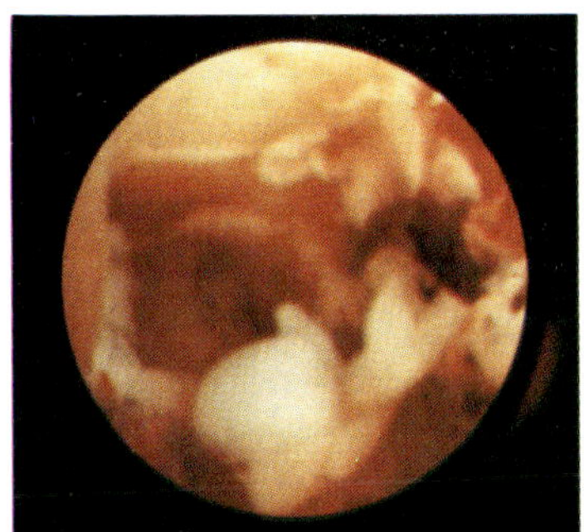

Fig. 4–15.

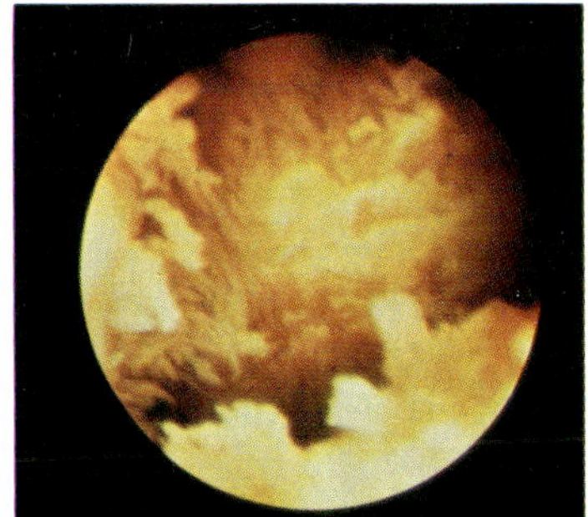

Fig. 4–16.

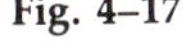

Fig. 4–17.

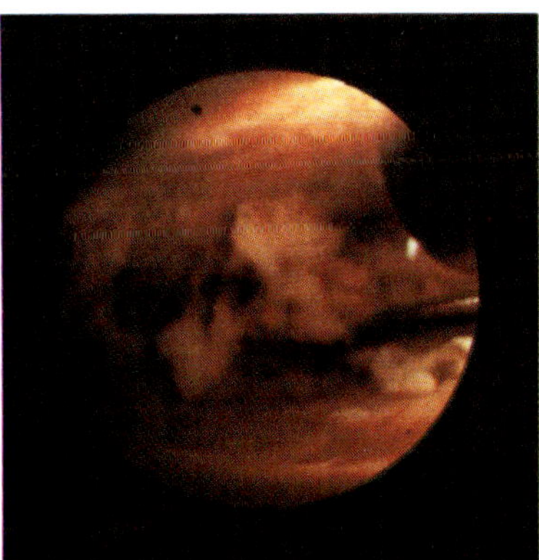

Fig. 4–13. Rheumatoid arthritis.

Fig. 4–14. Rheumatoid arthritis.

Fig. 4–15. Early stage of synovial osteochondromatosis.

Fig. 4–16. Synovium showing changes typical of hemophilia.

Fig. 4–17. Synovial appearance in a case of malignant synovioma.

The small crystalline deposits can be seen clearly because they reflect light from the arthroscope. Such specimens should not be sent to the laboratory in formalin because the crystals will dissolve. Rather, the crystals should be placed in alcohol. Figure 4–12 shows another case of gout with urate crystals deposited on the femoral condyle. Grossly, these crystals are similar to the calcium pyrophosphate crystals seen in pseudogout.

Figure 4–13 shows the suprapatellar pouch of a patient with early rheumatoid disease; note the chronic synovial hypertrophy. The synovium appears to be raised from the general level of the synovial lining in the bottom left-hand area of the illustration. The villi lack definition, and the delineation of the blood vessels is not clear. Note that normal areas appear alongside areas of inflammation, an important factor when considering a biopsy site because the error of a few millimeters can cause a false-negative result. Figure 4–14 shows another case of rheumatoid arthritis. Note the pannus in the bottom right-hand area of the illustration. These areas may bleed when biopsy is performed. Necrotic areas are often seen at the tips of the villi.

Figure 4–15 shows the suprapatellar pouch in a patient with multiple osteochondromatosis. The large, white, globular osteochondromata can be seen suspended from the wall of the distended pouch, and several hemorrhagic areas are noted. This finding is not uncommon in this condition. Figure 4–16 is a classic picture of hemophiliac synovium showing grossly hypertrophic synovitis. In hemophilia, the synovial cavity is usually large because of repeated hemarthroses. Apart from the chronic villous hypertrophy, note the extensive hemosiderin staining, which accounts for the unusual harvest colors in the picture. A large amount of fibrotic synovium can be seen at the bottom and on the right-hand side of the illustration.

In Figure 4–17, local hemorrhage and edema are clearly seen. This patient had a small mass in the superior portion of the suprapatellar pouch. On inspection, a friable area could be seen, although the lesion was ill defined. A biopsy specimen revealed malignant changes in the synovium typical of synovioma.

Chapter 5

LESIONS OF THE ARTICULAR CARTILAGE

S. Ward Casscells

In their zeal to diagnose meniscal tears, arthroscopists often overlook lesions of the articular cartilage, especially when such lesions are not located in the vicinity of the meniscus. When lesions of the articular cartilage are found, they are assumed to have been caused by a torn or damaged meniscus. In the past, meniscectomy was performed for minor tears in the hope that the lesion would not progress postoperatively. Based on investigations carried out in recent years, such a simple cause-and-effect relationship is probably untrue; it certainly remains to be proved. In this chapter, those lesions of the articular cartilage most commonly encountered by the arthroscopist are discussed, and some long-term results of the treatment of large lesions of the articular surface are presented.

Of all the structures within the knee or any other joint, the articular cartilage is certainly the most important, the most poorly understood, and the most difficult to treat. It is, therefore, important for arthroscopists to have some interest and some basic knowledge of the pathophysiology of this tissue, because they are in a position to see many more lesions than the average orthopedist or rheumatologist, and the burden of treatment will therefore fall upon them. Although many German writers of 50 years ago or more were pessimistic about the fate of articular cartilage,[1,2] recent work has shown their pessimism to be unfounded, and in the absence of trauma or malalignment of the joint, the articular cartilage is capable of remaining intact throughout a normal life span.[3] This opinion is supported by the work of a number of investigators, including Ekholm who stated in 1951 that present experiments demonstrate that "even in unfavorable circumstances, articular surfaces are very resistant to wear and tear, and it is possible under physiological conditions that there is so little loss of surface tissue in the healthy adult joint that no multiplication of cartilage cells need occur to sustain cartilage."[4] In 1969, Meachin found "surprisingly little evidence of a generalized aging change in properties of human articular cartilage 30 to 40 years of age."[5] He further stated: "in middle and later years of adult life, there is no evidence of generalized change with age." This is also my conclusion, based on a study of cadaver knees carried out some years ago.[3]

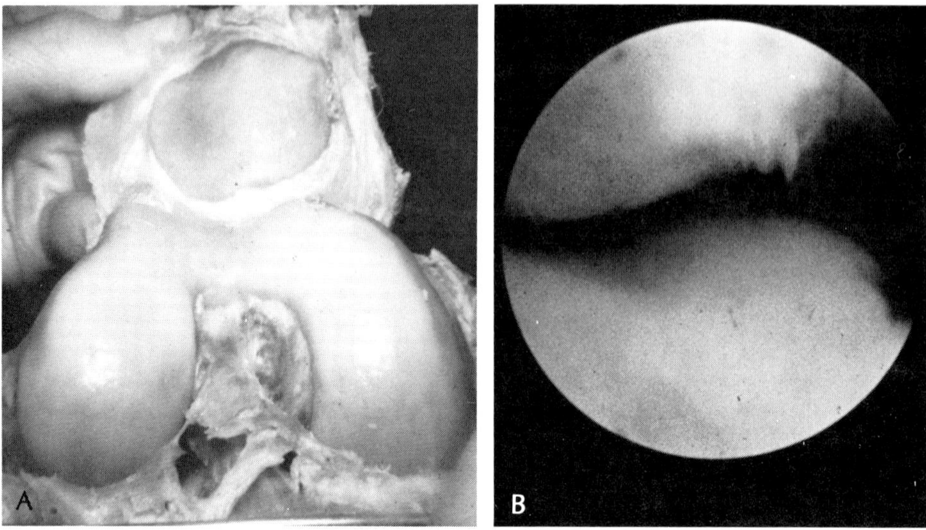

Fig. 5–1. *A,* A small area of chondromalacia patellae of the odd facet is seen in an 83-year-old cadaver joint that is otherwise normal. *B,* A small area of chondromalacia of the odd facet of the patella seen arthroscopically.

PATELLOFEMORAL JOINT

Pathologic lesions of the patella have usually been referred to as chondromalacia since Budinger first described this condition in 1906.[6] In recent years, however, the term has become almost synonymous with patellofemoral pain. This usage is unfortunate because most lesions of chondromalacia are not painful, except perhaps in advanced stages when bone is exposed, and then they are usually referred to as osteoarthritis or osteoarthrosis. Chondromalacia, or softened cartilage, is a pathologic condition and should not be used as a diagnosis for patients with idiopathic knee pain. Ficat and Hungerford also agree that the term should not be used to describe patellofemoral arthralgia.[7]

Inasmuch as the patella occupies an exposed portion of the body and is subject to a wider variety of forces than any other articular surface, it is not surprising that its articular surface is damaged more often than any other. When one does find a lesion of the patellar cartilage, it is important to determine the cause, if possible, because only then can proper treatment be instituted. At times, one can deduce the cause from the appearance of the lesion and its location. Almost all authors agree that lesions of the odd facet of the patella (Fig. 5–1) are nonprogressive, asymptomatic, and require no treatment.[7,9,13] Other lesions of the patella are more important and, in general, certain types of trauma produce recognizable lesions.

The articular surface of the patella, when

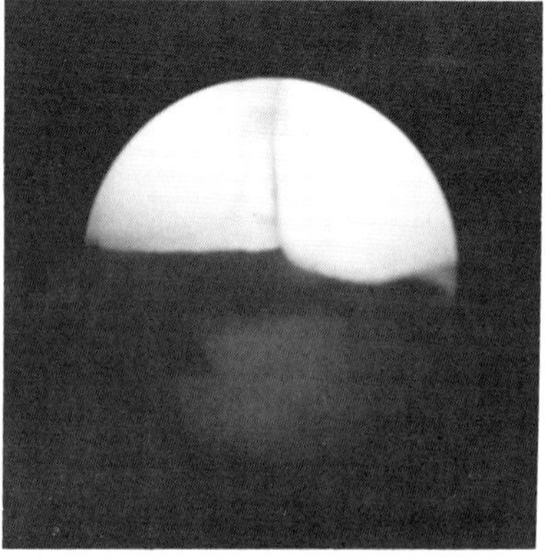

Fig. 5–2. Linear crack in the patellar surface of a patient who had a direct blow over the patella.

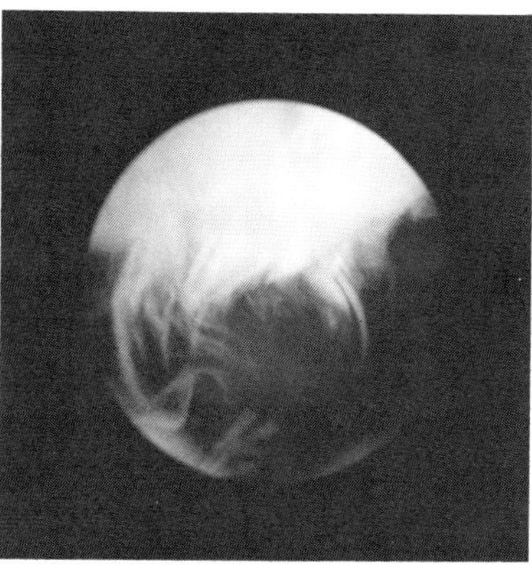

Fig. 5–3. Typical crabmeat appearance of an area of chondromalacia of the medial patellar facet.

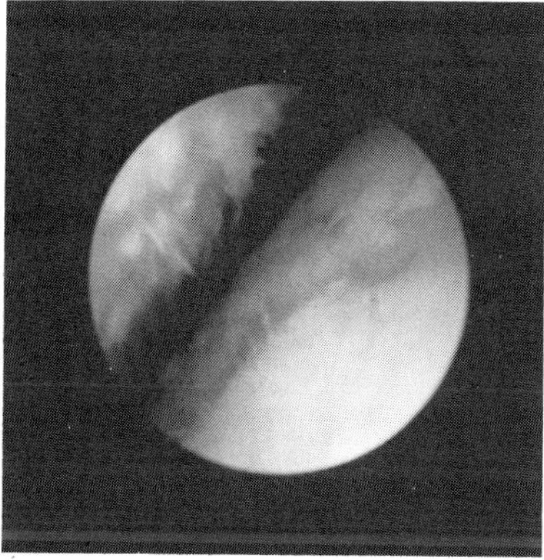

Fig. 5–4. Marked degenerative changes in the patella and lateral femoral condyle in a 62-year-old woman.

damaged by a direct blow, may result in a softened area with an intact surface that can be felt but not seen. In other cases, a linear crack in the cartilage may result (Fig. 5–2). Shearing-type forces often cause a lateral dislocation of the patella that may result in a chondromalacic defect on the medial facet with a typical crabmeat appearance (Fig. 5–3). Arthroscopically, one can duplicate this dislocation by pushing the patella laterally during the examination. An entirely different lesion is a wearing away or an abrasion of the lateral facet of the patella with a similar lesion on the opposing femoral surface (Fig. 5–4). This defect is typically seen in cases of malalignment when the lateral capsule is tight.

It is not yet known what determines the fate of the once-damaged cartilage; certainly, persistence of the malalignment usually results in a large area of cartilage loss. In other cases in which no malalignment is present, a lesion once established may remain stable for many years, and its fate may be determined in part by the physical activity of the patient in combination with an as yet poorly understood biochemical process. In the absence of trauma or malalignment, the available evidence suggests that patellar cartilage remains intact throughout life (Fig. 5–1*A*). This evidence is supported by the findings of Marrar and Pillay, in their study of 200 Chinese knees.[8] In this oriental people, who spend much of their lives in a squatting position, the incidence of chondromalacia of the patella was only 50% in those in the middle of their seventh decade. In my own study of cadaver knees, the average age of which was 70 years, 37% had a patellar cartilage that was essentially normal and an additional 25% had minor or clinically insignificant lesions. The patella has the highest incidence of damage to its articular surface. The prognosis for going through life unscathed of other joints in the body is considerably better.

WEIGHT-BEARING AREA OF THE TIBIOFEMORAL JOINT

Although of greater clinical significance, lesions of this area are less commonly seen than are those in the patellofemoral area. In the cadaver study already mentioned, the incidence of clinically significant lesions of the tibiofemoral area was only 23%. The weight-bearing surfaces of the knee joint, similar to those in the patellofemoral area, can also be damaged by a single traumatic incident (Fig. 5–5), as well as by long-standing malalignment (Fig. 5–6).

CHONDRAL AND OSTEOCHONDRAL FRACTURES

In sports injuries, as well as in other types of injuries, the joint surfaces are sometimes

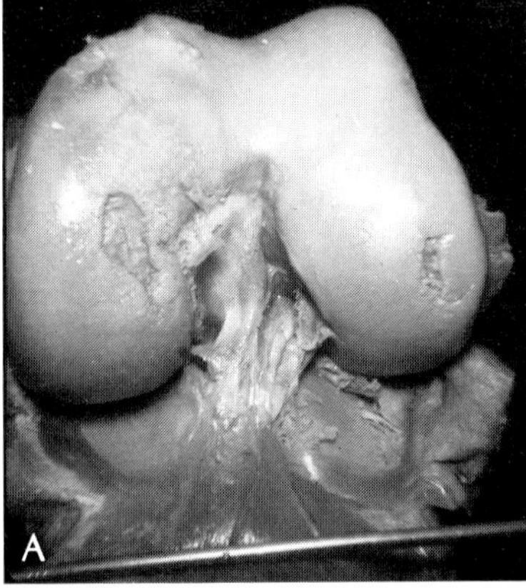

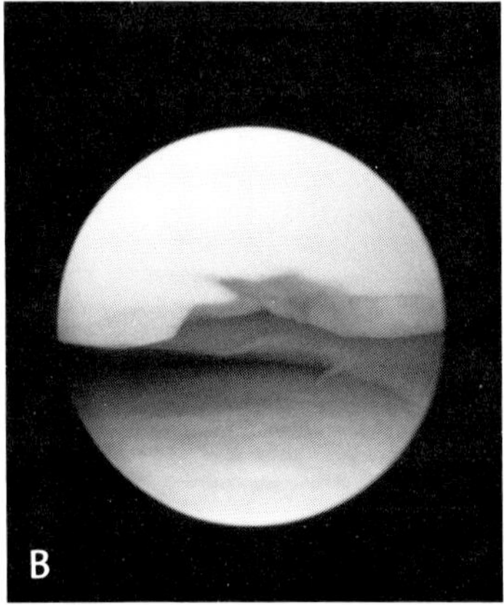

Fig. 5–5. *A,* **Punched out lesions of the femoral condyle typical of those seen following trauma.** *B,* **Arthroscopic view of a defect in the medial femoral condyle similar to** *A* **in which the patient is known to have jumped up in the air and landed on the extended knee.**

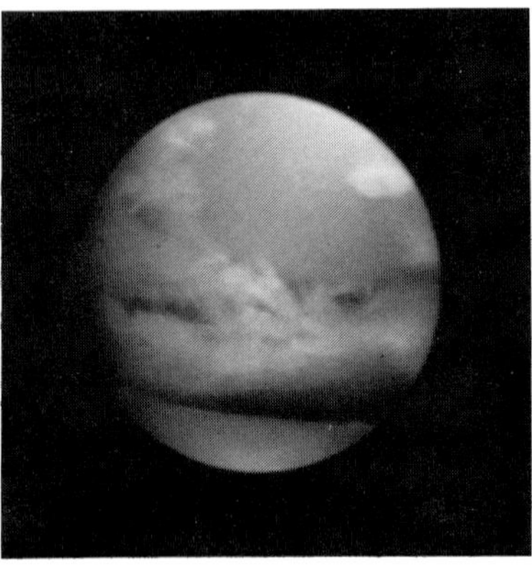

Fig. 5–6. Complete loss of articular cartilage in the lateral femoral condyle of a woman with valgus deformity.

brought forcefully together to cause a defect in the articular cartilage, usually of the femur. If the force is great enough, the underlying bone may be fractured. In patients with grossly displaced fractures, roentgenograms may give all the needed information, and arthroscopy is unnecessary.

More commonly, only the articular cartilage is damaged, and a sharply punched-out area of the articular cartilage results, with sharply defined vertical margins (see Fig. 5–5). This defect is often the result of force directed against the fully extended knee. If the knee is flexed, a shearing force will cause widespread damage to the articular cartilage (see Fig. 5–6). Such lesions are best evaluated by an arthroscopic examination.

DEGENERATIVE ARTHRITIS

Perhaps the most common lesion in the articular surfaces of the femur and tibia is degenerative arthritis, often the result of abnormal mechanics such as genu varum or genu valgum. When the traumatic lesions referred to in the previous paragraph are not seen until years after the initial

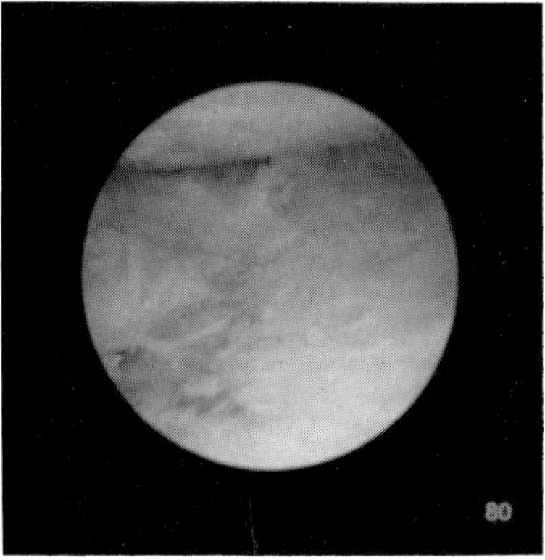

Fig. 5–7. Small area of degeneration of the articular cartilage of the medial femoral condyle in a patient whose roentgenograms taken in the weight-bearing position were normal.

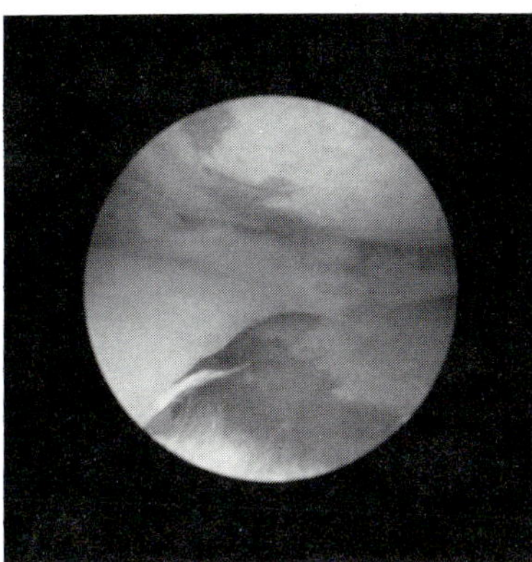

Fig. 5–8. Degenerative arthritis of the tibiofemoral area adjacent to the medial meniscus with little change in the meniscus.

injury, it may be difficult to distinguish traumatic lesions from those caused by malalignment. Lesions caused by malalignment start insidiously, and even when they reach the stage at which they produce pain, the roentgenogram may show little or no change (Fig. 5–7). By the time a weight-bearing x-ray film shows a detectable narrowing of the joint space, degenerative arthritis is moderately advanced. In my experience, this arthritis usually commences on the femoral surface, and only later is the tibia involved. The meniscus on the ipsilateral side of the joint may show little or no change in the early stages, but ultimately, the inner border of the meniscus degenerates, especially the posterior horn (Fig. 5–8).

Arthroscopy is the only method of detecting these lesions early; they are often seen accidentally because they do not usually cause pain at this stage, and patients do not see a physician for pain from these lesion until much later. Even then, it is surprising how often little discomfort occurs, even in patients with advanced arthritic changes. One of the greatest problems I have encountered is convincing active, middle-aged individuals with few symptoms that their athletic activities should be curtailed when these degenerative lesions are found arthroscopically.

RHEUMATOID ARTHRITIS

Although both the diagnosis and the treatment of rheumatoid arthritis are the concern of rheumatologists, the orthopedic surgeon may have more to offer the patient, at least when the knee joint is involved, as it frequently is. The latex fixation test is not aways positive when it should be, and blind biopsies of the synovium are not always reliably representative. Furthermore, nothing in the microscopic appearance of these lesions is pathognomonic of rheumatoid arthritis, but the lesions can be recognized grossly (Fig. 5–9) by the experienced arthroscopic surgeon. Prompt synovectomy may save a joint from ultimate destruction by the rheumatoid process. By the time the disease process has attacked the articular cartilage by invading and undermining it, it is too late to save the joint.

GOUT AND PSEUDOGOUT

Gout and pseudogout are usually treated by rheumatologists or internists. These diseases do involve the articular cartilage, but their potential for doing serious damage is not as great as that of rheumatoid arthritis. In my experience, gout seldom involves the larger joints, but pseudogout is frequently seen in the knee. Pseudogout may flare up after a traumatic episode and, at arthros-

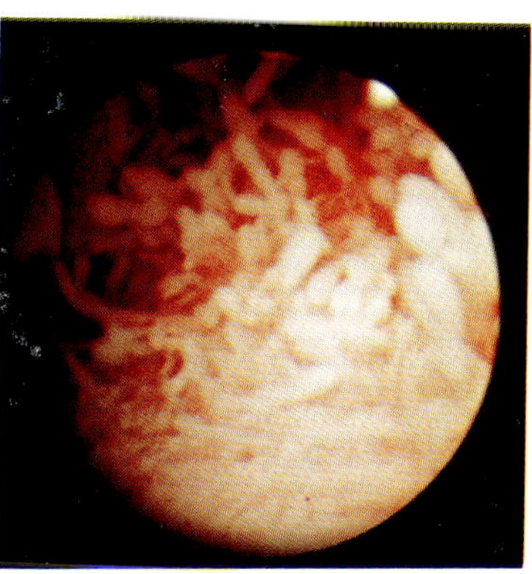

Fig. 5–9. Synovium in rheumatoid arthritis. This diagnosis can be made more easily arthroscopically than pathologically.

copy, one sees the typical calcium pyrophosphate crystals in the meniscus as well as in the articular cartilage.

FULL-THICKNESS DEFECTS OF THE ARTICULAR CARTILAGE

When a patient has a sizable defect in the femoral condyle, either from trauma or from osteochondritis dissecans, the orthopedic surgeon is required to treat these lesions. That defects created in the knees of young animal models, such as rabbits,

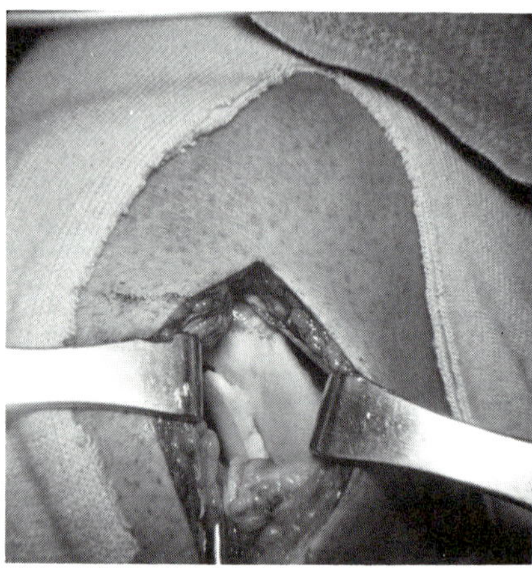

Fig. 5–10. Large defect of the medial femoral condyle in a patient with osteochondritis dissecans. These lesions are ideally suited to pinning.

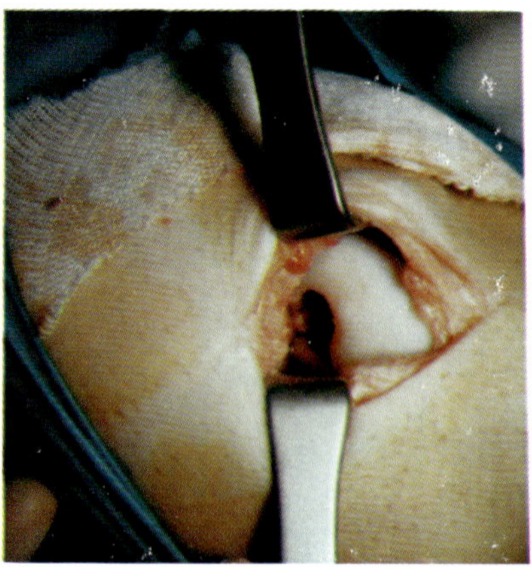

Fig. 5–11. Lesion of osteochondritis dissecans of medial femoral condyle drilled down to cancellous bone.

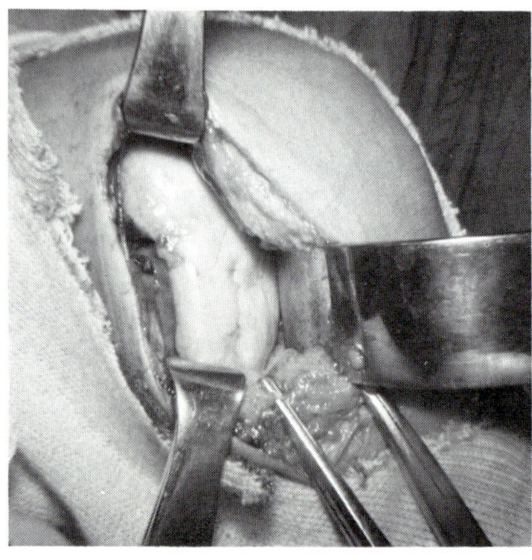

Fig. 5–12. A 7-year follow-up study of a 25-year-old man with a healed osteochondritic lesion of the medial femoral condyle. A large, calcified, loose body measuring 2 × 4 cm was removed from the suprapatellar pouch at the time this photograph was taken. The patient had no treatment following the initial injury and was never unable to walk.

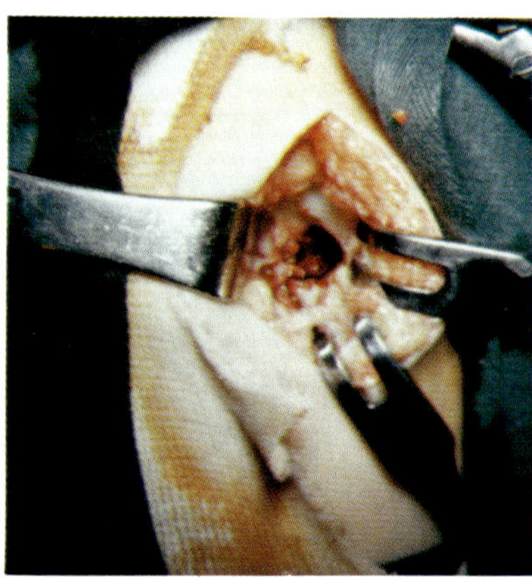

Fig. 5–13. Another osteochondritic lesion of medial femoral condyles taken down to the cancellous bone.

heal with hyaline cartilage has been known for many years. Shands showed this effect in 1931.[10] More recently, Salter and colleagues demonstrated the beneficial effects of continuous passive motion in the defects created in rabbit knees.[11] Those who have followed the lesions for a year or more report that the surface of these lesions breaks down and develops fissures at some time between 5 months and a year.[12] This change

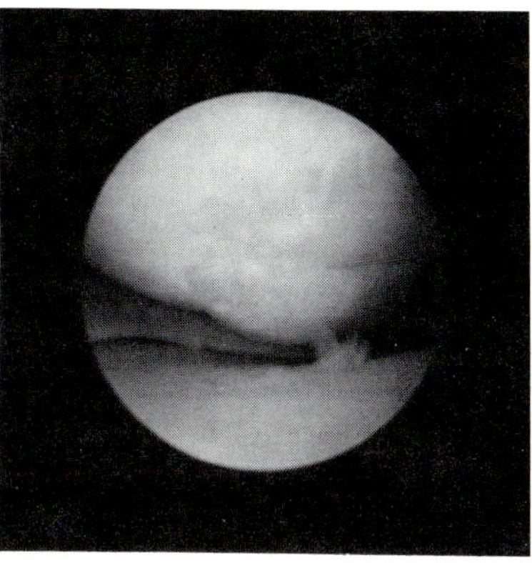

Fig. 5–14. **Arthroscopic view of the same patient in Figure 5–13 showing excellent healing 6 months later.**

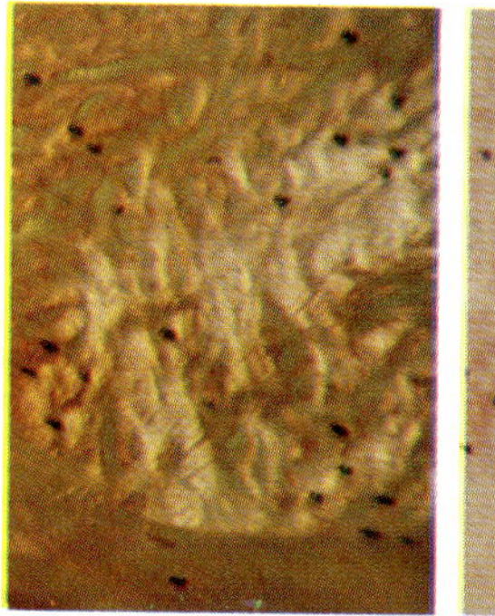

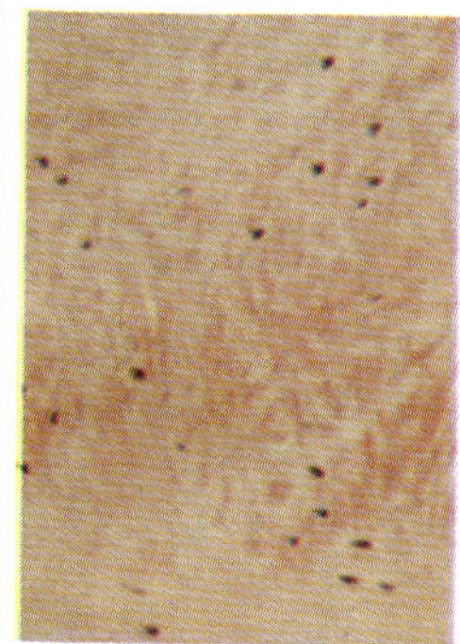

Fig. 5–16. **Biopsy of this area in Figure 5–15 showed fibrocartilage. On the left side of the figure are the collagen fibers seen under polarized light.**

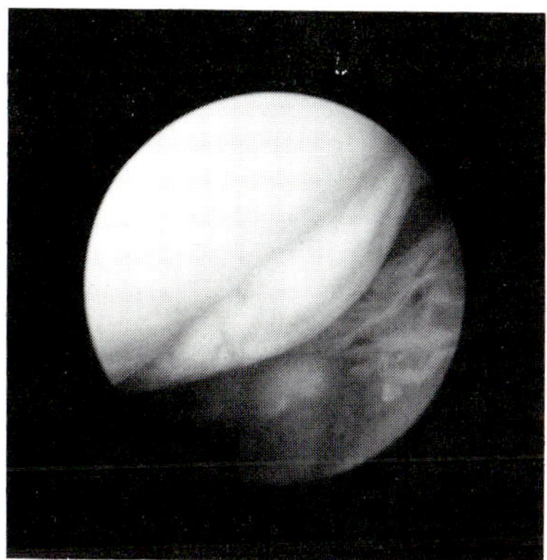

Fig. 5–15. **A 30-year-old man who, 5 years previously, had had a lesion similar to those seen in Figures 5–11 and 5–13. He had a twisting injury, and the fibrocartilaginous replacement separated from the underlying bone necessitating removal and curettement all the way down to bleeding bone.**

may be related to the preponderance of type 1 over type 2 collagen.

Almost everyone has expressed the opinion that early weight bearing of these joints should be avoided, although Furukawa, Eyre, Koide, and Glimcher have suggested that once the cartilage has developed, continuous mechanical loading may help to maintain its differentiated state.[12] Almost all reports pertain to experimental animal models. Unfortunately, little is known about similar problems in the human. The cases illustrated here may perhaps help one to understand and to treat lesions similar to those encountered by other orthopedic surgeons and may stimulate one to report his own successes and failures.

Large lesions of the condyle with the articular surface intact or nearly so should probably be pinned in situ because the fibrocartilaginous replacement (Fig. 5–10) does not withstand the same degree of wear and tear as hyaline cartilage. When replacement is not feasible, my practice is to remove the entire bed (Fig. 5–11) of cortical bone down to cancellous bone. This procedure is a radical form of the Pridie treatment. Early and repeated motion and full weight bearing are usually resumed within 2 or 3 weeks. Whether early weight bearing is wise is not yet known. The stimulus for this regimen came from observing several patients with excellent healing who never stopped walking (Figs. 5–12 to 5–16).

The only experimental evidence that advocates early weight bearing is the observation by Mitchell and Shepard on artificially created fractures in the condyles of rabbit knees.[14] They show that the fractures induced to heal by compression devices healed best with hyaline, not fibrocartilage, laid down. Mitchell and Shepard thought that chondrocytes were stimulated to heal the defect by the compressive forces. The healing of these defects in the articular cartilage, of course, is not analogous to the fractures that heal under compression.

Many more observations are needed to determine the best course to follow in the treatment of these defects in the human joint.

ABRASION ARTHROPLASTY

Abrasion arthroplasty, a new method of treatment for lesions of the articular cartilage, is based on the presence of tiny blood vessels under the cortical surface of the bone. By using a high-speed motorized bur, Johnson has demonstrated that it is possible to induce these vessels to bleed; the hope is that fibrous tissue will cover the bare area and will differentiate into a fibrocartilage. Thus far, no convincing evidence suggests that the fibrocartilaginous resurfacing will fill in to the level of the surrounding normal articular cartilage. The tiny cortical vessels appear to be too small and too few to provide a full-thickness resurfacing.

A more serious objection to abrasion arthroplasty is that most candidates for this procedure have angular deformity of the knee, most often genu varum. If the normal hyaline cartilage originally broke down because the load on the chondrocyte was too great, it is unrealistic to think that fibrocartilaginous replacement will survive for long. These patients would probably be better served by a high tibial osteotomy performed soon after the problem is diagnosed.

Abrasion arthroplasty, like any other arthroscopic procedure, has the advantage of being a minor operation, but the recommended two-month period of non-weight bearing on crutches nullifies many of the advantages of an arthroscopic procedure.

It will be some years before this type of arthroplasty can be properly evaluated. Perhaps the ultimate answer will be a combination of some type of arthroplasty and corrective osteotomy that will permit early and vigorous knee motion.

REFERENCES

1. Heine, J.: Arthritis deformans. Arch. Pathol. Anat., *260*:521, 1926.
2. Owre, A.: Chondromalacia of the patellae. Acta Chir. Scand., *77(Suppl.)*:41, 1936.
3. Casscells, S.W.: Gross pathological changes in the knee joint of the aged individual. Clin. Orthop., *132*:225, 1978.
4. Ekholm, R.: Relationship between articular changes and functions. Acta Orthop. Scand., *21*:81, 1951.
5. Meachin, G.: Age changes in articular cartilage. Clin. Orthop., *64*:33, 1969.
6. Budinger, K.: Uber Ablosung von Gelenkteilen und verwandte Prozesse. Dtsch. Z. Chir., *84*:311, 1906.
7. Ficat, R.P.,and Hungerford, D.S.: Disorders of the Patello-Femoral Joint. Baltimore, Williams & Wilkins, 1977.
8. Marrar, B.D., and Pillay, V.K.: Chondromalacia of the patella in Chinese: a post-mortem study. J. Bone Joint Surg. (Am.), *57*:342, 1975.
9. Radin, E.: A rational approach to the treatment of patello-femoral pain. Clin. Orthop., *144*:107, 1979.
10. Shands, A.R., Jr.: The regeneration of hyaline cartilage in joints: an experimental study. Arch. Surg., *22*:137, 1931.
11. Salter, R.B., et al.: The biological effect of continuous passive motion on healing of full-thickness defects and articular cartilage. J. Bone Joint Surg. (Am.), *62*, 1980.
12. Furukawa, T., Eyre, D.R., Koide, S., and Glimcher, M.J.: Biochemical studies on repair: cartilage resurfacing experimental defects in the rabbit knee. J. Bone Joint Surg. (Am.), *62*:79, 1980.
13. Goodfellow, J., Hungerford, D.S., and Woods, C.: Patello-femoral joint mechanics and pathology. 2. Chondromalacia patellae. J. Bone Joint Surg. (Br.), *58*:291, 1976.
14. Mitchell, N., and Shepard, N.: Healing of articular cartilage and intra-articular fractures in rabbits. J. Bone Joint Surg. (Am.), *62*:628, 1980.

Chapter 6

LESIONS OF THE MENISCUS

Bertram Zarins
Vincent K. McInerney

The purpose of this chapter is to describe the pathologic processes that affect knee menisci. The arthroscopist needs a clear understanding of meniscal lesions to be able to discern the nature of a tear when only a portion of the meniscus or tear is visible through the arthroscope. This knowledge is especially important when one is performing partial meniscectomy, which requires precise definition of the type, the size, and the location of a meniscal tear.

GENERAL PATHOLOGIC PROCESSES AFFECTING MENISCI

The pathologic processes responsible for most meniscal lesions are *trauma* and *degeneration*. As expected, traumatic meniscal lesions usually occur in young and athletic individuals as the result of injury. Degenerative changes are usually seen in older people without injury or with minor trauma.

Trauma

Traumatic tears result when excessive compression, tension, or shearing forces are applied to a meniscus.[1] The location, the direction, and the size of the tear depend on the magnitude and the direction of the forces and on the physical properties of the meniscus.

Degenerative Changes

Degenerative changes in menisci usually occur in association with similar changes in other parts of the knee joint. The result of these changes can be degenerative meniscal tears, cysts, or calcification.

Degenerative meniscal tears in older patients are caused by several age-related events. Changes in the knee that usually occur with advancing age include increased meniscal stiffness, decreased elasticity of capsular structures, and decreased thickness of articular cartilage.[2,3] Articular cartilage loss narrows the joint space, resulting in greater compressive forces being applied to the menisci. Irregular articular surfaces cause increased friction, which increases the shearing forces to which the menisci are subjected. The combination of gradually increased forces applied to a structurally weakened meniscus results in degenerative meniscal tears.

Solitary or multilocular cysts can result from degeneration of meniscal tissues, especially in the lateral meniscus. Small degen-

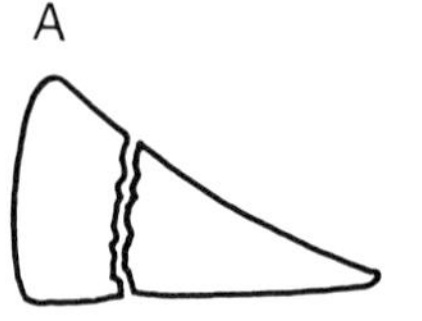

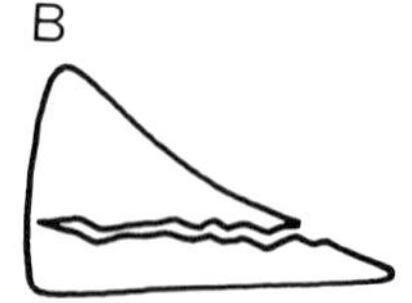

Fig. 6–1. Description of the direction of a tear with respect to the cross section of the meniscus. *A,* Vertical; *B,* horizontal.

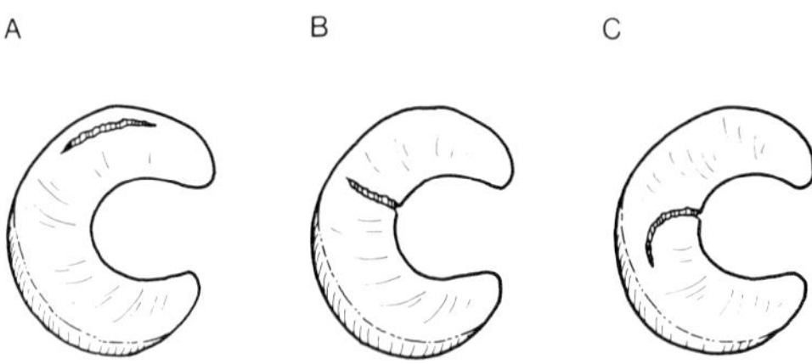

Fig. 6–2. Description of direction of a tear with respect to the circumference of the meniscus. *A,* Longitudinal; *B,* transverse; *C,* oblique.

erative cysts are often contained in the peripheral zone of the meniscus, whereas multilocular or single large cysts are usually parameniscal. Meniscal cysts frequently have an associated meniscal tear.[4]

Calcium salts in the form of *calcium pyrophosphate* dihydrate can be deposited in articular cartilage, menisci, and synovium. Rarely, hydroxyapatite and dicalcium phosphate dihydrate crystals cause articular calcification.[5]

Ossification of menisci can ocur as a primary event or secondary to calcification. Meniscal ossicles are extremely rare, but must be included in the differential diagnosis of loose bodies situated near the menisci.[6,7]

TERMINOLOGY OF MENISCAL TEARS

Tears in a meniscus can be described by direction, location, and size. In this chapter, the *direction* of a meniscal tear is described as vertical or horizontal with respect to the cross section of the meniscus (Fig. 6–1). The direction of the tear is called longitudinal, transverse, or oblique with

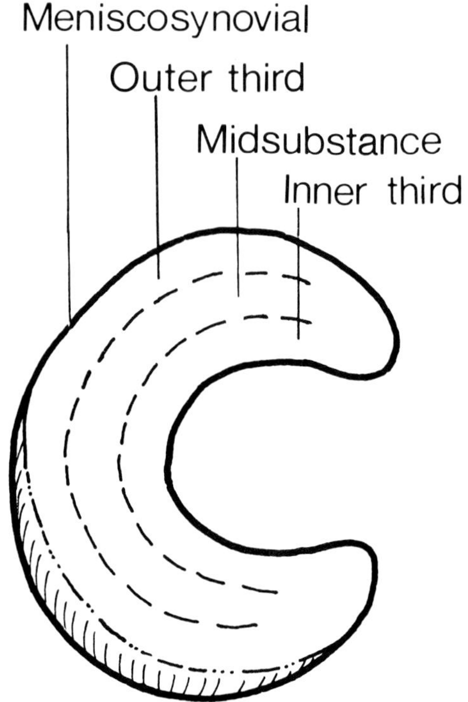

Fig. 6–3. Nomenclature for the division of the meniscus into circumferential thirds.

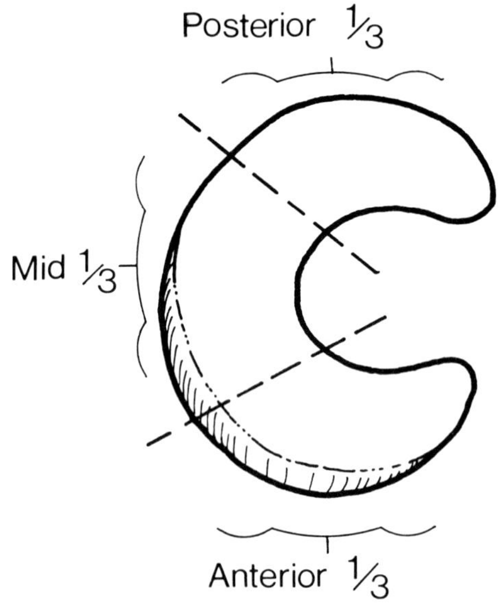

Fig. 6–4. Division of the meniscus into anterior, mid- and posterior thirds.

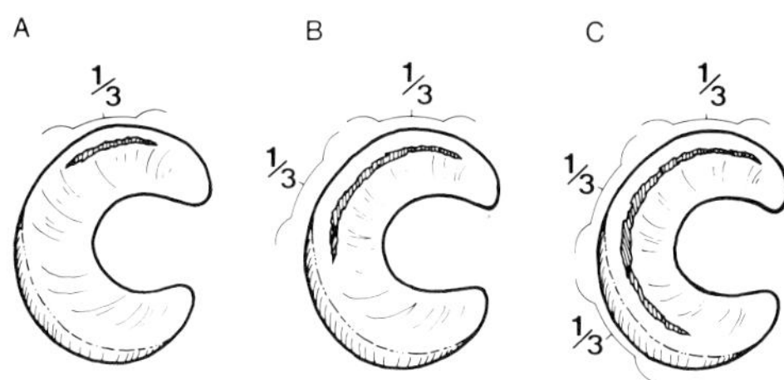

Fig. 6–5. Description of the size of a longitudinal tear. *A*, Small; *B*, medium; *C*, large.

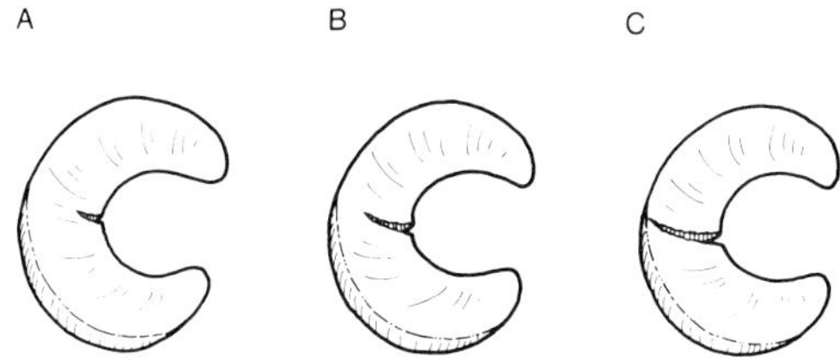

Fig. 6–6. Description of the size of a transverse tear. *A*, Small; *B*, medium; *C*, large.

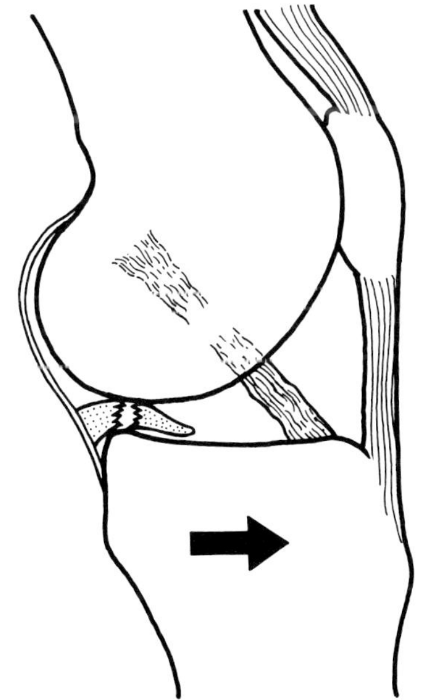

Fig. 6–7. Mechanism of a longitudinal vertical meniscal tear in the knee with a torn anterior cruciate ligament. The meniscus and tibia subluxate forward, and the posterior meniscus is sheared against the femoral condyle.

TABLE 6–1

CLASSIFICATION OF MENISCAL LESIONS
Vertical Longitudinal Tear (Circumferential)
Meniscal
Meniscosynovial Junction
Vertical Transverse Tear (Radial)
Horizontal Tear (Cleavage)
Oblique Tear (Flap)
Detachment of Meniscal Horns
Complex Tear
Cystic Degeneration
Miscellaneous Lesions
Partial-Thickness Tear
Postmeniscectomy Rim Tear
Discoid Meniscus
Calcification and Ossification

respect to the circumference of the meniscus (Fig. 6–2).

A vertical longitudinal tear can be *located* at the meniscosynovial junction or at the outer third, the midsubstance, or the inner third of the meniscus (Fig. 6–3). The meniscus can also be divided into anterior, middle, and posterior thirds for localization of a lesion (Fig. 6–4).

The *size* of a tear is referred to as small if it involves up to one-third, medium if it involves up to two-thirds, and large if it involves more than two-thirds of the meniscal length (Fig. 6–5) or width (Fig. 6–6).

For a classification of meniscal lesions, see Table 6–1.

VERTICAL LONGITUDINAL TEARS (CIRCUMFERENTIAL)

Vertical longitudinal tears are meniscal tears that are directed parallel to the circumference of the meniscus. Tears are commonly oriented in this direction because the collagen bundles in menisci are predominately arranged in a circumferential manner. Longitudinal tears lengthen because few fibers are radially directed. The scattered bundles of radial fibers are interspersed among the circumferential fibers and are usually located in the midportion and inferior surface of the meniscus.[8–10]

Vertical longitudinal tears are the most common meniscal tears in patients under age 40 and usually occur as the result of injury. The patient typically has a noncontact, deceleration, twisting injury of the knee. The anterior cruciate ligament tears, resulting in a hemarthrosis and instability of the knee.

The mechanism of tearing a meniscus in this manner can be explained readily. When the anterior cruciate ligament tears, the tibia subluxates anteriorly in relation to the femur. If the knee is under sufficient load at the time of this subluxation, the meniscus is compressed and tears[11] (Fig. 6–7). The torn meniscal fragment can remain displaced forward of the femoral condyle when the tibia relocates.

Circumferential tears also occur in stable knees. It is more difficult to explain the mechanism of meniscal injury in these cases. According to one theory, the meniscus becomes trapped between the femur and the tibia during an asynchronous knee motion.[12] The semimembranous tendon, which has an insertion into the posterior third of the medial meniscus by the posteromedial capsule,[13] pulls the medial meniscus posteriorly during knee flexion to prevent impingement of the meniscus between the femoral and tibial condyles. The popliteal tendon has an attachment to the posterior third of the lateral meniscus;[14] when the popliteal muscle contracts, it pulls the lateral meniscus posteriorly. If the semimembranous and popliteal muscles do not contract in synchrony with knee motion, the menisci may become wedged between the femur and the tibia and may tear.

The result of a vertical longitudinal tear is an unstable inner segment of meniscus. The degree of instability and displacement of the segment depend to a large extent on the length of the tear. Meniscal fragments are called *nondisplaceable* if the unstable segment cannot be pulled forward of the femoral condyle; such is usually the case with small tears. If the torn meniscus can be pulled forward of the femoral condyle with a probe, it is called *displaceable;* the tear is most likely medium or large in size. Large tears extend from the posterior to the anterior meniscal horn and are commonly *displaced* forward of the femoral condyle into the intercondylar area.

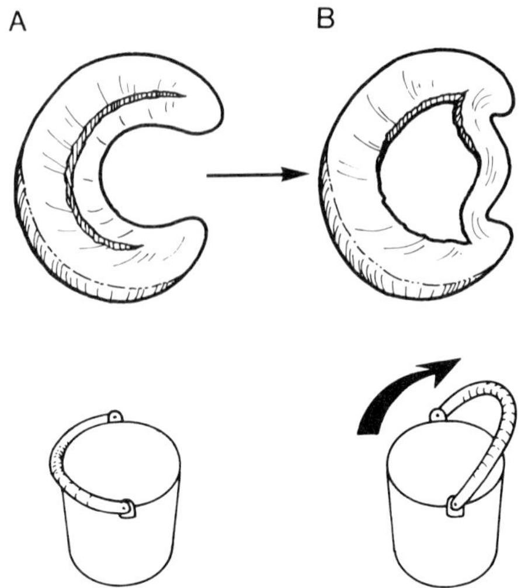

Fig. 6–8. ***A,* Nondisplaced vertical longitudinal meniscal tear. *B,* Displaced vertical longitudinal tear or displaced "bucket-handle" tear.**

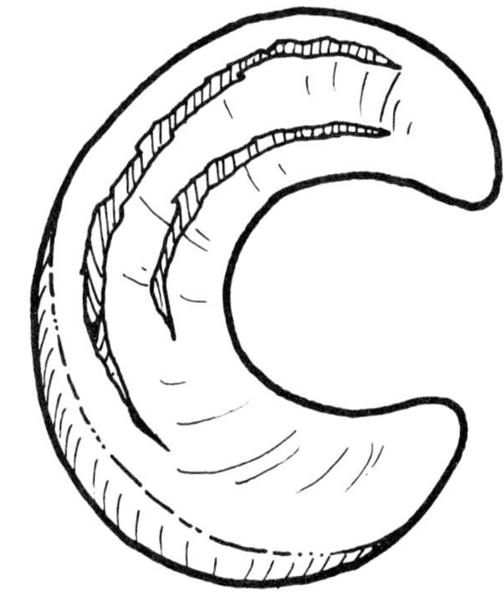

Fig. 6–9. Double vertical longitudinal meniscal tear.

The term "bucket-handle tear" is commonly used to describe a vertical longitudinal meniscal tear. The configuration of this type of tear is likened to a bucket and its handle (Fig. 6–8). This term is commonly misunderstood, so we prefer the terms "vertical longitudinal tear" or "circumferential tear."

The most common location for a vertical

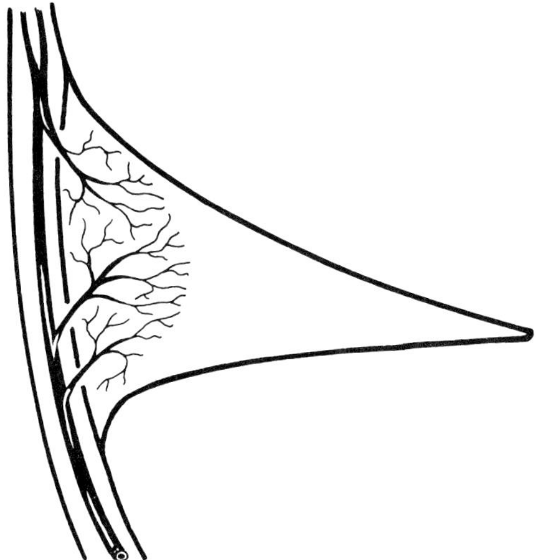

Fig. 6–10. Cross section of meniscus showing the vascular supply of the peripheral third.

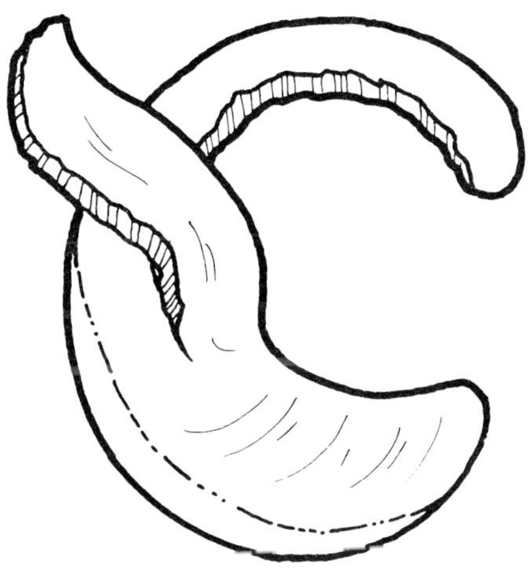

Fig. 6–11. Vertical longitudinal meniscal tear, which has torn from its posterior attachment to form an anteriorly based flap.

longitudinal tear is the thick outer third of the meniscus. The meniscus tears less frequently in its midsubstance or inner third. When the meniscus tears in its central two-thirds, it is likely to have a second or even a third peripheral tear (Fig. 6–9). Moreover, the meniscus can be torn from its capsular and synovial attachments and may cause the same symptoms as a tear in the meniscal body.

Recognition of the exact location of a tear in a meniscus is important in planning treatment. Tears in the outer third and meniscosynovial junction have the potential to heal because of the vascular supply that extends from the capsule into the peripheral third of the meniscus[15–22] (Fig. 6–10).

The posterior attachment of a vertical longitudinal tear can become detached and can form a large pedunculated flap (Fig. 6–11). The free end of the torn meniscus can displace toward the joint line, to produce a tender mass. In other patients, the meniscal fragment tears in the middle, resulting in two meniscal flaps similar to a "T-shaped" tear. Tearing of the anterior attachment of a vertical longitudinal tear, resulting in a posteriorly based flap, occurs more rarely.

A torn meniscus can change in size and appearance as the tear propagates within the meniscus. Such a change usually occurs with repeated knee injuries, especially in the unstable knee.

The clinical symptoms of a meniscal tear depend on the mobility of the unstable fragment. An undisplaceable tear may cause pain, swelling, catching, or popping when the mobile fragment momentarily catches between the femoral and tibial condyles. Pain is not caused by force exerted on the meniscus itself because the meniscus is aneural. When the unstable fragment becomes caught in the joint interface, however, traction on the synovial and capsular attachments of the meniscus causes pain. Locking or a sudden inability to extend the knee occurs if the meniscal fragment remains displaced anterior to the femoral condyle.

Arthroscopic Diagnosis

One should inspect and probe the superior and inferior surfaces of both menisci to diagnose vertical longitudinal tears. The posterior third of the medial meniscus is best seen when the knee is held in approximately 10° of flexion while abduction and external rotational forces are applied

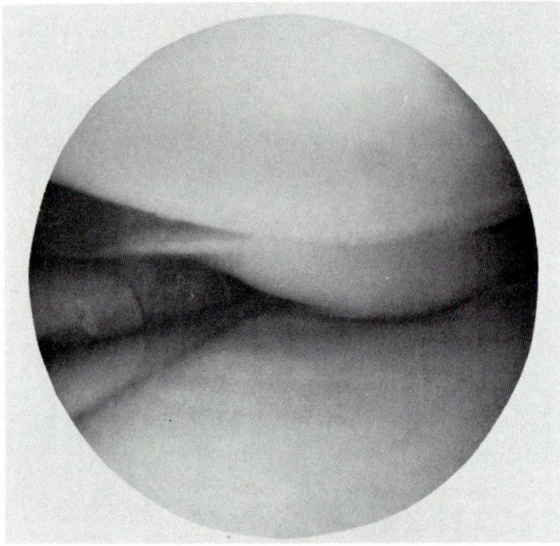

Fig. 6–12. Vertical longitudinal tear of the posterior third of the medial meniscus (left knee). The tear cannot be seen, but the probe demonstrates excessive mobility of the meniscus. This is an unstable meniscus, but would be classified as nondisplaceable because the segment cannot be pulled *forward* of the femoral condyle.

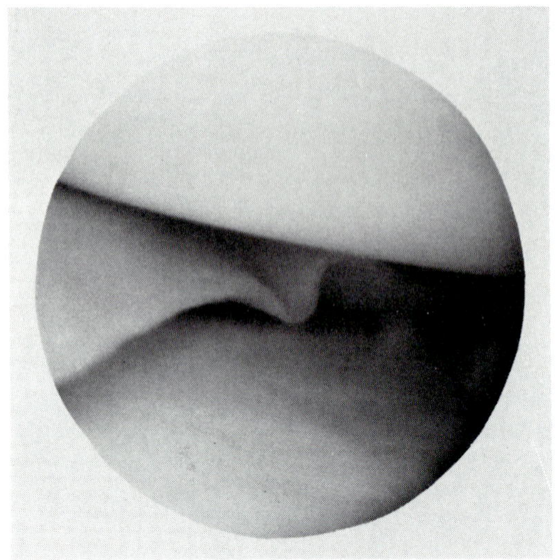

Fig. 6–14. A normal fold of the inner edge of the posterior third of the medial meniscus that occurs with tibial rotation is called a "flounce" (left knee).

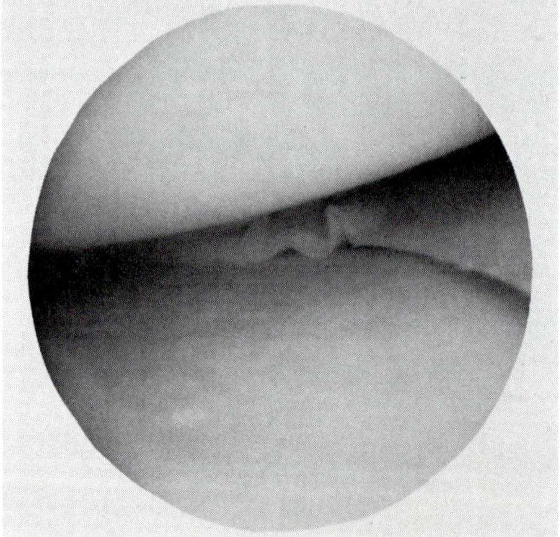

Fig. 6–13. Excessive folding of the inner edge of the posterior aspect of the medial meniscus suggesting a hidden tear (right knee).

to the tibia. The posterior third of the lateral meniscus is best visualized when the hip is externally rotated and the knee is flexed to 90° with a varus force applied (the figure-4 position).

A vertical longitudinal tear located in the posterior horn of the medial meniscus may

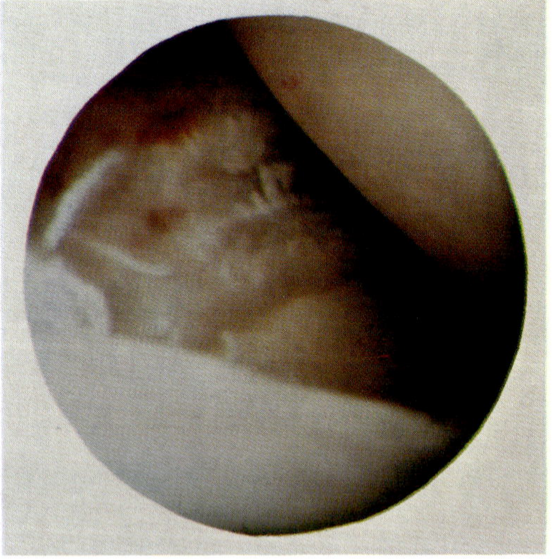

Fig. 6–15. Displaced vertical longitudinal tear of the medial meniscus that can block the view from the anterolateral portal. If the meniscal rim appears to be small in a knee that has not undergone surgical correction, one should assume the presence of a displaced meniscal fragment in the intercondylar notch until proved otherwise.

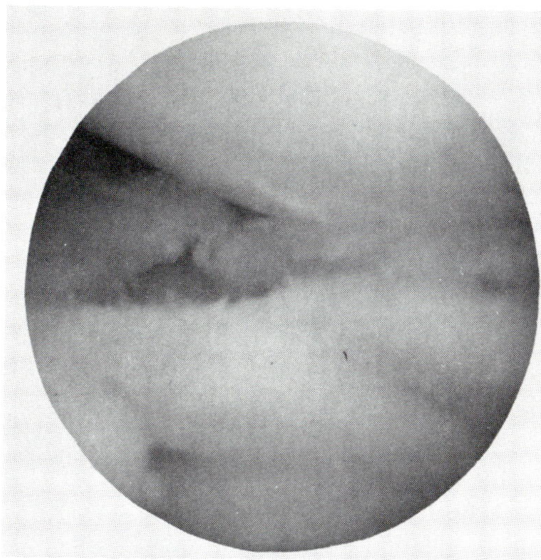

Fig. 6–16. Double vertical longitudinal tear of the left medial meniscus, both displaced. The medial femoral condyle is on top and the tibia is below.

be difficult to see because of the large medial femoral condyle. Recognition of secondary meniscal signs should raise one's suspicions and should lead to identification of the tear. An area of articular cartilage fibrillation in the weight-bearing portion of the medial femoral condyle is frequently associated with a posterior meniscal horn tear. If the posterior third of the meniscus is easily seen, one should suspect a tear allowing the meniscus to be displaced anteriorly ("pouting"). The tear can be confirmed by using a probe to pull the meniscus anteriorly (Fig. 6–12).

Excessive folding or waviness of the free edge of the meniscus often occurs as the result of a torn meniscus (Fig. 6–13) and should be differentiated from a flounce, which is a single, symmetrical fold in the free edge of the normal meniscus (Fig. 6–14).

If a vertical longitudinal meniscal tear is seen, one should suspect a torn anterior cruciate ligament and look for it. Conversely, when a torn anterior cruciate ligament is visualized, one should assume the presence of a torn meniscus until proved otherwise.[23,24]

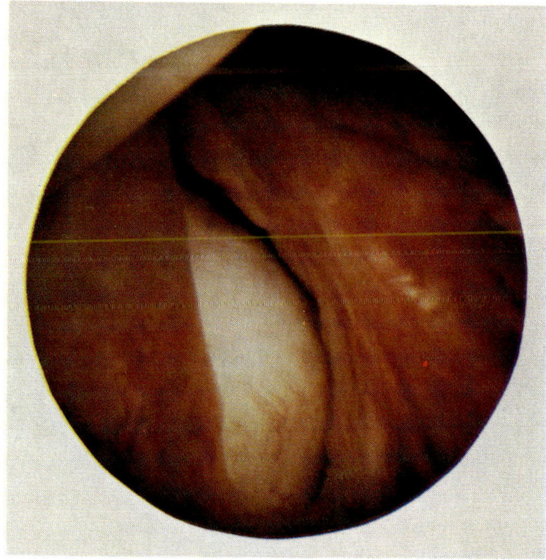

Fig. 6–17. Posteromedial corner of the right knee viewed through the intercondylar notch by the anterolateral portal. The synovium and capsule, seen on the right, are torn from the posterior third of the medial meniscus, seen on the left. The medial femoral condyle is at the extreme upper left. The tibial plateau is seen through the tear.

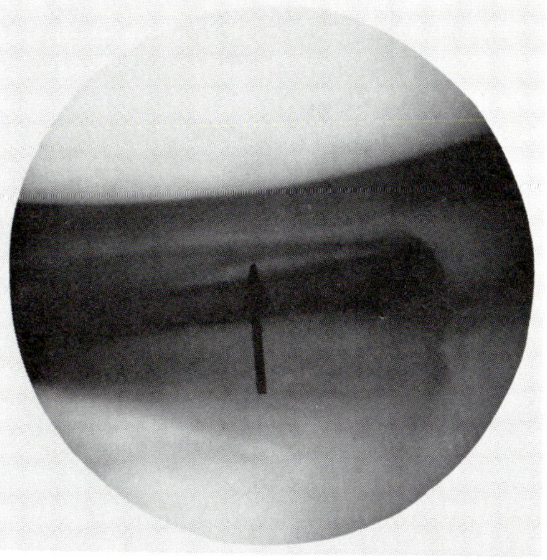

Fig. 6–18. Small vertical longitudinal tear of the posterior third of the left lateral meniscus (arrow). This tear can be confused with a normal space that occurs at the popliteus recess.

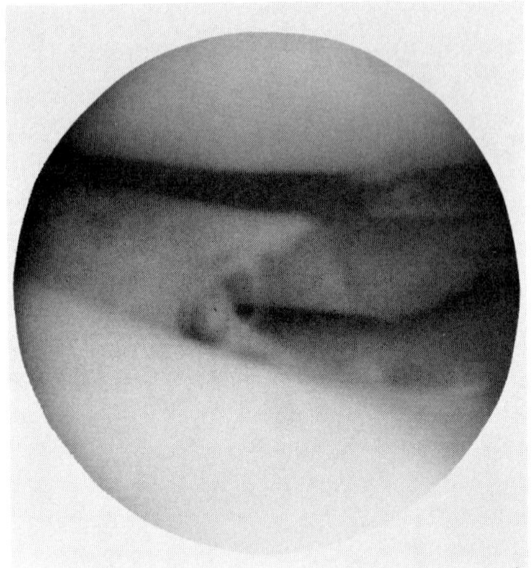

Fig. 6–19. Excessively wavy appearance of the free edge of right lateral meniscus due to a vertical transverse tear.

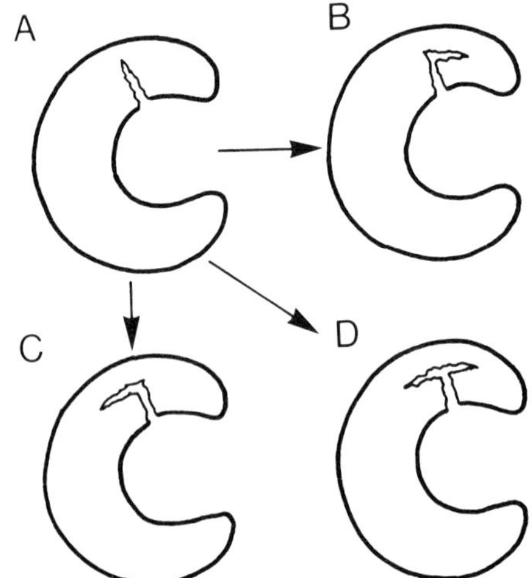

Fig. 6–20. *A,* A radial tear in the posterior meniscus can propagate in a longitudinal direction and become: *B,* an "L-shaped" tear with posterior flap; *C,* an "L-shaped" tear with anterior flap, or *D,* a "T-shaped" tear.

Arthroscopic visualization of a displaced, vertical longitudinal tear can be frustrating because the displaced meniscal fragment occupies most of the anterior joint space. One should suspect this type of tear if the meniscal rim appears more narrow than normal (Fig. 6–15). Viewing from another portal may help to identify the meniscal lesion. It is best to reduce the displaced fragment with a probe to determine the exact size and nature of the tear.

Double or triple vertical longitudinal tears must be suspected if the inner meniscal fragment is narrow[25] (Fig. 6–16). The second tear may not be visible until the first meniscal fragment is resected.

Meniscosynovial junction tears are diagnosed by noting a disruption of the normal continuity of the synovium with the outer portion of the meniscus. The best view of a meniscosynovial tear of the posterior third of the medial meniscus is through the intercondylar notch (Fig. 6–17). Any separation of the synovium

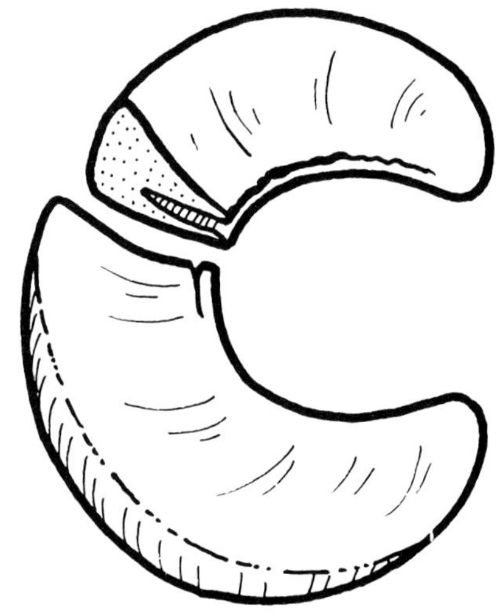

Fig. 6–21. Horizontal (cleavage) meniscal tear.

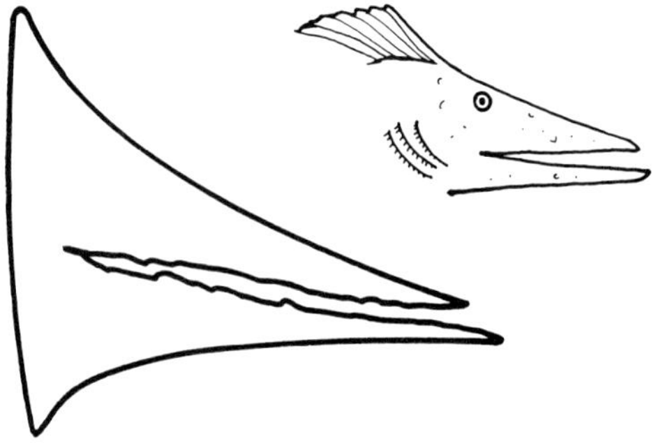

Fig. 6–22. Horizontal "fishmouth" tear of the lateral meniscus.

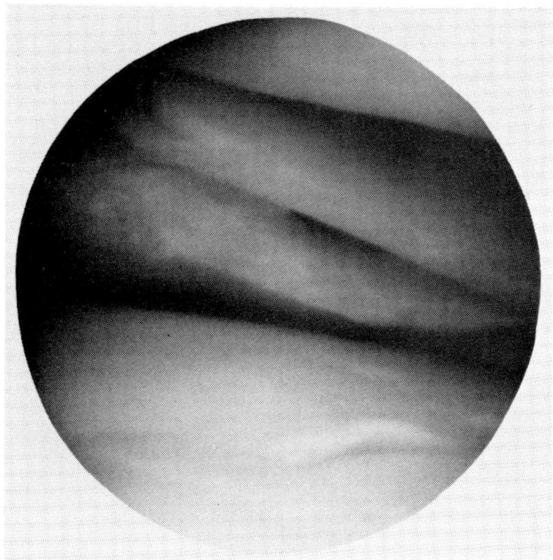

Fig. 6–23. Horizontal "fishmouth" tear of the left lateral meniscus.

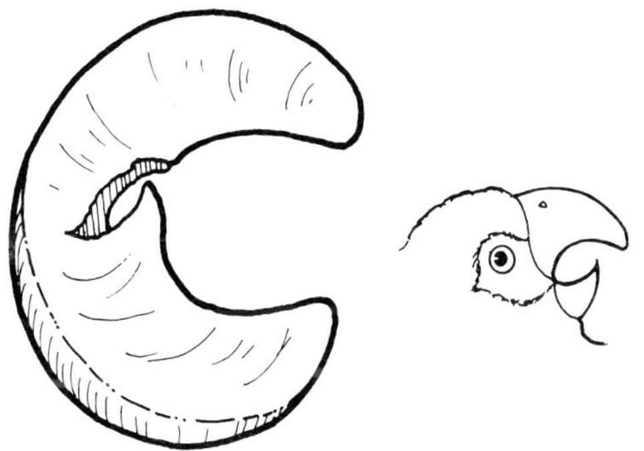

Fig. 6–24. Oblique tear, also called a "parrot-beak" tear.

from the medial meniscus is abnormal. Laterally, however, normal space exists between the peripheral attachment of the meniscus and the capsule in the posterior third at the popliteal tendon recess. This space should not be misinterpreted as a peripheral tear, which appears as a disruption in the substance of the lateral meniscus itself (Fig. 6–18). The distinction can be made by palpation with a probe.

VERTICAL TRANSVERSE TEAR (RADIAL)

Vertical transverse meniscal tears occur in a plane perpendicular to the tibial plateau and the inner edge of the meniscus. The most common location of transverse tears is the middle third of the lateral meniscus. This tear can be difficult to see from the standard anterolateral arthroscopy portal and can be mistaken for a normal fold in the meniscus (Fig. 6–19). When a lateral meniscal tear is suspected, but not seen, the meniscus should be visualized from an anteromedial portal and should be probed.

Occasionally, radial tears propagate in a longitudinal direction causing "L-shaped" or "T-shaped" tears (Fig. 6–20). These patterns usually occur in the posterior third of the meniscus.

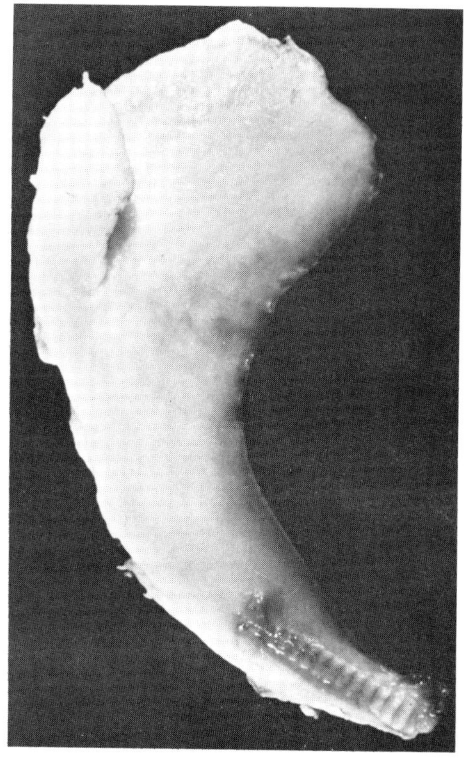

Fig. 6–25. Superior flap tear of the medial meniscus.

HORIZONTAL TEAR (CLEAVAGE)

Such tears are either degenerative or nondegenerative.

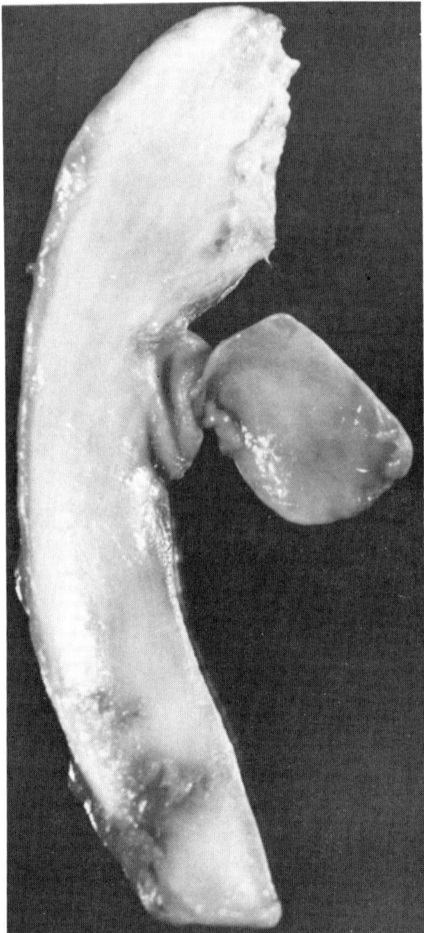

Fig. 6–26. Inferior flap tear of the medial meniscus. Note the flattened appearance and rounded edge of the flap secondary to compression between the condyles.

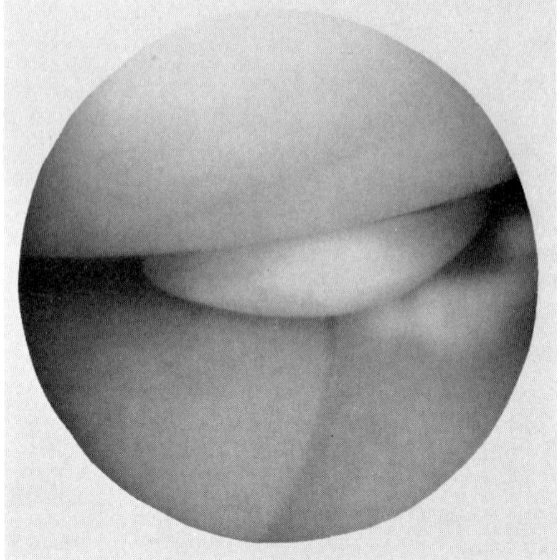

Fig. 6–27. Anteriorly based flap tear of the medial meniscus. If this type of tear is seen, one should inspect the posterior horn for a second flap (See Fig. 6–28). This meniscal tear may in fact be an old longitudinal tear that has split in the middle.

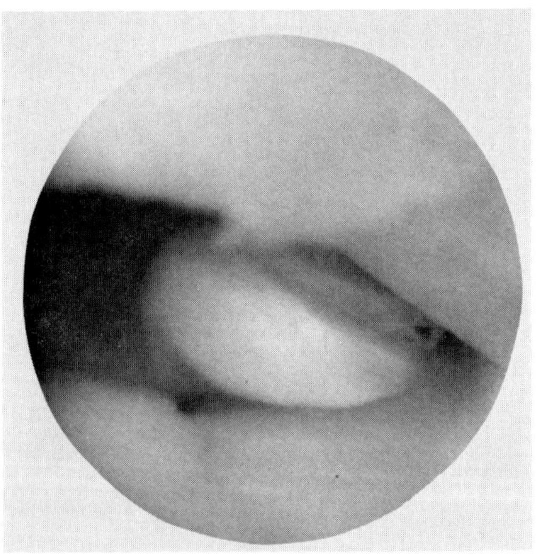

Fig. 6–28. Posteriorly based flap tear in the same medial meniscus as in Figure 6–27 with an anteriorly based flap tear.

Degenerative Horizontal Tear

Horizontal meniscal tears occur in a plane parallel to the tibial plateau and inner meniscal edge (Fig. 6–21). These tears are common in vigorous middle-aged athletes and in the elderly population and are associated with degenerative changes of the meniscus and articular cartilage.[2]

Most cleavage tears occur in the posterior third of the medial meniscus. Although the major component of degenerative tears is in the horizontal plane, multiple tears in different planes can occur.

Nondegenerative Horizontal Tear

Menisci in otherwise healthy knees can tear in a horizontal plane. These tears are most often found in the lateral meniscus of young and middle-aged patients and are sometimes referred to as "fishmouth tears" (Figs. 6–22 and 6–23).

The stability of the upper and lower flaps of the horizontal tear is determined by palpation with a probe. Arthroscopic resection of the entire upper and lower flaps may not be necessary because the peripheral attachments are often intact.

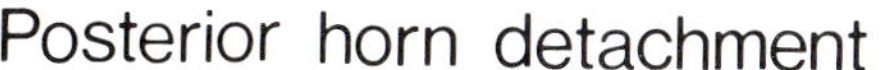

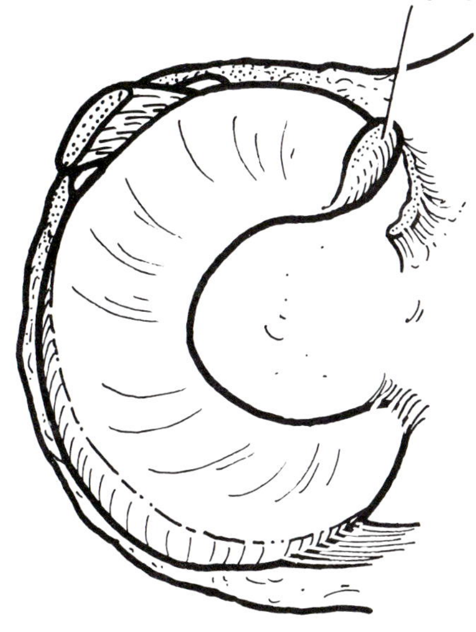

Fig. 6–29. Tear of the posterior attachment of the lateral meniscus from the tibia.

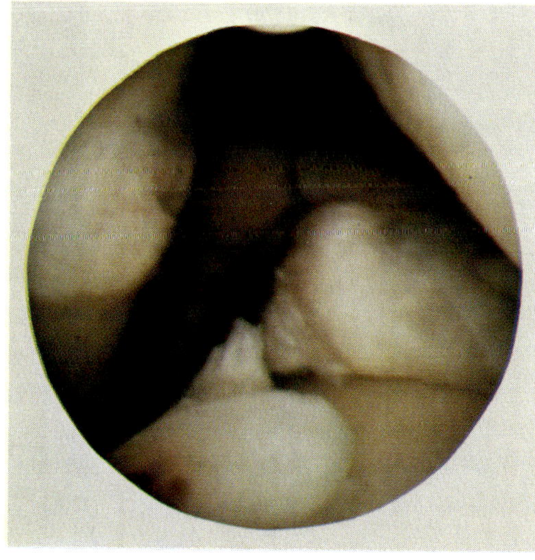

Fig. 6–30. Posteromedial corner of the left knee seen through the intercondylar area showing the posterior horn of the medial meniscus (in center) detached from the tibia. (Medial femoral condyle is at upper right and posterior cruciate ligament at left.)

OBLIQUE TEAR (FLAP)

An oblique tear is a combination of longitudinal, transverse, and horizontal tears that produces a pedunculated fragment attached to the remainder of the meniscus. Oblique tears commonly occur in all age groups and in both menisci. Clinically, oblique tears produce symptoms of clicking, catching, and popping of the knee. Occasionally, a meniscal flap may be displaced and may appear as a joint-line mass.

The term "parrot-beak tear" has been used to describe certain oblique tears that resemble the beak of a parrot (Fig. 6–24). This confusing term should probably be avoided.

Superior flap tears result from partial-thickness, oblique tears in the superior portion of the meniscus (Fig. 6–25). *Inferior flaps* arise from oblique tears in the inferior surface of the meniscus (Fig. 6–26). An inferior flap tear must be suspected if the edge of the meniscus appears rounded rather than tapered.[26] Both these tears usually occur in the posterior third of the menisci.

Numerous other types of oblique tears can occur and are described by the appearance and location of the flaps. Anteriorly and posteriorly based double flaps are common (Figs. 6–27 and 6–28). In general, lateral meniscal flaps are more irregular and varied because of extension of the tears into the popliteal tunnel.

DETACHMENT OF MENISCAL HORNS

The posterior meniscal horn can tear from its tibial attachment as an isolated lesion or in association with a torn anterior cruciate ligament (Figs. 6–29 and 6–30). In our experience, anterior horn tears or detachments are rare and are usually associated with posterior instability of the knee.

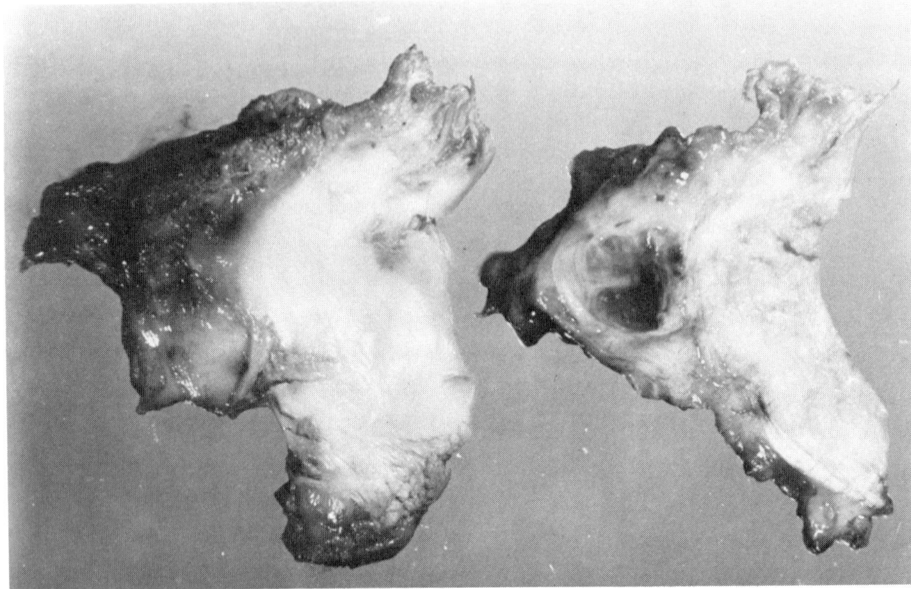

Fig. 6–31. Section through a large solitary cyst connected to the lateral meniscus.

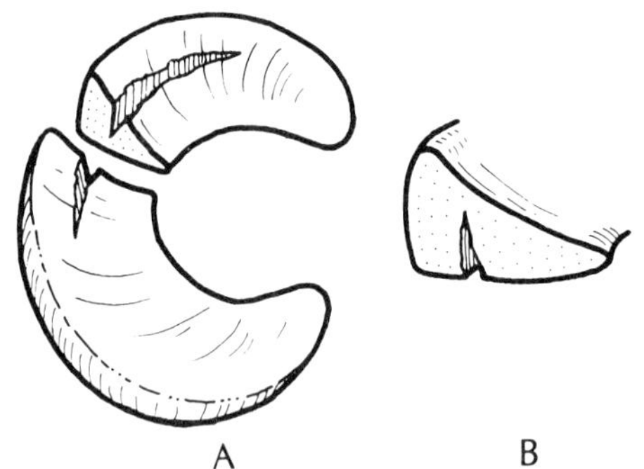

Fig. 6–32. Partial-thickness meniscal tears: *A*, Superior; *B*, inferior.

Smillie also reports a low incidence of anterior meniscal tears.[3]

COMPLEX TEARS

Combinations of the previously mentioned tears are classified as complex tears. Some menisci are so completely disrupted that the predominant tear patterns cannot be categorized.[27] These lesions are usually seen in unstable knees and are the result of repeated trauma to the menisci.

CYSTIC DEGENERATION

Menisci can undergo cystic degeneration resulting in multilocular or unicameral cysts (Fig. 6–31). The lateral meniscus is most commonly involved, and patients usually have a joint-line mass and tenderness. The cysts are rarely seen during arthroscopy. Probing usually reveals a concomitant horizontal tear in the meniscus.

MISCELLANEOUS LESIONS

Partial-Thickness Tears

Tears that do not extend completely through the meniscus are most often longitudinal tears involving the superior or inferior surface of the posterior third of the meniscus (Fig. 6–32). Partial-thickness tears do not result in meniscal instability and rarely cause severe enough symptoms to warrant resection. Probing determines the depth of the tear and the stability of the meniscus. Anterolateral rotary instability is a common cause of these tears.

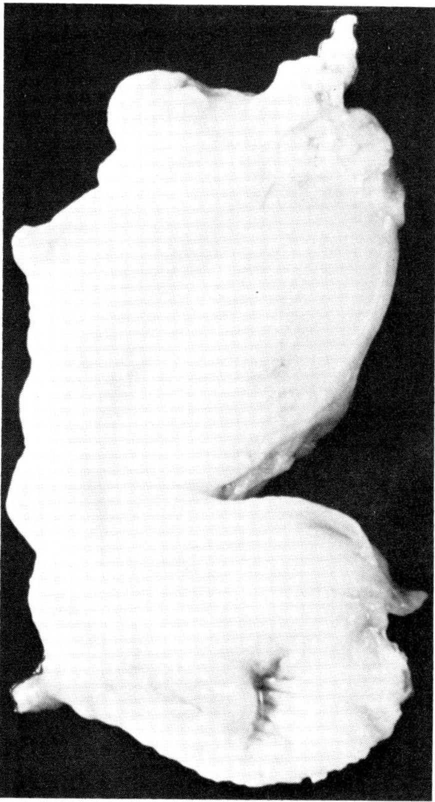

Fig. 6–33. Vertical transverse tear in the mid-third of the discoid lateral meniscus.

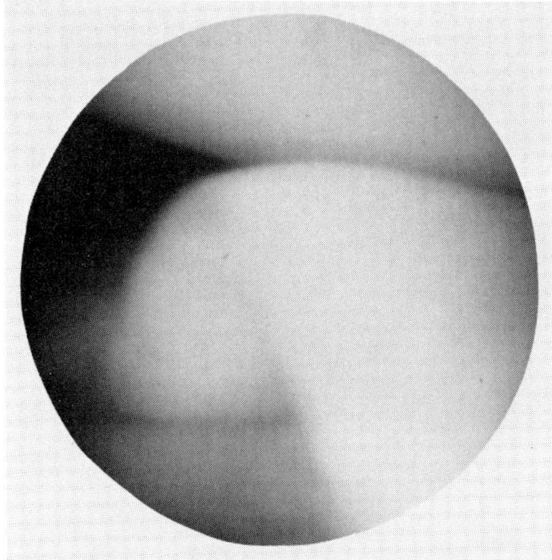

Fig. 6–34. Free edge of the left discoid lateral meniscus can be mistaken for a displaced "bucket-handle" tear of the lateral meniscus. (Lateral femoral condyle is above and tibia is at lower left.)

Postmeniscectomy Meniscal Rim Tears

Tears can occur in the meniscal rim, which remains after partial meniscectomy, especially in the unstable knee. The rim tear can represent either a new tear not present at the time of meniscectomy or a component of a double or triple longitudinal tear that was not recognized at the time of meniscectomy.

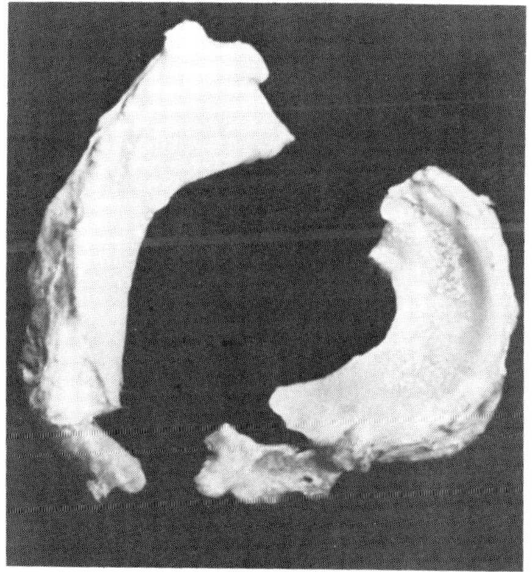

Fig. 6–35. Calcium pyrophosphate crystal deposition in lateral and medial menisci of the same knee.

Discoid Meniscus

Smillie reported discoid lateral menisci in 4% of male and 11% of female patients who underwent meniscectomy. Discoid medial menisci comprised only .07% of Smillie's series.[3]

Because a discoid meniscus occupies almost the entire joint space, the meniscus is more susceptible to damage between the femoral and tibial condyles. Longitudinal, radial, and oblique tears frequently occur (Fig. 6–33).

Visualization of a discoid meniscus is often difficult. The free edge of a discoid meniscus is located near the intercondylar notch (Fig. 6–34) and can be mistaken for the edge of a displaced vertical longitudinal meniscal tear. To make the distinction, one

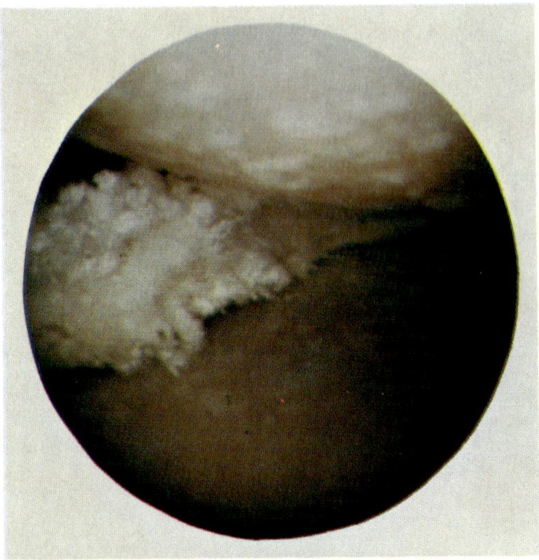

Fig. 6–36. White calcium pyrophosphate crystals in the rim of a previously excised medial meniscus.

should determine the size of the meniscus on the other side of the free edge by following the superior surface toward the periphery.

Calcification and Ossification

Several clinical presentations of calcium pyrophosphate deposition disease may be seen, including chondrocalcinosis, crystal-induced synovitis (pseudogout), and pyrophosphate arthropathy.[5,28–30] One or more of these patterns can occur in the same patient. Arthroscopic visualization of chondrocalcinosis reveals small, white calcium deposits in the menisci (Fig. 6–35) or articular cartilage. Crystal deposits can also occur in the synovium or rim of a previously excised meniscus (Fig. 6–36). Other causes of articular chondrocalcinosis, either occurring alone or concomitantly with calcium pyrophosphate deposition disease, include hyperparathyroidism, hemochromatosis, Wilson's disease, and ochronosis. An association between certain collagen vascular diseases and calcium pyrophosphate deposition disease has been suggested.[5]

Ossification of menisci is extremely rare and is most likely a result of trauma rather than an embryologic defect. Most ossicles occur in the posterior horn of the medial meniscus and are difficult to distinguish radiologically from loose bodies.[31]

ACKNOWLEDGMENT

We would like to thank Drs. Carter R. Rowe and Edwin F. Cave for use of their photographs and Laurel L. Cook for the artwork.

REFERENCES

1. Mathur, P.D., McDonald, J.R., and Ghormley, R.K.: A study of the tensile strength of the menisci of the knee. J. Bone Joint Surg. (Am.), *31*:650, 1949.
2. Noble, J., and Hamblen, D.L.: The pathology of the degenerate meniscus lesion. J. Bone Joint Surg. (Br.), *57*:180, 1975.
3. Smillie, I.S.: Injuries of the Knee Joint. 5th Ed. Edinburgh, Churchill Livingstone, 1978.
4. Hartlepool, M.F., and Kelly, J.P.: Local excision of cyst of lateral meniscus of knee without recurrence. J. Bone Joint Surg. (Br.), *58*:88, 1976.
5. McCarty, D.J. (ed.): Arthritis and Allied Conditions. 9th Ed. Philadelphia, Lea & Febiger, 1979.
6. Cave, E.F.: Calcification in the menisci. J. Bone Joint Surg., *25*:53, 1943.
7. Mariani, P.P., and Puddu, G.: Meniscal ossicle: a case report. Am. J. Sports Med., *9*:392, 1981.
8. Bullough, P.G., Munuera, L., Murphy, J., and Weinstein, A.M.: The strength of the menisci of the knee as it relates to their fine structure. J. Bone Joint Surg. (Br.), *52*:564, 1970.
9. Ghadially, F.N., Thomas, I., Yong, N., and Lalonde, J-M.A.: Ultrastructure of rabbit semilunar cartilages. J. Anat., *125*:499, 1978.
10. O'Connor, B.L.: The histological structure of dog knee menisci with comments on its possible significance. Am. J. Anat., *147*:407, 1976.
11. Kennedy, J.C.: The Injured Adolescent Knee. Baltimore, Williams & Wilkins, 1979.
12. Hughston, J.C.: A simple meniscectomy. J. Sports Med., *3*:179, 1975.
13. Warren, L.F., and Marshall, J.L.: The supporting structures and layers on the medial side of the knee: an anatomical analysis. J. Bone Joint Surg. (Am.), *61*:56, 1979.
14. Last, R.J.: Some anatomical details of the knee joint. J. Bone Joint Surg. (Br.), *30*:683, 1948.
15. Annandale, T.: An operation for displaced semilunar cartilage. Br. Med. J., 779, 1885.
16. Cabaud, H.E., Rodkey, W.G., and Fitzwater, J.E.: Medial meniscus repairs: an experimental and morphologic study. Am. J. Sports Med., *9*:129, 1981.
17. Cassidy, R.E., and Shaffer, A.J.: Repair of peripheral meniscus tears: a preliminary report. Am. J. Sports Med., *9*:209, 1981.
18. Heatley, F.W.: The meniscus—can it be repaired? An experimental investigation in rabbits. J. Bone Joint Surg. (Br.), *62*:397, 1980.

19. King, D.: The function of semilunar cartilages. J. Bone Joint Surg., *18*:1069, 1936.
20. Scapinelli, R.: Studies on the vasculature of the human knee joint. Acta Anat., *70*:305, 1968.
21. Schneider, D.A., and Johnson, L.L.: Peripheral detachment of the meniscus: arthroscopic and clinical correlations. Orthop. Rev., *6*:55, 1977.
22. Stone, R.G.: Peripheral detachment of the menisci of the knee: a preliminary report. Orthop. Clin. North Am., *10*:643, 1979.
23. DeHaven, K.E.: Diagnosis of acute knee injuries with hemarthrosis. Am. J. Sports Med., *8*:9, 1981.
24. Noyes, F.R., Bassett, R.W., Grood, E.S., and Butler, D.L.: Arthroscopy in acute traumatic hemarthrosis of the knee. J. Bone Joint Surg. (Am.), *62*:687, 1980.
25. Andrews, J.R., Norwood, L.A., and Cross, M.J.: The double bucket handle tear of the medial meniscus. J. Sports Med., *3*:232, 1975.
26. Hansen, F.W.: Underside lesions of the meniscus. Acta Orthop. Scand., *49*:610, 1978.
27. Dandy, D.J.: Arthroscopic Surgery of the Knee. Edinburgh, Churchill Livingstone, 1981.
28. Bjelle, A., and Sunden, G.: Pyrophosphate arthropathy: a clinical study of fifty cases. J. Bone Joint Surg. (Br.), *56*:246, 1974.
29. McCarty, D.J., Hogan, J.M., Gatter, R.A., and Grossman, M.: Studies on pathological calcifications in human cartilage. J. Bone Joint Surg. (Am.), *48*:309, 1966.
30. Moskowitz, R.W., and Katz, D.: Chondrocalcinosis and chondrocalsynovitis (pseudogout syndrome): analysis of twenty-four cases. Am. J. Med., *43*:322, 1967.
31. Lonon, W.D., and Crawford, A.H.: Ossicle of the medial meniscus in a child. Orthop. Rev., *10*:129, 1981.

Chapter 7

ANTERIOR CRUCIATE LIGAMENT INJURIES

R.W. Jackson

It has been said that the anterior cruciate ligament is the "watch-dog" of the knee. When the ligament is disrupted, problems inevitably occur; however, arthroscopy has revealed a spectrum of disorders affecting the anterior cruciate ligament and has led to the concept that the treatment of such disorders should be specifically directed toward the degree of functional disability. This chapter reviews the anatomic and pathologic findings at arthroscopy and outlines a selective approach to treatment based not only on this fundamental knowledge, but also on clinical observations regarding the natural history of untreated anterior cruciate ligament injuries.

CLINICAL PICTURE

Rupture of the anterior cruciate ligament occurs when forces generated by the individual in either decelerating or changing direction exceed the tensile strength of the ligament itself. This phenomenon can occur, for example, when a running athlete stops suddenly, changes direction, or lands from a jump. Characteristically, the femur is externally rotated on the tibia in a knee that is in slight flexion, with the tibia fixed to the ground on a planted foot. Another classic way of tearing the anterior cruciate ligament is by applying an extraneous valgus, varus, or anterior displacement force to the flexed knee. When such an extraneous force is applied as in North American football, the injury is usually associated with a concomitant tear of the medial or lateral collateral ligament, either of the menisci or the posterior capsule.[1] The individual classically feels a "popping" sensation in the knee, followed by pain and dysfunction due to a feeling of instability.[2,3] The knee rapidly swells as a result of hemorrhage from rupture of the vascularized synovium overlying the cruciate ligament. Noticeable swelling due to bleeding usually occurs within 2 to 3 hours. It can be differentiated, therefore, from a traumatic effusion, which is a reaction to injury of a nonvascular structure within the joint and which usually occurs in the ensuing 24 hours. Pain from a torn anterior cruciate ligament is often experienced posterolaterally or may be difficult to localize.

Physical examination demonstrates a swollen joint, usually held in a slightly flexed position. If a torn anterior cruciate ligament is the only major injury in the joint, tenderness may be present posterolaterally at or superior to the joint line. If associated collateral ligament or capsular injuries are present, findings related to these deranged structures may be more prominent.

The anterior cruciate ligament should always be clinically assessed by performing both the Lachman's test,[4] in which anterior displacement of the tibia on the femur is assessed with the knee in 15 to 20° of flexion, and the drawer test, in which similar displacement is assessed with the knee at 70 to 90° of flexion. In addition, the various tests for anterolateral rotatory instability, such as the pivot shift,[5–7] flexion-rotation drawer,[8] Slocum,[9] Losee,[10] or jerk tests,[11] should be performed. Special investigations include plain roentgenograms, stress roentgenograms if indicated, examination under anaesthesia, and arthroscopic examination of the interior of the joint.

SPECTRUM OF PATHOLOGIC LESIONS

Numerous studies have shown that in substantial injuries to the knee that result in a hemarthrosis, a 72 to 75% chance exists that a torn anterior cruciate ligament is the cause of the hemorrhage within the joint.[8,12–14] Coincidentally, the possibility also exists that a meniscus torn at its periphery, an osteochondral fracture, or a capsular tear is the cause of the bleeding. Therefore, in cases of traumatic hemarthrosis secondary to a substantial injury, a significantly high probability exists that the lesion within the joint is amenable to surgery. It behooves the orthopedic surgeon, therefore, to make an accurate and complete diagnosis in the early stages following the injury because the ideal opportunity to repair any torn ligament or capsule is during these stages, a time previously referred to as the "golden period" by Palmer.[15]

In the past, many of these injuries were treated "expectantly," with conservative splinting and a "wait-and-see" attitude about whether any significant disability would result. With the capability of making a precise early diagnosis through arthroscopy, however, it is reasonable for the modern orthopedic surgeon to approach the problem in a more aggressive way. He should find out exactly what the lesion is and then decide whether to continue with conservative management or to attempt an operative repair.

Arthroscopic examinations of a consecutive series of traumatic hemarthroses have revealed the full spectrum of pathologic disorders involving the anterior cruciate ligament[16] (Figs. 7–1 to 7–7). On the minimal end of the scale is isolated partial rupture of the anterior cruciate ligament. At the most severe end of the scale is total rupture of the anterior cruciate ligament combined with some other ligamentous or meniscal disorder within the joint. Through the correlation of the findings at clinical examination with the isolated partial ruptures, significant information regarding the function of the component parts of the anterior cruciate ligament has been obtained.

FUNCTIONAL ANATOMY

Fetto and Marshall,[5] van Dyke,[17] and others[18–20] have shown that the anatomy of the anterior cruciate ligament is more complex than previously thought. The crescentic origin and a "functional" banding of the cruciate ligament lead to a degree of tension in certain fibers of the ligament in every position of flexion and extension. When the knee is in full extension, the posterolateral component of the anterior cruciate ligament is tight and the anteromedial component is loose. As the knee progressively moves towards flexion, the anteromedial component becomes tight and the posterolateral component becomes loose. Anatomic dissections suggest that these two main functional bands do exist and that stress is progressively passed from one band to the other during the flexion and extension movements of the knee.

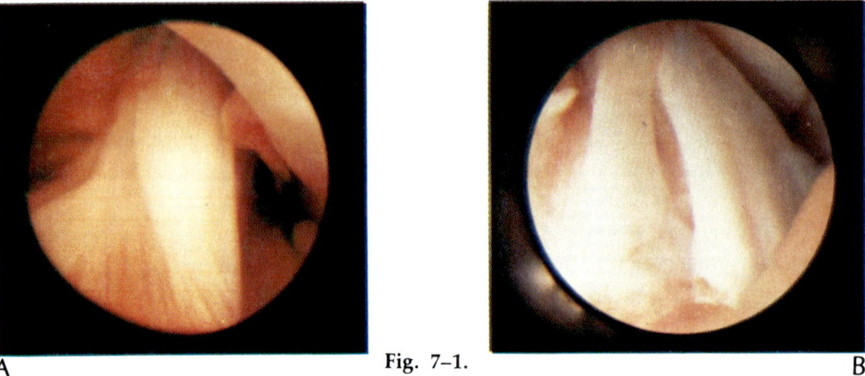

Fig. 7–1.

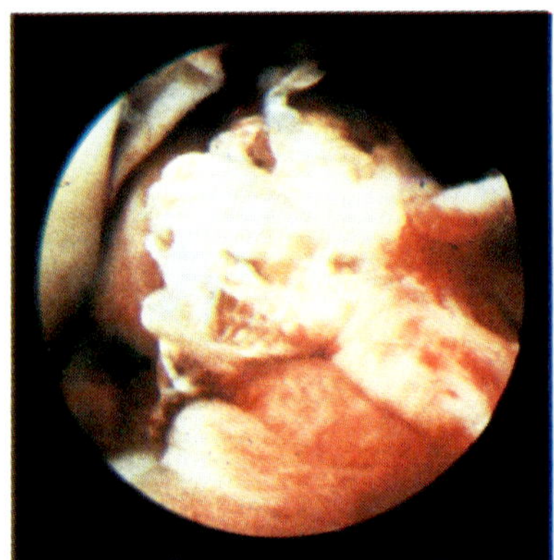

Fig. 7–2.

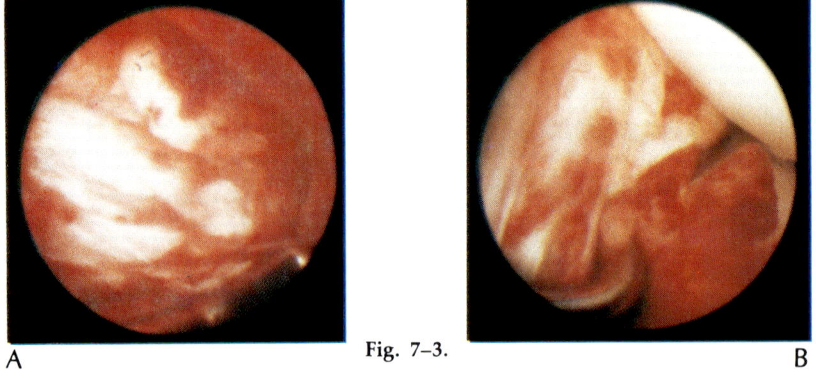

Fig. 7–3.

Fig. 7–1. *A* and *B*, Intact anterior cruciate ligaments clearly showing the functional banding, that is, anteromedial and posterolateral bands.

Fig. 7–2. Complete tear of both bands of the anterior cruciate ligament, with rupture of the synovial sheath.

Fig. 7–3. *A* and *B*, Incompetent anterior cruciate ligament, with an intact synovial sheath and marked subsynovial hemorrhage. Note the use of the probe to assess the competence of the ligament.

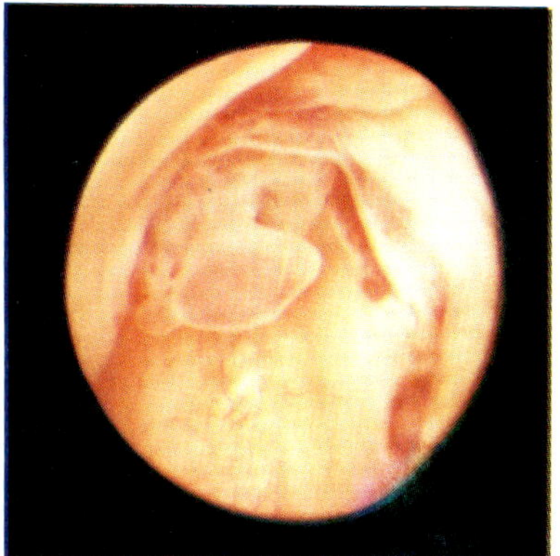

Fig. 7–4.

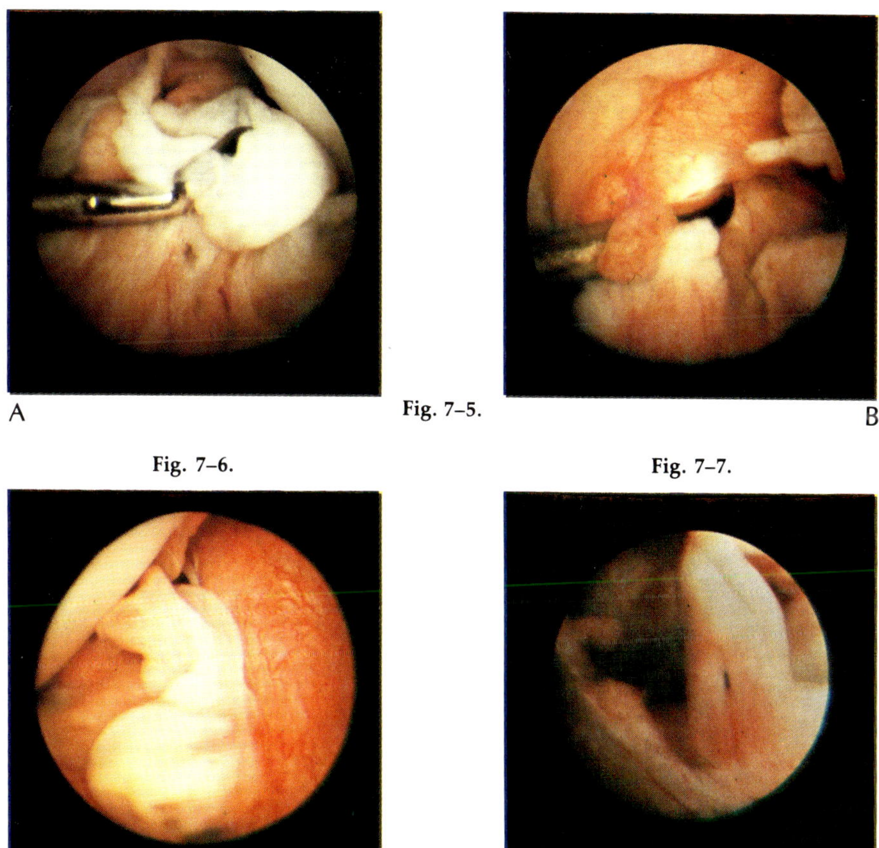

Fig. 7–5.

Fig. 7–6.

Fig. 7–7.

Fig. 7–4. Partial rupture of the anterior cruciate ligament with subsynovial hemorrhage.

Fig. 7–5. *A* and *B,* Partial rupture of the anterior cruciate ligament of the left knee. The posterolateral band has ruptured, with an intact anteromedial band.

Fig. 7–6. Partial rupture of the anterior cruciate ligament of the right knee. The posterolateral band has ruptured, with an intact anteromedial band.

Fig. 7–7. Old tear of the anterior cruciate ligament. The posterior cruciate ligament is visible in the background.

No question exists that many anterior cruciate ligament injuries went undiagnosed in the past because of the inability of the examining surgeon clinically to detect any significant degree of instability within the joint shortly after the initial injury. The common instability tested for was neither functional nor dynamic. For example, a positive anterior drawer test with the knee at 70 to 90° of flexion may not have any great significance in terms of functional disability if the adjacent musculature and secondary restraints are intact and functioning. Recently, attention has been drawn to the clinical test attributed to Lachman,[4] which is essentially a drawer test in 20 to 30° of flexion. It is said to be a more sensitive clinical indicator of anterior cruciate ligament rupture, and if positive, has more significance than the classic drawer test, in terms of functional disability.

CORRELATION WITH CLINICAL FINDINGS

Considering the anatomic features, it is obvious that the anteromedial band of the anterior cruciate ligament is tense in 90° of flexion. Theoretically, therefore, its integrity should be assessed by means of the drawer test. If the anteromedial band is torn, the drawer test should be positive.

As the knee is brought into extension, the posterolateral band becomes taut. Its integrity then, should be assessed by the Lachman test, and if this band is torn, the Lachman test should be positive.

Correlating the clinical findings with isolated partial ruptures of the anterior cruciate ligament, I have been able to identify the Lachman test with the lack of integrity of the posterolateral band and the drawer test with a similar deficiency in the anteromedial band.[16] If both bands are torn, then both tests are usually positive. Associated with this clinical evaluation, however, is the finding that anterolateral rotatory instability, as evidenced by pivot shift, jerk, and flexion-rotation drawer tests, is associated *only* with the posterolateral band tear. Such tests are not positive with isolated, partial anteromedial band tears. The key anatomic structure, therefore, in regard to the prevention of anterolateral rotatory instability is the posterolateral band of the anterior cruciate ligament. If this band is torn or insufficient due to stretching, then anterolateral rotatory instability can result.[16]

BIOMECHANICAL AND ANATOMIC CORRELATIONS

The mechanism of injury of the two main functional band deficiencies is postulated to be different. An isolated anteromedial band tear occurs when that portion of the ligament is stretched, such as in the flexed knee position, and a displacement force occurs to the back of the tibia, causing the already taut anteromedial band fibers to be ruptured. This rupture typically occurs in the clipping type of injury in football. Conversely, the isolated posterolateral band tear normally occurs when the knee is in full extension. This injury is usually self-generated and occurs when the individual is running hard, plants his foot to decelerate or change direction ("cut"), and thus creates an internal rotation of the tibia on the femur. This movement puts the posterolateral band on maximum tension, and with the sudden deceleration or cutting movement, or landing from an extended position following jumping, in addition to the forward pull of the quadriceps muscles on the tibia, the posterolateral band can rupture. A total rupture can be caused by either mechanism, if the magnitude of the force is so great that the "other" band fails after rupture of the first. It can also occur with the classic valgus strain that ruptures the medial collateral ligament, the capsule or the medial meniscus, and finally, the anterior cruciate ligament.

When the integrity of the posterolateral band is compromised, a degree of anterolateral rotatory instability can occur on any repetition of that type of stress. For example, when the individual attempts to decelerate after jumping or to change direction when cutting in football or soccer, the tibia shifts anteriorly on the femur to produce a momentary subluxation of the lateral compartment, and as the body's momentum carries the individual forward, the knee flexes, the tibial femoral articulation reduces with a sudden and dynamic "clunk" or "jerk," and the patient's knee gives way.[6,7,9,10,21–22]

The isolated anteromedial band deficiency is of little consequence unless a similar injury, such as a forward thrust on the back of the tibia, occurs with the knee in the flexed position. The anteromedial band deficiency by itself can easily be compensated for by well-developed muscles. Posterolateral band deficiency *cannot* be compensated for by muscular activity, however, because the instability occurs with the knee in an extended position, a position in which the muscles have minimal control, owing to their mechanical disadvantage.

INCIDENCE OF ANTERIOR CRUCIATE LIGAMENT RUPTURES

It is not yet known what the incidence of injury to the anterior cruciate ligament is in relation to the overall population engaged in sporting or work activities. In a consecutive personal series of 1000 knee problems, however, I found 119 anterior cruciate ligament ruptures.[23] In 61 instances, the rupture was complete, with both bands of the cruciate ligament visibly and clinically torn. Partial ruptures of the anterior cruciate ligament were seen in 42 patients, with 34 of the partial ruptures involving the posterolateral band and 8 involving the anteromedial band. In 16 instances, the ligament appeared to be superficially intact, but on probing and on clinical examination, it was judged to have been stretched beyond its elastic limit and therefore was considered to have an insubstance tear. In these instances, some subsynovial hemorrhage always surrounded the anterior cruciate ligament, and this hemorrhage could be taken as confirmatory evidence of loss of integrity. It would appear, therefore, that anterior cruciate ligament ruptures occur frequently (12% of knees seen) and, when a rupture is present, a 51% chance exists that both bands of the cruciate ligament will be grossly separated. A partial rupture occurs in 35% of patients, with the posterolateral band injured 4 times as frequently as the anteromedial band. Lesions in continuity occurred in 14% of patients.

UNTREATED ANTERIOR CRUCIATE LIGAMENT RUPTURES

Early disillusionment with the final results of surgical repair of midsubstance ruptures of the anterior cruciate ligament led to the belief that suturing this ligament was invariably unrewarding and that the surgical time could best be spent in repairing other torn structures in the traumatized knee joint. Therefore, in my practice, for almost 15 years, patients with clinical disruptions of the capsular or ligamentous structures would be taken to the operating room for arthroscopic evaluation and documentation of the disorder, followed by surgical repair of the torn medial or lateral ligaments and capsule and surgical removal of any mobile fragments of meniscus. Whenever possible, however, I repaired the torn meniscus if it was damaged near its peripheral attachments. The cruciate ligament injury was deliberately ignored, except when it was disrupted by virtue of avulsion of a fragment of bone from its distal attachment. These exceptions were repaired; the others were left untreated. Therefore, over the years, a number of traumatized knees were seen in which no repair of the anterior cruciate was attempted. Included were many knees with an isolated anterior cruciate lesion, with the term "isolated" applied to those in which arthroscopic and clinical evaluation showed no other significant disorder. The isolated lesions showed equal numbers of partial as well as total ruptures of the anterior cruciate ligament. If any other pathologic process was detected, the anterior cruciate lesion was considered a "combined" lesion.

A recent study of the late results of these untreated but arthroscopically proved anterior cruciate ligament lesions revealed 63 knees for which no surgical treatment had been undertaken and in which sufficient follow-up information was available.[24] The results clearly fell into 2 groups. The "combined" injury group consisted of 43 knees, of which 37 knees had associated meniscal disorders, 15 had collateral ligament instability, and 3 were associated with osteochondral fractures of the medial femoral condyles. Most of these injuries were caused by sporting activity. Disruption of the anterior cruciate ligament was complete and total in 65% of the knees and partial in 35%. The follow-up period ranged from 1 to 23 years. This group demonstrated a reinjury rate of 35%, with 25% of the knees requiring further surgical treatment. Functionally, these individuals were more severely disabled, and because of the instability in their knees, only 10% of the patients had attempted to resume competitive sports. Almost half of this group (45%) had given up all sporting activity and felt that the condition of their knees was still deteriorating.

On the other hand, the group with isolated anterior cruciate injuries was different. Although interstitial damage to the joint capsule and other minor soft tissue disorders may accompany such injuries, it was believed that these minor injuries had the potential for soundly healing. It was considered, however, that the anterior cruciate ligament would not demonstrate such healing potential. In other words, although the prime stabilizer of the knee, that is, the anterior cruciate ligament, was disrupted, the secondary restraints of the knee were essentially intact or only minimally damaged and could be expected in time to regain their normal function unless further traumatized. Hence these injuries were considered isolated anterior cruciate lesions. All the injuries in the isolated group were due to sporting activity. In one-third of the instances, the diagnosis was established only at arthroscopy because physical examination failed to reveal the presence of cruciate ligament injury. Moreover, in the early days of this study, the Lachman test was not routinely performed, and clinical evaluation depended largely on the drawer and pivot shift tests.

In this group of patients with isolated injuries, there were as many partial as total ruptures. The follow-up period was from 1 to 10 years. It was obvious that this group were entirely different from the group with combined injuries. Of the patients in the isolated injury group, 80% were still involved in sports, and several were still functioning at a high level of professional athletics. Significant reinjury had occurred in only 5 of 22 patients (approximately 25%), and only 5% had required further surgical procedures.

When comparing the 2 groups, results were excellent in only 12% of the combined injury group, whereas 35% of the isolated injury group had excellent results. Moreover, the majority (80%) of the group with isolated injuries were still participating in sports, although 50% of them wore a brace for protective purposes. Those of the combined injury group who had a positive pivot shift test had predictably poor results.

RELATION OF MENISCAL TEARS TO ANTERIOR CRUCIATE LESIONS

In recent years, with the diagnostic accuracy of arthroscopy and the increasing capability of performing partial meniscectomy arthroscopically, a new situation has arisen. Patients identified as having combined lesions, both acute and chronic, with a recognizable disruption of the anterior cruciate ligament and a tear of one or both of the menisci, were initially treated by partial arthroscopic meniscectomy followed by knee rehabilitation. In some instances, open surgical procedures were performed to remove the meniscal remnants. The theory was that the real or potential instability might be due to the unstable meniscus, rather than to the ligament's insufficiency.

Thirty-nine patients with this combination were reviewed.[25] Fifteen of the 39 patients (38%) continued to experience episodes of "giving way" and ultimately required reconstructive procedures for their anterior cruciate ligament instability. If reconstruction was considered necessary, it was usually indicated at an early stage following the original injury and the reconstruction was performed at an average of 8 months following the primary arthroscopic examination. Of these patients, however, 62% (24 cases) had *not* required reconstruction at the time of follow-up, and the average time elapsed since injury was 25 months. The nonreconstructed group had a high incidence of flap tears of the meniscus and consisted of predominantly male patients. In contrast, patients in the reconstructed group were predominantly female, were injured at a younger age, and initially had a peripheral tear or a major bucket-handle tear of the meniscus in addition to a complete anterior cruciate ligament disruption. This group, therefore, had not only significant damage to the prime stabilizer of the knee, that is, the anterior cruciate ligament, but also major damage to one of the secondary restraints, that is, the meniscus.

In summary, almost two-thirds of the patients in this small series were improved by arthroscopic meniscectomy and were subsequently able to function well without any surgical treatment of the anterior cruciate ligament. One-third of the patients in this series deteriorated rapidly, however, probably because of more serious injuries to both the meniscus and the anterior cruciate ligament at the time of the "original injury." The obvious message is that, whenever possible, the bulk of the meniscus should be retained for its function as a secondary restraint, although arthroscopic resection of smaller fragments of meniscus may benefit the patient by increasing stability and by avoiding a major operative procedure.

ACUTE INJURIES

Rational Approach to Treatment

As with any treatment, it is important to perform the right procedure at the right time in the right patient. Selection of patients is therefore important. Arthroscopy is helpful in determining the type and degree of disorder within the joint. The surgeon's initial decision, then, is whether to treat the lesion conservatively or surgically. If one decides to operate, a second decision must then be made, and that is whether a repair alone is sufficient or whether augmentation of the repair is necessary.[20,26–29]

Based on the previously reported studies, the following considerations have proved useful in my practice when making these decisions:

Because 80% of patients with isolated lesions of the anterior cruciate ligament function at an acceptable level, my initial treatment of such a lesion is usually nonoperative. This category includes both total and partial ruptures. If a patient has a partial rupture of the anteromedial band, the function of this band can be replaced by muscle action because the knee is potentially unstable only in the flexed position. If a partial rupture of the posterolateral band exists, the chance of an annoying or a disabling instability in the future is greater. Instability in such instances occurs when the knee is almost straight, that is, in the position in which muscular control is minimal. The secondary restraints and the type of activities engaged in by the patient must also be considered. If the individual is extremely active, the secondary restraints (the joint capsule and the menisci) might be compromised or stretched, and the chances of functional instability developing at a later date are increased.

If the injury is a total, isolated rupture, the degree of instability is similar to that with an isolated posterolateral band tear. An isolated rupture of the cruciate ligament, whether partial or total, is analogous to a dislocating shoulder, surgical repair of which is recommended when episodes of dislocation recur frequently. Similarly, in the knee, recurrent episodes of anterolateral subluxation lead one to consider surgical repair. In many instances, however, protective bracing and modification of activities, as outlined in the next section of this chapter, are sufficient, and surgical reconstruction is not necessary.

If the lesion is combined, such as an anterior cruciate rupture and a torn meniscus, a capsular tear, or a collateral ligament injury, the treatment of choice appears to be the repair of all injured structures. If the meniscal lesion is small, the mobile fragment may be removed. If it is a peripheral tear or a large bucket-handle tear, one should attempt to repair the meniscus or at least to preserve the periphery of the meniscus because it is an important secondary restraint. The joint capsule and the collateral ligaments should be repaired because these vascular structures have the potential for healing. The anterior cruciate ligament, if torn from its proximal or femoral end (10 to 15% of patients), should be repaired using an "over-the-top" procedure.[28] If the ligament is torn in its midsubstance (75 to 80% of cases), one should try to approximate the torn ends, but because the results of midsubstance repairs have been unpredictable in the past, one should also consider "augmenting" the repair by some other method.[26] Augmentation is performed using either the medial third of the patellar tendon,[30] theoretically replacing anteromedial band function, or a lateral substitution reconstruction as described by Galway and MacIntosh,[22] Ellison,[21] or Losee.[10] The semitendinosus tendon may also be used through the center of the joint instead of a portion of the patellar tendon, or a strip of fascia lata may be brought "over-the-top" as in the lateral-substitution over-the-top procedure described by Galway and MacIntosh.

Nonoperative Treatment

Nonoperative treatment does not mean *no treatment*. Patients that one elects to treat nonsurgically must be fully rehabilitated, with particular attention paid to the hamstring musculature. One must educate the individual regarding which sports he can engage in with minimal risk. The patient should be advised not to engage in sports that involve jumping, cutting, and fast stops or starts. Sports in which the knee is mainly functioning in the semiflexed position, such as skiing, bicycling, and skating are acceptable, whereas volleyball, basketball, and football are not. A brace may be helpful as a reminder to the individual to work in the flexed-knee position. Indeed, an extension stop limiting the final few degrees of full extension might be of value.

Using the selection criteria described, only 35 out of 100 recent, consecutive, fresh anterior cruciate ligament ruptures were treated primarily by operative measures. Two-thirds (65%) were managed conservatively.

Operative Treatment

If the individual who was initially treated conservatively has repeated episodes of giving way of the knee, surgical stabilization should be considered. Evidence of increasing degenerative change within the joint or of a developing meniscal disorder also leads one to a decision to stabilize the knee. It is always better for the patient to take part in the decision-making process and to request a secondary procedure.

Choice of Secondary Operative Procedure. No question exists that the lateral substitution reconstruction as described by MacIntosh has proved to be a reliable and acceptable operative procedure for anterolateral rotatory instability.[6,7,31–32] The variations of this operative procedure as described by Ellison,[21] Losee and colleagues[10] and others all have one element in common, which is an extra-articular tenodesis to stabilize the lateral compartment of the knee from anterior subluxation in the extended position. The unstable, isolated partial rupture of the posterolateral band of the cruciate ligament is ideal for this type of repair. The next best case is the isolated total rupture. This procedure must be combined with maximum rehabilitation of the musculature to stabilize the knee when it is flexed.

In combined lesions, I believe that an extra-articular repair should be performed in all instances and an associated intra-articular repair[27,30,33–34] added if the medial collateral ligament is still lax, if anteromedial rotatory instability is present, or if significant meniscal tissue was removed following the initial injury. In essence, this condition would be an unstable or "sloppy" knee because of the loss of both primary and secondary restraints. A combined intra- and extra-articular repair is then indicated.

In all instances, the age of the patient and the expected demands on the knee should be considered. The young physical education student or professional athlete has a greater expectation for knee function in the future than the aging secretary who is not specifically oriented toward athletics.

Postoperative Management

Following a repair of the extra-articular type, the limb should be immobilized in 60 to 90° of flexion with the tibia in external rotation. If intra-articular and extra-articular repairs are both conducted, the limb should be immobilized at approximately the midpoint of function, at 45 to 60° of flexion. The period of protective immobilization should be long enough for sound soft tissue healing to occur, approximately 5 weeks. Early studies on the use of hinged casts, applied approximately 2 weeks postoperatively and permitting motion of the knee from 30 to 90°, are encouraging and suggest that rehabilitation may be more rapid by this method, without jeopardizing stability. Following removal of all external immobilization, active movements are used to regain the full range of knee motion. Quadriceps muscle exercises are delayed because strenuous efforts at rebuilding the quadriceps muscles pull the tibia anteriorly and may compromise the repair process. Rehabilitation is largely directed toward the hamstring musculature. Unprotected weight bearing is allowed when the knee is almost straight. Protective bracing is encouraged for a minimum of 6 months for routine daily activities and for more than a year if the individual wishes to resume sporting activities. Although primary healing occurs quickly, remodeling of the repair occurs slowly, and the biomechanical strength of the repair does not reach a maximum for at least a year following the surgical procedure.

Results of Secondary Treatment

Thirty-one lateral extra-articular reconstructions were available for review from 2 to 12 years postoperatively.[32] Fifteen of the procedures were MacIntosh operations and 16 were Ellison's. Good to excellent results were recorded in 89%, with 19 knees (63%) classified as having excellent results (asymptomatic) and 8 knees (26%) classified as having good results (minimal symptoms only). Only 4 knees (11%) were unchanged or worse postoperatively.

Future Prospects

Much work is being done at present on vascularized grafts using microsurgical techniques and on ligament augmentation devices of carbon fiber[35] or braided polyester and other synthetic materials. Whether the results achieved by these methods will prove superior to those already obtainable by extra-articular procedures will only be known with the passage of time. It is expected, however, that this aggressive approach toward accurate diagnosis and early repair, with augmentation when indicated, will improve the overall statistics.

In summary, anterior cruciate ligaments are frequently damaged, either alone or in combination with other structures within the knee. Treatment must be individualized. Partial ruptures and isolated ruptures may well be treated conservatively. Combined ruptures must be treated by repair of all salvageable tissues and augmentation of the cruciate ligament as a primary procedure. Aggressive postoperative management and protective bracing are also important. The keystone to treatment, however, is accurate diagnosis and appropriate selection of patients. Arthroscopy plays a large role in this selection process.

REFERENCES

1. Chick, R., and Jackson, D.: Tears of anterior cruciate ligaments in young athletes. J. Bone Joint Surg. (Am.), *60*:970, 1978.
2. Feagin, J.A.: The syndrome of the torn anterior cruciate ligament. Orthop. Clin. North Am., *10*:81, 1979.
3. Fetto, J.D., and Marshall, J.L.: The natural history and diagnosis of anterior cruciate ligament insufficiency. Clin. Orthop., *147*:29, 1980.
4. Torg, J.S., Conrad, W., and Kalen, V.: Clinical diagnosis of anterior cruciate ligament in the athlete. Am. J. Sports Med., *4*:84, 1976.
5. Fetto, J.F., and Marshall, J.L.: Injury to the anterior cruciate ligament producing the pivot shift sign. J. Bone Joint Surg. (Am.), *61*:710, 1979.
6. Galway, R.D., Beaupre, A., and MacIntosh, D.L.: Pivot shift: a clinical sign of symptomatic anterior cruciate ligament insufficiency. J. Bone Joint Surg. (Br.), *54*:763, 1972.
7. MacIntosh, D.L.: The lateral pivot shift. *In* Symposium on Knee Injuries. ACS Clinitape, C73-OR3, 1973.
8. Noyes, F.R., Bassett, R.W., Grood, E.S., and Butler, D.L.: Arthroscopy in acute haemarthrosis of the knee. J. Bone Joint Surg. (Am.), *62*:687, 1980.
9. Slocum, D.B., James, S.L., Larsen, R.L., and Singer, K.M.: A clinical test for antero-lateral rotatory instability of the knee. Clin. Orthop., *118*:63, 1976.
10. Losee, R.E., Johnson, T.R., and Southwick, W.O.: Anterior subluxation of the lateral tibial plateau. J. Bone Joint Surg. (Am.), *60*:1015, 1978.
11. Hughston, J.C., Andrews, J.R., Cross, M.J., and Moschi, A.: Classification of knee ligament instabilities. Part II. The lateral compartment. J. Bone Joint Surg. (Am.), *58*:173, 1976.
12. DeHaven, K.: Diagnosis of acute knee injuries with haemarthrosis. Am. J. Sports Med., *8*:9, 1980.
13. Gillquist, J., Hagberg, G., and Oretorp, N.: Arthroscopy in acute injuries of the knee joint. Acta Orthop. Scand., *48*:190, 1977.
14. O'Connor, R.L.: Arthroscopy in the diagnosis and treatment of acute ligament injuries of the knee. J. Bone Joint Surg. (Am.), *56*:333, 1974.
15. Palmer, I.: On the injuries to the ligaments of the knee joint. Acta Chir. Scand. (Suppl.), 53, 1938.
16. Jackson, R.W., and Campbell, A.J.: Diagnosis of partial ruptures of the anterior cruciate ligament. Orthop. Trans., *5*:441, 1981.
17. Van Dijk, R.: The behavior of the cruciate ligaments in the human knee. Doctoral thesis, University of Nijmegen, Netherlands, 1983.
18. Horne, J.G.: The anterior cruciate ligament: its anatomy and a new method of reconstruction. Can. J. Surg., *20*:214, 1977.
19. Kennedy, J.C., Weinberg, H.W., and Wilson, A.S.: The anatomy and function of the anterior cruciate ligament. J. Bone Joint Surg. (Am.), *56*:223, 1974.
20. Larson, R.L.: Injuries of the ligaments of the knee. *In* Fractures. Edited by C.A. Rockwood and D.P. Green. Philadelphia, J.B. Lippincott, 1975.
21. Ellison, A.E.: The pathogenesis and treatment of anterolateral rotatory instability. Clin. Orthop., *147*:51, 1980.
22. Galway, R.D., and MacIntosh, D.L.: The lateral pivot shift: a symptomatic sign of anterior cruciate insufficiency. Clin. Orthop., *147*:45, 1980.
23. Gomes, J., and Jackson, R.W.: Incidence of rupture of the anterior cruciate ligament. Unpublished data, 1981.
24. Jackson, R.W., and Peters, R.I.: Late results of untreated anterior cruciate ligament lesions. Presented at Annual Meeting of the Canadian Orthopaedic Association, 1977.
25. Jackson, R.W., and Johnson, R.G.: Results following arthroscopic meniscectomy in anterior cruciate deficient knees. Presented at the Annual Meeting of the Arthroscopy Association of North America, 1982.
26. Cabaud, H.E., Feagin, J.A., and Rodkey, W.G.: Experimental studies of the anterior cruciate ligament injury and augmented repair. Am. J. Sports Med., *8*:395, 1980.
27. Marshall, J.L., Warren, R.F., and Wickiewicz, T.L.: The anterior cruciate ligament: a technique of repair and reconstruction. Clin. Orthop., *143*:97, 1979.
28. MacIntosh, D.L.: Acute tears of the anterior cruciate ligament. Over the top repair. Presented at the AAOS Meeting in Dallas, Texas, 1974.
29. Palmer, I.: Injuries to the cruciate ligaments of the knee joint as a surgical problem. Reconstr. Surg. Traumatol., *4*:181, 1957.
30. Lam, S.J.S.: Reconstruction of the anterior cruciate ligament using the Jones' procedures and Guy's Hospital modification. J. Bone Joint Surg. (Am.), *50*:1215, 1968.
31. Ireland, J.: MacIntosh tenodesis for antero-lateral instability of the knee. J. Bone Joint Surg. (Br.), *62*:340, 1980.
32. Jackson, R.W., and Mullan, G.B.: Anterior cruciate insufficiency. J. Bone Joint Surg. (Br.), *60*:287, 1978.
33. Eriksson, E.: Reconstruction of the anterior cru-

ciate ligament. Orthop. Clin. North Am., *7*:167, 1976.

34. Jones, K.G.: Reconstruction of the anterior cruciate ligament using the central one-third of the patellar ligament. J. Bone Joint Surg. (Am.), *52*:1302, 1970.
35. Jenkins, H.R.: The repair of cruciate ligaments with flexible carbon fibre. J. Bone Joint Surg., *60*:520, 1978.
36. Alm, A., Ekstrom, H., and Gillquist, J.: The anterior cruciate ligament. A clinical and experimental study of tensile strength, morphology, and replacement by patellar ligament. Acta Chir. Scand. (Suppl.), 445, 1974.
37. Feagin, J.A., and Curl, W.W.: Isolated tear of the anterior cruciate ligament: five year follow-up study. Am. J. Sports Med., *4*:3, 95, 1976.
38. Hey-Groves, E.W.: The cruciate ligaments of the knee joint: their function, rupture and the operative treatment of the same. Br. J. Surg., *7*:505, 1920.
39. Hey-Groves, E.W.: Operation for the repair of the cruciate ligaments. Lancet, *2*:674, 1917.
40. Jackson, R.W.: Lesions of the ligaments. *In* Arthroscopy and Arthrography of the Knee. American Academy of Orthopaedic Surgeons. St. Louis, C.V. Mosby, 1978.
41. Kennedy, J.C., and Fowler, P.J.: Medial and anterior instability of the knee. J. Bone Joint Surg. (Am.), *53*:1257, 1971.
42. McDaniels, W., and Dameron, T.: Untreated ruptures of anterior cruciate ligament. J. Bone Joint Surg. (Am.), *62*:696, 1980.

Chapter 8

EVALUATION OF THE ACUTELY INJURED KNEE

Kenneth E. DeHaven

This chapter considers the role of arthroscopy in the diagnosis and evaluation of acute knee injuries. The history of a significant traumatic episode, usually from athletic, occupational, or vehicular injury, with immediate disability and the early onset of hemarthrosis frequently indicates disruption of one or more important structures within the knee, including collateral or cruciate ligaments and the extensor mechanism as well as displaced meniscal tears, and intra-articular fractures. A return to optimal levels of knee function following such injuries may depend upon early, definitive diagnosis and appropriate surgical treatment, and it is the orthopedic surgeon's task to identify specific disorders so that proper treatment can be initiated.

CLINICAL EVALUATION

The definitive diagnosis can be made clinically or with roentgenograms in many of these cases, and arthroscopy plays little or no role. The diagnosis of an acutely torn ligament is based upon the demonstration of pathologic laxity on clinical stress testing, and particularly in the case of significant disruption of the medial or lateral collateral ligament, arthroscopic examination is *not* recommended. Because the capsular system is no longer closed, irrigation fluid extravasates into the tissues, which subsequently will be repaired, and the edema from the irrigating fluid makes the repair more difficult. Moreover, because of the extravasation, it can be difficult to clear the blood from the joint to ensure adequate visualization. The potential also exists for massive extravasation of fluid into the adjacent soft tissues, resulting in neurovascular compression syndromes, some of which cause permanent neurovascular deficits. For these reasons, along with the probability of adequate visualization of the interior of the knee using the surgical exposure to repair the torn collateral ligament, arthroscopic examination is *not* recommended when the collateral ligament injury is severe enough to warrant surgical repair.

The diagnosis of torn cruciate ligaments also depends upon the clinical tests for integrity of these ligaments, and arthroscopic examination is *not* necessary to make the diagnosis in most cases. A significant percentage of cases of anterior cruciate ligament tears, however, have associated meniscal disorders, and arthroscopic examination is useful to document the location of the lesion, to determine whether it is complete or partial, and to evaluate the status of the menisci and articular surfaces.

Extensor mechanism disruption is entirely a clinical diagnosis demonstrated by the patient's loss of ability to extend the knee actively into the last 45° of full extension. This diagnosis is frequently missed in emergency rooms, but arthroscopy plays little or no role in the evaluation of these injuries.

If intra-articular fractures are obvious on routine roentgenograms with unquestionable displacement or lack of displacement, arthroscopy is not necessary for deciding between operative and nonoperative treatment. Arthroscopic visualization of the intra-articular fracture line may, however, help to resolve questionable cases of displacement, may identify intra-articular fragments to be removed arthroscopically if nonoperative treatment is otherwise opted, or may guide reduction of depressed tibial plateau fractures. In other cases, the osseous fragment of an osteochondral fracture may be so small that it is not visible on a roentgenogram, and arthroscopic examination provides the definitive diagnosis, and frequently the definitive treatment as well.

ARTHROSCOPIC EVALUATION WHEN CLINICAL EVALUATION NOT DEFINITIVE

The remainder of this discussion focuses on patients with acute knee injuries who have the same history of significant trauma, immediate disability, and early onset of hemarthrosis, but who are stable when the usual clinical tests are performed in the emergency room or office setting without anesthesia, and whose roentgenograms are negative or nondiagnostic. The damage in these injuries has often been considered insignificant, and a "wait-and-see" attitude is followed. Evaluation under anesthesia and arthroscopic examination in these patients, however, frequently substantiate the presence of serious injuries, and indications for definitive surgical treatment may be present in as many as 90%.[1] In analyzing 145 consecutive personal cases collected over nearly a 5-year period, anterior cruciate ligament tears were present in 73% of patients, many of whom also had associated meniscal tears, major meniscal tears without cruciate ligament injury were present in 14%, osteochondral fractures in 6%, posterior cruciate ligament tears in 2%, and no significant internal derangement in 5%. These figures are similar to those reported by others in similar cases.[2–4]

Technical Considerations

Hemarthrosis presents problems for arthroscopic visualization, and some modifications of standard techniques may be necessary to perform an adequate examination. Open surgical procedures frequently follow arthroscopy in these cases, and every attempt is made to avoid using the tourniquet, usually possible because significant active bleeding is rarely encountered. The arthroscope's sheath is inserted, and the bloody effusion is flushed out through the large, 5- or 6-mm sheath until the returning fluid has cleared (Fig. 8–1). A high-flow, constant irrigation system is used during the procedure with the inflow through the arthroscope's sleeve and the outflow through a large, multiply perforated outflow cannula located in the suprapatellar pouch. This irrigation system almost always permits an adequate arthroscopic examination, but inflation of the tourniquet is sometimes necessary. When proceeding to an open surgical procedure following arthroscopy, the leg should be reprepared and redraped, the surgical team regowned and regloved, and a new set of sterile instruments should be used to minimize the risk of infection. I routinely use prophylactic antibiotics if a ligament operation is to be performed.

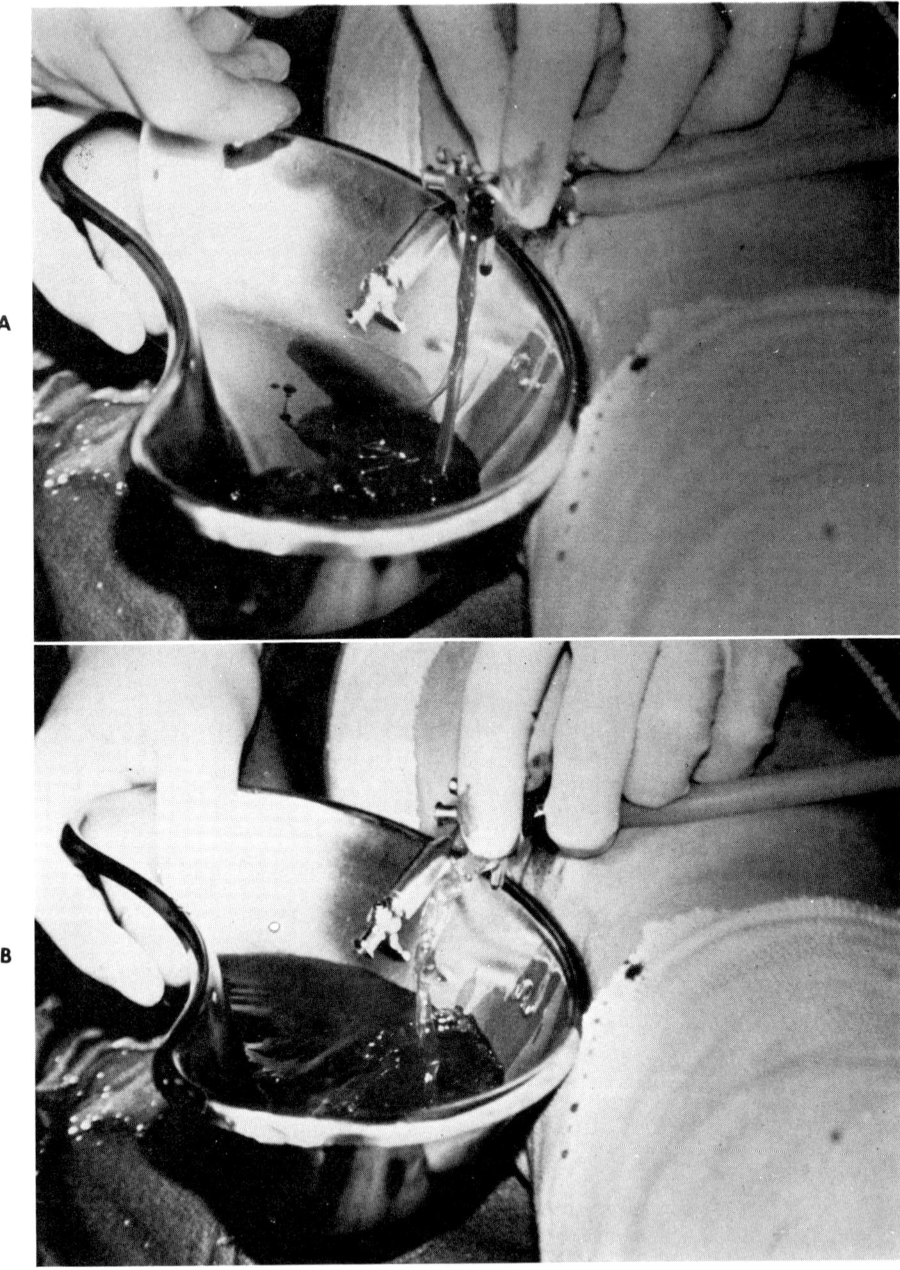

Fig. 8–1. *A,* Grossly bloody synovial fluid is encountered initially as the arthroscope sleeve is inserted into the acutely injured knee. *B,* Copious irrigation is continued until the fluid becomes sufficiently clear of blood to provide adequate arthroscopic visualization. (From DeHaven, K.E.: Acute injury to the knee: arthroscopy. *In* American Academy of Orthopaedic Surgeons: Symposium on Arthroscopy and Arthrography of the Knee. St. Louis, C.V. Mosby, 1978.)

Anterior Cruciate Ligament Tears

When nearly 75% of these patients have tears of the anterior cruciate ligament, the obvious question is why this condition could not be more easily diagnosed clinically. The classic clinical test for anterior cruciate ligament integrity is the anterior drawer sign, performed at 90° of flexion. In acute, "isolated" tears of the anterior cruciate ligament, this test is negative without anesthesia in approximately 90% of patients; even under anesthesia, the test is clearly positive in only 60% (Table 8–1). The anteromedial rotatory instability test of Slocum and Larson[5] is negative with or without anesthesia in 75% of the cases of isolated tear of the anterior cruciate ligament.

The lateral pivot-shift sign, as described by Galway, Beaupré, and MacIntosh,[6] and the closely related flexion-rotation drawer sign, described by Noyes and co-workers,[4] are much more sensitive. These tests are positive in 85 to 90% of patients under anesthesia, but they require relaxation to demonstrate the sign, and an adequate examination cannot usually be performed without anesthesia. The Lachman sign, however, popularized by Torg and associates,[7] is helpful in these acute injuries. It is positive without anesthesia in 84% of patients, and it is virtually 100% reliable under anesthesia. Using all these clinical tests, with patients awake as well as under anesthesia, it is almost always possible to make the clinical diagnosis of torn anterior cruciate ligament with certainty prior to insertion of the arthroscope.

The arthroscopic examination is important to document the location and extent of the lesion (Fig. 8–2), however, and to demonstrate associated lesions. In 50 to 70% of patients, an associated meniscal tear is present, whereas in approximately 25 to 30% the anterior cruciate ligament injury is "isolated," meaning that no other ligament is completely torn and neither meniscus is torn, but interstitial damage has been done to the capsular secondary restraints. In addition, a few partial tears of the anterior cruciate ligament are present. It is important to recognize these tears, so that adequate protection can be provided to let them heal (Fig. 8–3).

Two points are important with regard to associated meniscus tears. First, the relative incidence of lateral meniscal tears is high, approximately 1:1 medial versus lateral, as compared to the usual situation in which medial meniscal tears are more frequent than lateral. Second, these tears are usually located posteriorly and may be difficult to demonstrate arthroscopically with-

TABLE 8–1

CLINICAL TESTS FOR ANTERIOR CRUCIATE LIGAMENT INTEGRITY IN 25 CONSECUTIVE, ACUTE, COMPLETE, "ISOLATED" TEARS

Test	Without Anesthesia	Under Anesthesia
Anterior Drawer Sign		
Positive	24%	60%
Negative	76%	40%
Anteromedial Rotatory Instability		
Positive	12%	24%
Negative	72%	76%
Unable to test	16%	
Lateral Pivot-Shift		
Positive	16%	84%
Negative	4%	15%
Unable to test	80%	
Lachman		
Positive	84%	100%
Negative	16%	0%

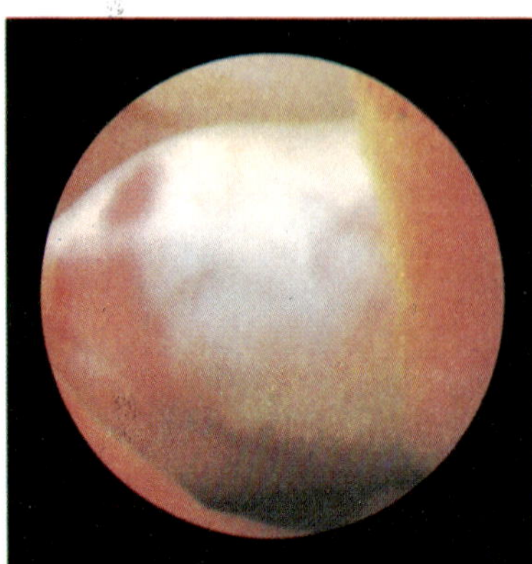

Fig. 8–2.

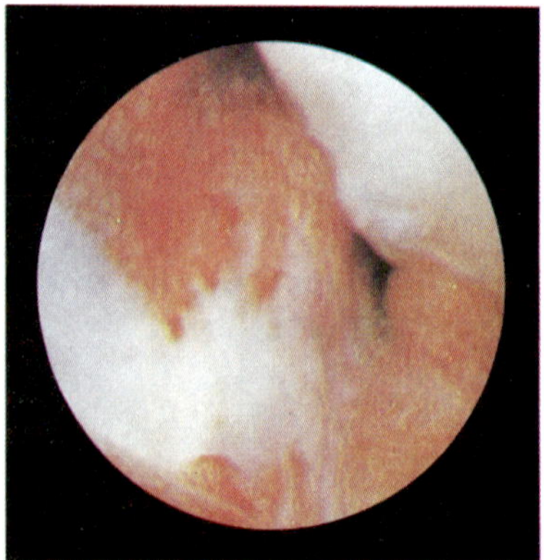

Fig. 8–3.

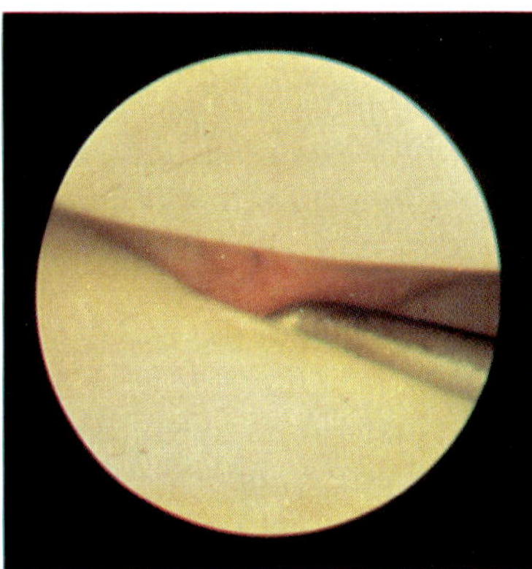

Fig. 8–4.

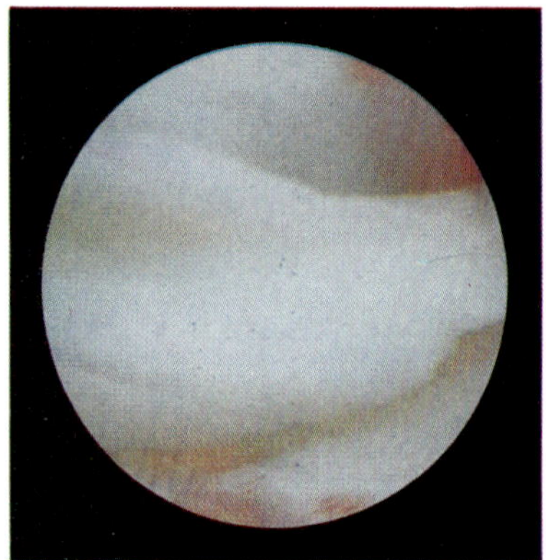

Fig. 8–5.

Fig. 8–2. Acute anterior cruciate ligament tear from the femur. A hemorrhagic edematous ligament is seen lying horizontally in the intercondylar notch. (From DeHaven, K.E.: Acute injury to the knee: arthroscopy. *In* American Academy of Orthopaedic Surgeons: Symposium on Arthroscopy and Arthrography of the Knee. St. Louis, C.V. Mosby, 1978.)

Fig. 8–3. Acute partial anterior cruciate ligament tears are recognized arthroscopically by the appearance of hemorrhage within the synovial sheath around the anterior cruciate ligament, which remains in continuity and in its normal anatomic position. This needs to be confirmed by probing. (From DeHaven, K.E.: Acute injury to the knee: arthroscopy. *In* American Academy of Orthopaedic Surgeons: Symposium on Arthroscopy and Arthrography of the Knee. St. Louis, C.V. Mosby, 1978.)

Fig. 8–4. This lateral meniscus was normal to arthroscopic visualization until probing with the nerve hook demonstrated a complete posterior peripheral tear.

Fig. 8–5. Displaced bucket-handle tear of the medial meniscus, with the displaced portion occupying the medial portion of intercondylar notch, blocking arthroscopic visualization of the medial compartment. (From DeHaven, K.E.: Acute injury to the knee: arthroscopy. *In* American Academy of Orthopaedic Surgeons: Symposium on Arthroscopy and Arthrography of the Knee. St. Louis, C.V. Mosby, 1978.)

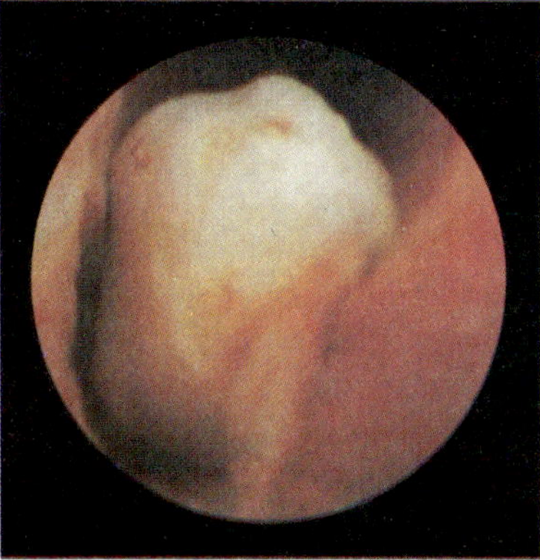

Fig. 8–6.

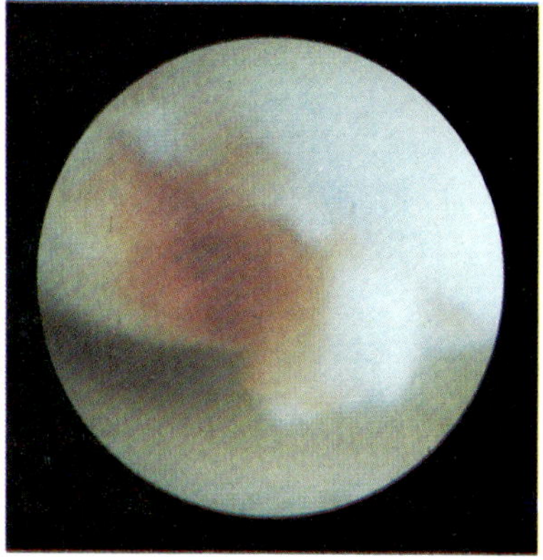

Fig. 8–7.

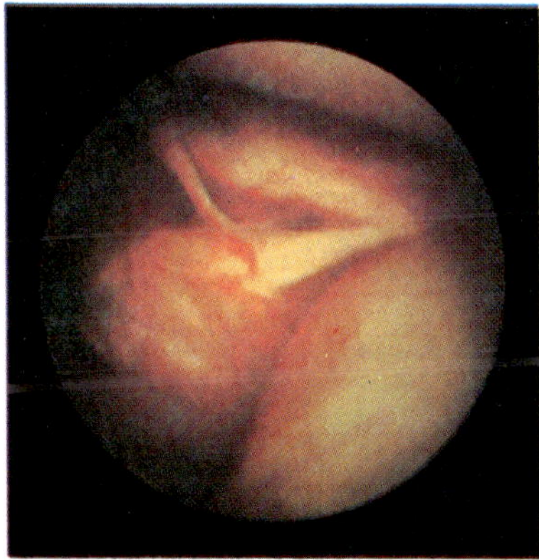

Fig. 8–8.

Fig. 8–6. Loose body from an acute patellar dislocation with an osteochondral fracture lying in the lateral sulcus between the lateral femoral condyle and the lateral capsule. (From DeHaven, K.E.: Acute injury to the knee: arthroscopy. *In* American Academy of Orthopaedic Surgeons: Symposium on Arthroscopy and Arthrography of the Knee. St. Louis, C.V. Mosby, 1978.)

Fig. 8–7. Arthroscopic appearance of an acute osteochondral fracture involving the weight-bearing portion of the medial femoral condyle. (From DeHaven, K.E.: Acute injury to the knee: arthroscopy. *In* American Academy of Orthopaedic Surgeons: Symposium on Arthroscopy and Arthrography of the Knee. St. Louis, C.V. Mosby, 1978.)

Fig. 8–8. "Isolated" tear of the posterior cruciate ligament from the tibia as visualized arthroscopically from the posteromedial approach. A corner of the posterior medial femoral condyle is seen in the upper portion of the photograph, and the periphery of the posterior horn of the medial meniscus is seen below. (From DeHaven, K.E.: Acute injury to the knee: arthroscopy. *In* American Academy of Orthopaedic Surgeons: Symposium on Arthroscopy and Arthrography of the Knee. St. Louis, C.V. Mosby, 1978.)

out careful evaluation and probing with a nerve hook (Fig. 8–4).

Meniscal Tears Without Cruciate Ligament Lesions

The injuries in this category are almost all major displaced or displaceable bucket-handle tears, and the medial meniscus is involved much more frequently than the lateral (3:1) (Fig. 8–5).

Osteochondral Fractures

Osteochondral fractures difficult to visualize radiographically are usually the result of patellar dislocation or major subluxation, with the osteochondral fracture occurring to the patella or to the lateral femoral condyle. The free fragment is frequently found lying in the lateral capsular sulcus adjacent to the lateral femoral condyle (Fig. 8–6) and can be retrieved arthroscopically. Occasionally, the osteochondral fracture occurs in the weight-bearing surface of the femoral condyle (Fig. 8–7), and an associated meniscal tear may be present.

Posterior Cruciate Ligament Tears

I have seen three unusual cases of isolated tears of the posterior cruciate ligament. The posterior drawer sign was positive in two of these patients, but in one it was not demonstrated until examination under anesthesia and in another it remained negative under anesthesia even when the test was repeated when the diagnosis had been made arthroscopically. Posterior visualization by posteromedial puncture or through the intercondylar notch with an angled arthroscope was necessary to visualize the lesion in two of the three cases (Fig. 8–8).

Absence of Significant Internal Derangement

In a few patients, no significant internal derangement can be identified, and the diagnosis is that of a stable sprain of the collateral ligament with synovial bleeding that accounts for the hemarthrosis.

CONCLUSIONS

In summary, patients with acute knee injuries with hemarthrosis frequently have disruptions of important structures within the knee, and prompt definitive diagnosis and primary surgical treatment may be required for optimal functional recovery. For many of these patients, clinical or roentgenographic findings provide the definitive information, and arthroscopy plays little or no role (collateral ligament tears, extensor mechanism disruption, intra-articular fractures). For patients who have acute injuries with early hemarthrosis that are stable to ligament testing without anesthesia (except for the Lachman sign) and have negative roentgenograms, however, arthroscopy plays an important role in providing direct visualization of the disorder, demonstrating associated pathologic processes that may be unsuspected, and adds no significant morbidity to that of the injury itself. Armed with the additional information gained from arthroscopic examination, a more informed decision can be made regarding treatment, and one either can intervene surgically or treat the patient conservatively with a much higher degree of confidence. Casscells's statement that "seeing is no substitute for thinking" is certainly true, but on the other hand, no substitute exists for seeing the full extent of an existing disorder so that the best possible decision can be made for treating each individual patient.

REFERENCES

1. DeHaven, K.E.: Diagnosis of acute knee injuries with hemarthosis. Am. J. Sports Med., *8*:9, 1980.
2. Eriksson, E.: Sports injuries of the knee ligaments: their diagnosis, treatment, rehabilitation and prevention. Med. Sci. Sports, *8*:133, 1976.
3. Gillquist, J., Hagberg, G., and Oretorp, N.: Arthroscopy in acute injuries of the knee joint. Acta Orthop. Scand., *48*:190, 1977.
4. Noyes, F.R., Bassett, R.W., Grood, E.S., and Butler, D.L.: Arthroscopy in acute traumatic hemarthrosis of the knee. J. Bone Joint Surg. (Am.), *62*:687, 1980.

5. Slocum, D.B., and Larson, R.L.: Rotatory instability of the knee: its pathogenesis and a clinical test to demonstrate its presence. J. Bone Joint Surg. (Am.), *50*:211, 1968.
6. Galway, R.D., Beaupré, A., and MacIntosh, D.L.: Pivot-shift. A clinical sign of symptomatic anterior cruciate ligament insufficiency. *In* Proceedings of the Canadian Orthopaedic Association. J. Bone Joint Surg. (Br.), *54*:763, 1972.
7. Torg, J.S., Conrad, W., and Kalen, V.: Clinical diagnosis of anterior cruciate ligament instability in athletes. Am. J. Sports Med., *4*:84, 1976.

Chapter 9

ARTHROSCOPY OF JOINTS OTHER THAN THE KNEE

Nils Oretorp

In the rapid development of arthroscopy during the last 10 years, the primary interest has been focused on the knee. Strong reasons exist to believe that the interest in scientific study with this excellent tool will extend to other joints. Today, most joints can be examined arthroscopically. From scientific and clinical points of view, however, the joints that are of most interest depend on the integrity of soft tissue for stability and are often exposed to trauma. Such joints are the shoulder, the elbow, and the ankle.

SHOULDER

The shoulder joint has the same features that allowed successful development of knee arthroscopy. It is a large and biomechanically complex joint dependent on its soft tissues for stability. The shoulder is therefore sensitive to external trauma, and the variety of injuries is wide. Moreover, as with the knee, most of these injuries are not demonstrable on ordinary roentgenograms, and many are difficult to differentiate even when a contrast medium is used in arthrography.

Technique of Examination

The patient is placed in a lateral decubitus position. When the patient is draped, his arm should be left free to allow full or nearly full mobility during the examination (Fig. 9–1). The anesthetist's area should be draped obliquely for the same reason.

The examination can be performed under local anesthesia, with infiltration at puncture sites and a bolus injected into the joint cavity (Fig. 9–2). Local anesthesia is not always enough to allow the patient full relaxation, however. If the patient is not relaxed or is trying to help the surgeon by keeping the arm in certain positions, the contact between the humeral head and the glenoid cavity will limit the maneuverability of the telescope within the joint. In most patients, general anesthesia is therefore preferred.

The surgeon stands behind the patient for a posterior puncture. The nurse is on the opposite side of the operating table. A separate assistant to manipulate the patient's arm facilitates the visualization process for the surgeon. The role of the assistant in shoulder arthroscopy is even more important than in knee arthroscopy

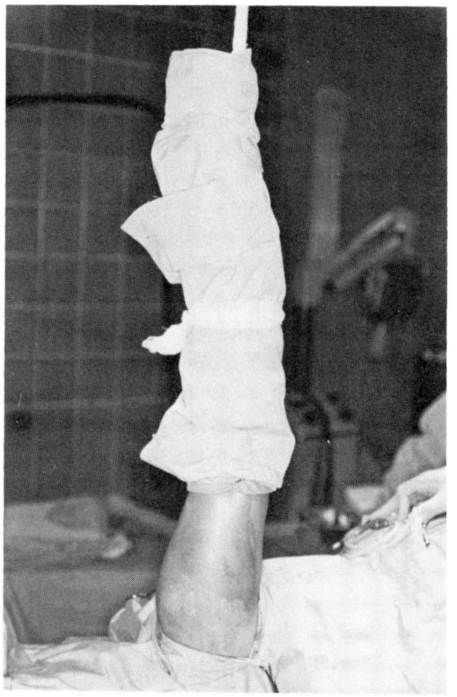

Fig. 9–1. Patient in lateral decubitus position with arm draped and overhead traction applied. Some surgeons rely on an assistant instead of on traction.

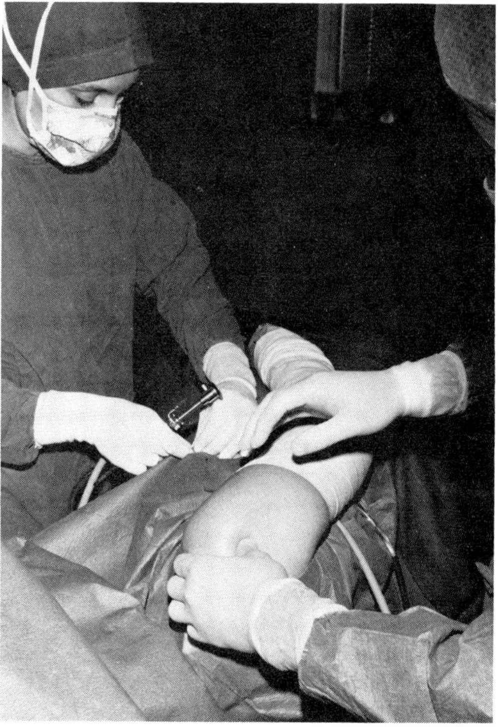

Fig. 9–2. Some surgeons prefer to have the arm at the side with an assistant applying traction and, when necessary, rotating the arm and shoulder. Here, the surgeon is palpating the soft spot behind the acromium prior to making the incision for the arthroscope.

and cannot be performed by a mechanical device.

A standard arthroscope is used for both diagnosis and surgical procedures, as in the knee. A foreoblique, 4.0-mm telescope is generally used in adults, temporarily replaced for special purposes by the 70° lens through the same 5.0-mm trocar sheath. In exceptionally small patients, an arthroscope with the outer diameter of 3.8 mm is used.

Adequate visualization of the joint capsule is provided by the flow of saline solution through the arthroscope's sheath; a separate outflow cannula, smaller than for the knee, is inserted anteriorly. The joint can be distended by using a syringe directly on the telescope or, more efficiently, by an infusion pump. If an infusion pump is used, it should be directly controlled by the surgeon, so that the intra-articular pressure is not raised uncritically.

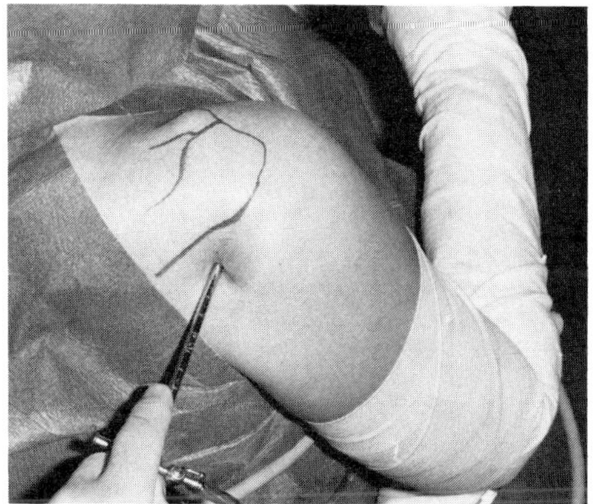

Fig. 9–3. Sharp trocar introduced from the posterior approach.

Steps for Visualization. Two punctures are needed for adequate visualization of all areas; the posterior is generally more useful than the anterior. Palpation is important for optimal location of the puncture sites. The anatomic landmarks are the sharp posterior angle of the acromion posteriorly and the coracoid process anteriorly.

Posteriorly, a short incision is made just distal to the spine of scapula and 2 cm medial to the angle of the acromion. The arthroscope with the sharp trocar is inserted just through the skin (Fig. 9–3). Then the instrument is directed toward a point proximal and medial to the center of the posterior convexity of the humeral head. The patient's arm is held in neutral rotation along the trunk. The instrument is gently pushed until direct contact with the head of humerus is felt. The arm is then abducted and is elevated posteriorly 30°, with the instrument continuously in contact with the posterior surface of the humeral head. The tip of the instrument, then, follows the same movements as the humeral head in a proximal and medial direction, until it glides off tangentially inside the joint. Force should be avoided. Studies on cadavers have shown that, when this maneuver is performed correctly, the instrument's tip enters the joint between the supraspinatus and infraspinatus muscles. Posteriorly, this entry point combines the benefits of excellent instrument mobility for the arthroscopist with minimal trauma to the joint. Clinically, therefore, the postoperative discomfort is minor.

The anterior puncture is made just lateral to the palpated coracoid process. The instrument is introduced with the patient's arm in neutral rotation. Entry is facilitated by distension of the joint with saline solution and concomitant slight traction of the arm. Within the joint, the trocar is changed to the telescope (Fig. 9–4). By the posterior approach, the biceps tendon comes directly into sight. Rotation of the telescope permits visualization of the upper anterior glenoid lip and of the anterior recess. By anterior elevation of the patient's arm, the biceps tendon can be followed all the way to its outlet in the bicipital groove. Close to this area is the insertion of the superior glenohumeral ligament and the biceps tendon (Fig. 9–5). To examine the deep subcoracoid part of the recess, however, one must use the 120° lens. Without it, free fragments cannot be ruled out from the posterior approach. Even when examined from the anterior approach, loose bodies may escape in a pouch. The whole anterior glenoid lip and glenoid cavity are visualized from the posterior approach when the surgical assistant distracts the humeral head from the glenoid cavity (Fig. 9–6). This maneuver allows the surgeon to follow the glenoid cartilage with the arthroscope's tip, scanning this area superiorly to inferiorly. To study details in the most distal pouch of the joint, the instrument's tip should be at the posterior edge of the lower labrum.

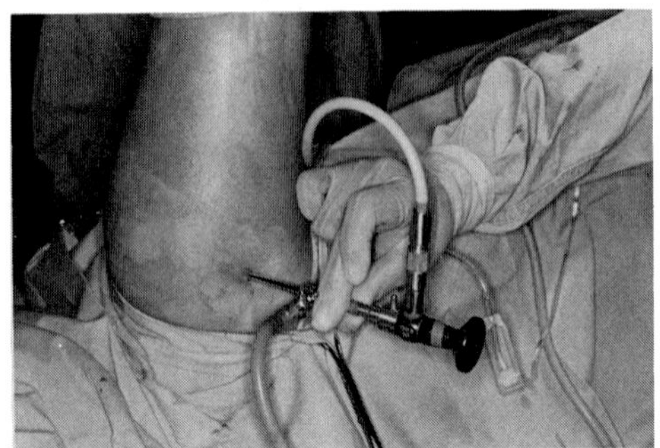

Fig. 9–4. Arthroscope inserted into the shoulder joint posteriorly.

Clinical Value

Arthroscopy of the shoulder is not a difficult procedure, and it can provide important and detailed information on all areas of this joint. Information about the integrity of the glenoid rim and lip (Fig. 9–6*B*), as well as that of the glenohumeral ligaments, is of interest in patients with joint instability. Hill-Sacks lesions can be seen and evaluated (Fig. 9–7), and the planning of operative procedures can be

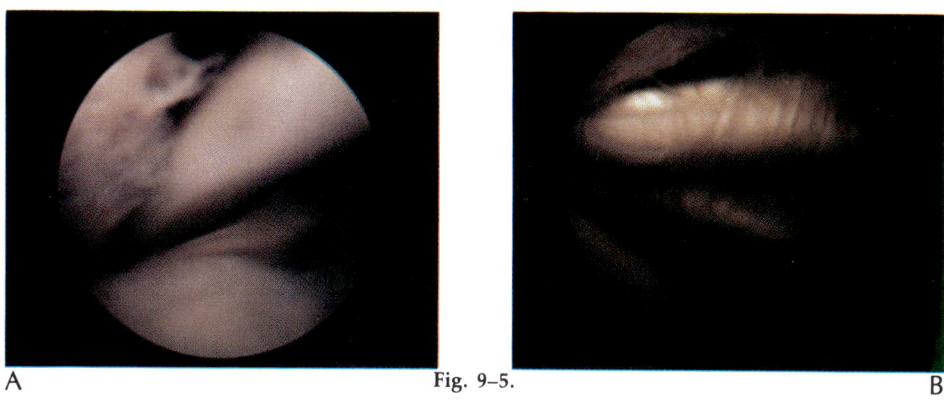

Fig. 9–5.

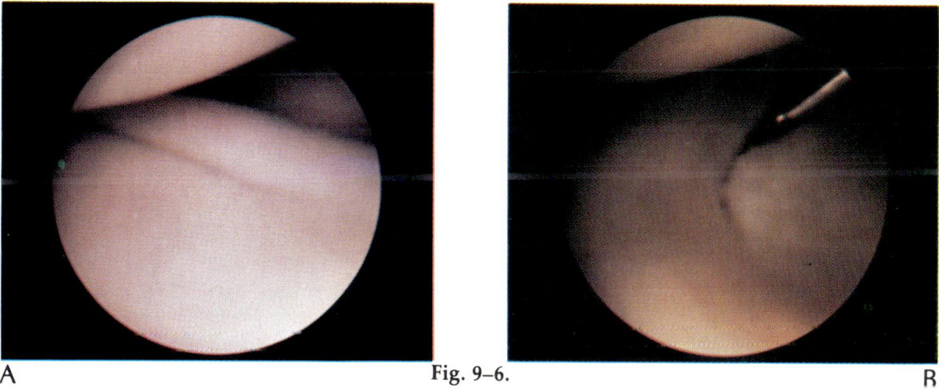

Fig. 9–6.

Fig. 9–5. Anterior and lateral anatomy from the posterior portal. ***A,*** **Biceps tendon.** ***B,*** **Glenoid humeral ligament.**

Fig. 9–6. ***A,*** **Normal glenoid labrum.** ***B,*** **Glenoid rims tested by a probe introduced from an anterior portal.**

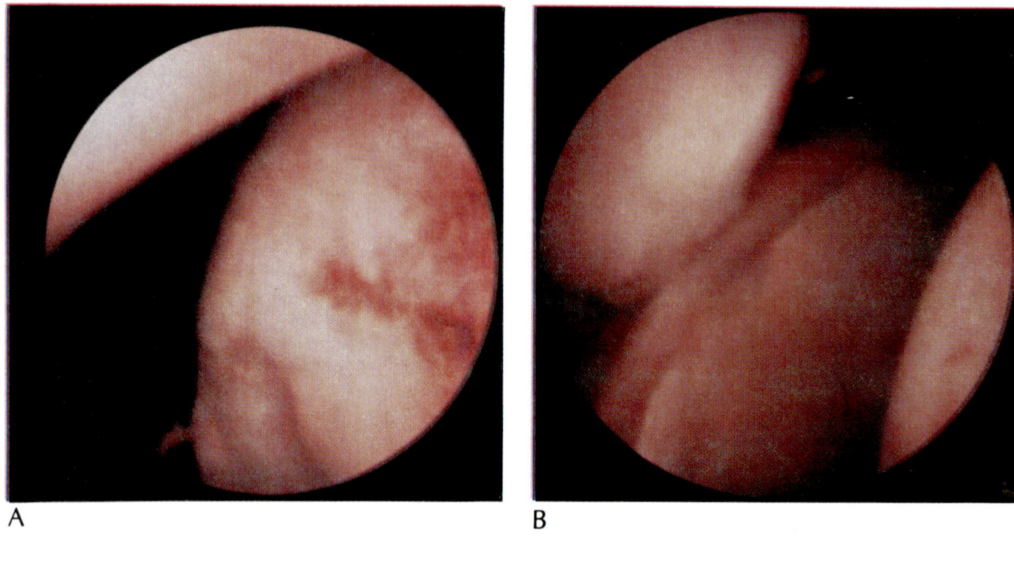

A B

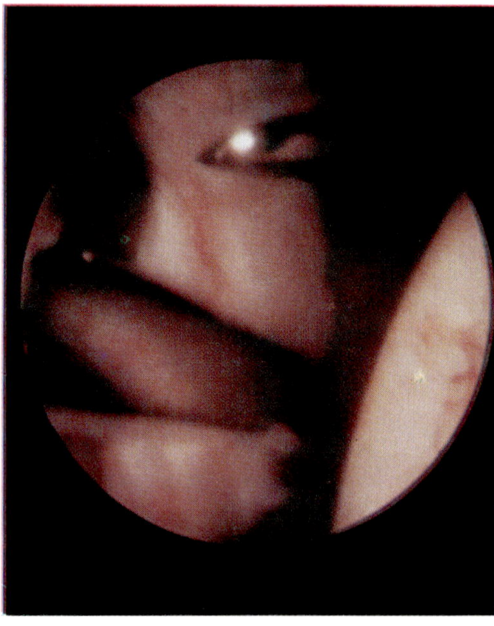

C

Fig. 9–7. *A,* Right shoulder seen from the posterior approach in a patient with a history of dislocation. A Hill-Sachs lesion is visible on the humeral head. *B,* The fragment is displaced from the humeral head. *C,* A fragment is manipulated by an instrument introduced from an anterior portal.

made more accurate. In addition to diagnostic arthroscopy of the shoulder, there is a place for arthroscopic surgery, although so far only a few orthopedic surgeons use this technique. Whenever indicated, one can easily extract loose fragments from the head of the humerus or from the glenoid cavity from both anterior and posterior portals by triangulation; degenerated and torn biceps tendon stumps can be removed; and localized synovial derangements can be repaired.

ELBOW

Technique of Examination

The patient is placed supine on the operating table, and an arm support is attached. The patient's arm is draped to allow full mobility of the elbow and at least 90° abduction of the shoulder. Axillary plexus anesthesia is preferred; a tourniquet is not used routinely. Intravenous analgesia is less useful because the lower tourniquet restricts the use of the telescope from a posteroradial portal.

Foreoblique telescopes with a diameter under 4 mm are most suited for the elbow. A 5-mm arthroscope can be used without difficulties anteriorly, but it requires a certain skill in posterior portals. Two insertion sites are needed for adequate examination of the elbow. To facilitate an atraumatic insertion, the joint is first punctured anterior to the radial epicondyle and is distended by 10 to 20 ml saline solution; backflow through the cannula should be checked. A proximal anteroradial puncture gives access to the entire anterior compartment of the joint. The skin incision is made 1 to 1.5 cm anterior and proximal to the radial epicondyle with the elbow flexed 90°. The arthroscope with the sharp trocar is directed toward the radioulnar joint and should follow close to the humerus. This procedure is to ensure that the instrument will pass directly into the joint without interfering with structures anterior to the joint capsule. The joint is entered about 1 cm proximal to the radial head. This proximal anteroradial portal allows full visualization of all anterior joint structures (Fig. 9–8).

The location of the posteroradial puncture is critical for adequate posterior examination (Fig. 9–9*A*). The skin incision should be placed over the palpated sulcus between the humerus and the ulna and just proximal to a line connecting the radial epicondyle with the tip of olecranon. The joint is adequately distended, and the instrument is directed toward the humeral fossa to enter the joint. Correctly used, this portal gives an adequate view not only of the posterior area of the humerus all the way to the ulnar side (Fig. 9–9*B*), but also of the ulnar cartilage, radioulnar joint, sacciform recess, and posterior attachment of the annular ligament. These structures cannot be examined from any other portal.

An anterior puncture on the ulnar side is superfluous unless the anteroradial portal is located too close to the radial head. The ulnar puncture is needed only when a wide overview of the radiohumeral joint is necessary. Posterior punctures on the ulnar side are contraindicated because they injure the ulnar nerve.

Clinical Value

Several clinical conditions produce pain in the elbow. When pain is located laterally, it is sometimes difficult to differentiate lateral epicondylitis or nerve entrapment from disorders affecting the radiohumeral or, especially, the radioulnar joint. Several patients diagnosed and treated without success for tennis elbow have been found by arthroscopy to have disorders of the annular ligament and proximal radioulnar articulation. Tears of the annular ligament have been found at arthroscopy, sometimes with tiny fragments of bone avulsed from the ulna. Today, little is known about the true incidence of injuries to this important joint.

My own observations indicate that synovitis of the elbow is often restricted to the radioulnar portion of the joint. Proximal

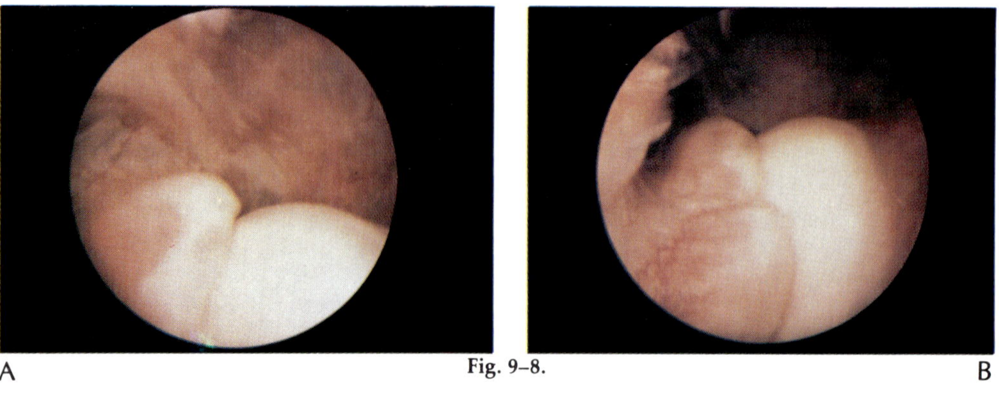

A Fig. 9–8. B

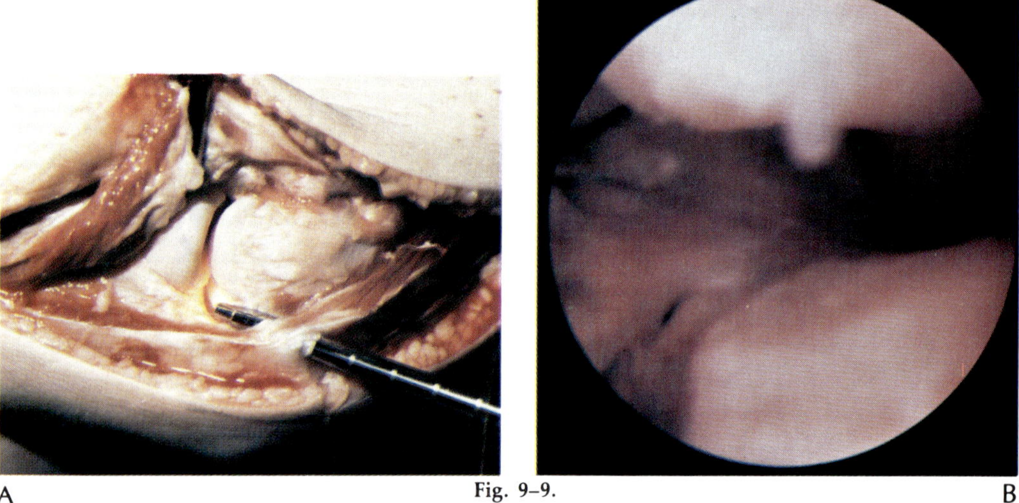

A Fig. 9–9. B

Fig. 9–8. *A,* Anterior aspect of the elbow from the proximal anteroradial approach to the ulnar and capsular wall. *B,* Anteroradial approach showing the coronoid process of the ulna.

Fig. 9–9. *A,* Cadaver specimen for location of insertion of the arthroscope to view the radioulnar joint. The sacciform recess has been longitudinally opened; forceps hold the annular ligament away. *B,* Normal anatomic features are seen from the posteroradial entry to the joint showing the distal end of the humerus with the head of the radius barely visible in the upper left and the ulnar cartilage below.

radioulnar joint synovitis is a clinical entity that, when suspected, needs arthroscopic or arthrotomic confirmation. Today, we do not know the full significance of traumatic and other disorders of the radioulnar articulation, but we have reasons to believe that arthroscopy will widen our knowledge considerably.

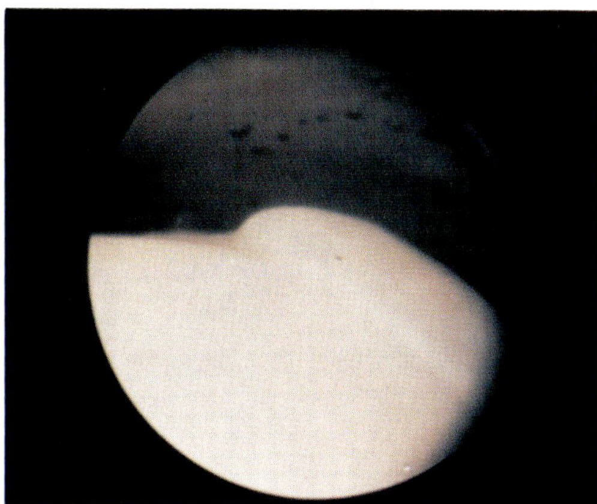

Fig. 9–10. Osteochondritic lesion of the talus.

ANKLE

Ankle joint injuries are most common in orthopedic practice. The joint is easy to examine clinically, radiologically, and arthroscopically. For arthroscopic examination, two anterior portals are used. The joint capsule is thin and often leaks when distended for arthroscopy. Therefore, when distension is ineffective, it is practical to examine the joint diagonally, the medial portion from a lateral portal and vice versa. The central area between the tibia and the talus can only be examined with the smaller arthroscopes because the normal concavity of the lower tibia blocks penetration by larger instruments. A 2.2-mm (1.7-mm telescope) needlescope or a 3.8-mm arthroscope is therefore preferred.

Technique of Examination

The skin in infiltrated with 0.5% lidocaine after careful palpation of the joint line between the talus and the tibia. The sites selected are the medial and lateral corners of the talus. A bolus of 10 to 15 ml saline solution is injected into the joint to distend it. Before the arthroscope is inserted, the patient's foot is dorsiflexed. This maneuver opens the space between the joint capsule and bone and protects the talus from damage at insertion. A short skin incision is made, the arthroscope is introduced directly, and the talotibial border is followed for 1 or 2 cm to secure the instrument tip's position inside the joint cavity. The inflow is through the arthroscope, the outflow is separate, through a cannula placed in the posterior joint cavity posterolaterally.

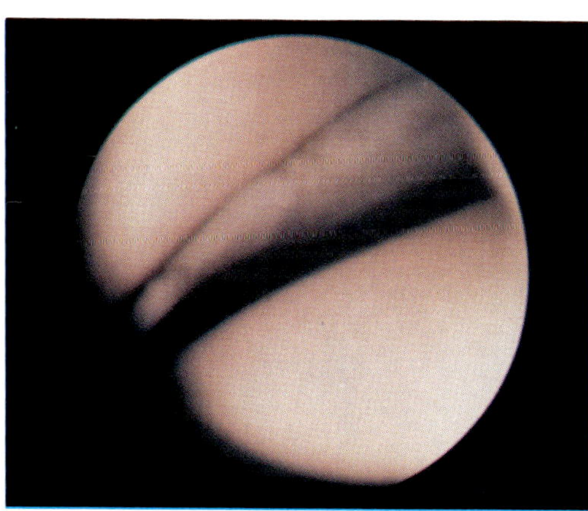

Fig. 9–11. Synovial impingement between the talus and the tibia.

From the anterior portals, more than half the talus can be seen without difficulty.

Even more can be visualized when the foot is forcibly plantarflexed and is distracted inferiorly, the lower end of the table flexed to allow effective traction against the patient's thigh resting on the table. To visualize the posterior process of the talus as well, a posterior puncture is made posterior to the peroneal tendons. The ligaments can be seen when they are not obscured by an excess of thickened synovium. The tibiofibular syndesmosis is integrated into the capsular tissues and, usually only its most medial fibers can be seen from the anteromedial portal.

Clinical Value

Ankle joint arthroscopy is indicated in selected cases in which clinical examination and roentgenograms have not established a reliable basis for treatment. One may be surprised by the arthroscopic findings, such as articular cartilage injuries, synovial impingement lesions, and loose bodies (Figs. 9–10 and 9–11). Arthroscopy is also of value to plan or to carry out treatment in selected patients with unilateral or bilateral osteochondritis of the talus. In the ankle, as in other joints, arthroscopic surgical procedures can be performed. Although important in certain patients, the benefits of arthroscopic surgical procedures in the ankle are generally not as great as in the knee, shoulder, and elbow.

Chapter 10

PROBLEMS AND COMPLICATIONS IN ARTHROSCOPY

Ralph T. Lidge

Diagnostic arthroscopy is an important and demanding procedure that requires visual as well as motor skills to permit formulation of a plan of therapy. Problems and complications annoy and frustrate the arthroscopist. Often, such difficulties can be anticipated and prevented. When such is not possible, however, one must learn to overcome these problems.

PROBLEMS

Extra-Articular

The problems often begin with an ill-prepared patient. He may have a poor understanding of the procedure and may have unrealistic expectations. He may fail to comprehend the difference between a diagnostic procedure and one in which a surgical procedure is contemplated. So much publicity has been given to arthroscopy in the lay press in recent years, with varying degrees of accuracy, that the patient could easily expect too much or too little of the procedure. The patient may not listen carefully to the surgeon who explains the procedure. The surgeon himself may give an inadequate explanation. Written instructions and explanations, therefore, are most helpful and minimize the possibility for misunderstanding that could present medicolegal difficulties, especially if some type of arthroscopic operation is contemplated. Because of problems within the knee, which are enumerated later, the possibility always exists that the surgical procedure cannot be accomplished arthroscopically, and an arthrotomy may be the best way of treating the patient's disorder. The patient should be made to realize this possibility and should give his permission not only for an arthroscopic procedure, but also for an arthrotomy, if necessary. The surgeon should also discuss the possibilities of performing the procedure under local or general anesthesia.

At times, patients arrive at the hospital with an inadequate preoperative work-up. How much of a preoperative work-up is required depends, of course, on the age and the physical condition of the patient, as well as on other factors, such as choice of anesthesia. Although arthroscopy is a minor procedure, it frequently requires a general anesthetic. Some point in the patient's medical history may be overlooked in the preoperative work-up, but discovered by the anesthesiologist just prior to the surgical procedure. This situation is most embarrassing to surgeon and patient alike and can be prevented by careful preoperative planning.

Equipment Failure

In this era of fiberoptic arthroscopes, equipment failure is infrequent, unlike a few years ago, when the light system in the Watanabe arthroscope often failed. A tendency exists, however, for the fiberoptic light cord gradually to lose its brilliance owing to rupture of the tiny glass fibers. The eye does not perceive this loss of light for a long time, but the camera does, and dark photographs are often the result.

Tourniquets, of course, are occasionally faulty, but this problem is not unique to arthroscopy and need not be mentioned further. Many surgeons prefer to work without the tourniquet inflated, but it is best to have it available if needed.

The increasing tendency among arthroscopists is to employ an assistant who is familiar with the instruments. This practice, in turn, will prevent instrument failure. A magnifying lens can be employed to examine the various instruments, particularly those with a mobile part, to avoid intra-articular breakage (Fig. 10–1).

Physician's Level of Skill

The many problems in this category are inversely proportional to the experience of the surgeon. Probably, no orthopedic procedure is as difficult to learn as arthroscopy. Even after performing 50 to 100 or more arthroscopic examinations, the arthroscopist often experiences difficulty with some cases, a fact he finds puzzling. Some surgeons, especially younger ones, seem to master the necessary skills faster than those who are older and perhaps less patient. Some difficulties are inherent in learning the various portals of entry for the arthroscope and the optimal position of the patient's leg for viewing certain areas of the knee joint. These techniques are discussed in Chapter 3. How to interpret what one sees through a 3- or 4-mm aperture cannot be taught and must be learned. This factor is perhaps the major reason that some are much more successful than others in performing arthroscopy.

Intra-Articular

Intra-articular problems are discussed in more detail in Chapter 3 and are mentioned here only briefly. When viewing through any telescopic instrument, one obviously needs a clear field, whether the medium is gas or water. Cloudy or bloody joint fluid does not permit a clear view of the interior of the joint, and to obtain such a view is often time-consuming. Even after the joint fluid appears to be clean, some turbidity may remain in the posterior recesses of the joint, when using saline solution. Some

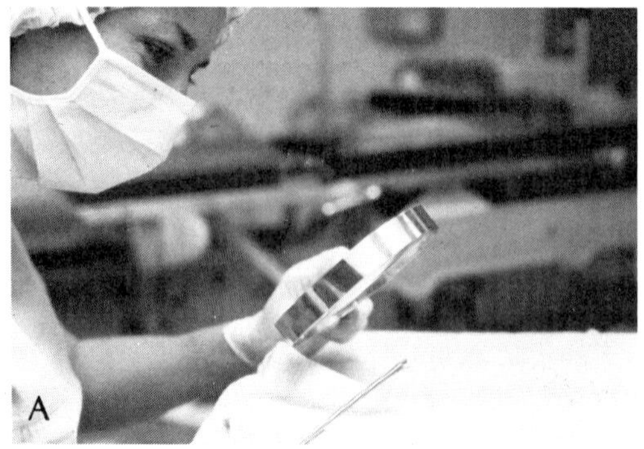

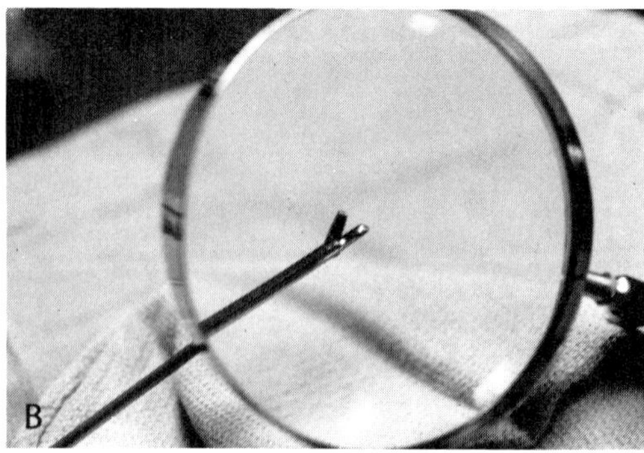

Fig. 10–1. *A* **and** *B***, Magnifying lens used to examine instruments and to detect defects that may result in breakage of the instruments inside the knee.**

have found that the temporary use of water in the joint hydrolyzes the blood cells and makes it possible to obtain a clearer joint fluid more quickly. Saline solution is more physiologic both for the synovium and the joint cartilage, however, and should be substituted for water as soon as possible.

Enlarged fat pads, hypertrophied synovial villi, and occasionally, adhesions, often prevent adequate visualization of the interior of the knee joint. Often, one is confronted with the decision whether to try to push the fat pad against the synovium by increased fluid pressure within the joint or to excise the fat pad using the motorized shaver. If one must excise the fat pad, it is important to realize that this procedure promotes bleeding and possibly adhesion formation. No solution is ideal. Up to now, no satisfactory fat pad retractor has become available.

No doubt exists that a tight knee joint presents a real problem, and again, no solution may be satisfactory. Certain positions of the leg permit slightly better visualization of the posterior recess of the joint than others. Occasionally, it is not possible to obtain even a fair view of the posterior horn of either the medial or lateral meniscus. The use of auxiliary approaches such as the posteromedial or posterolateral or the alternative of passing the scope through the intercondylar notch are often helpful, but they do not permit visualization of the main body of the meniscus. Even experienced arthroscopists have ruptured the medial collateral ligament in an effort to obtain a better view posteriorly. Sometimes one has to be satisfied with an incomplete view of certain areas in the knee joint. A knowledgeable assistant can be of greatest help in any arthroscopic procedure.

The telescope is a magnifying lens, and this property is always a problem when one attempts to evaluate lesions within the joint. Even when one knows that at 1 mm, the magnification is approximately tenfold, the tendency still exists to overestimate the size of the lesion and, therefore, the importance of the pathologic process.

COMPLICATIONS

Complications in arthroscopy can be divided up into those that involve the instruments and, more important, those that involve the patient.

Postoperative Bleeding and Effusion

Usually, this problem is minor and resolves itself. The joint, of course, should be emptied of fluid before the arthroscope is withdrawn. Occasionally, a bleeding synovial vessel causes some hemorrhaging to the joint; rarely, it is necessary to aspirate the joint postoperatively.

Infection

For some years and for many thousands of cases, it was thought that intra-articular infection never occurred following arthroscopy. It appeared that the technique prevented large numbers of bacteria from entering the joint, and constant irrigation would wash out most, if not all, bacteria that did manage to enter the joint. In recent years, several cases of intra-articular infections have been reported after operative and diagnostic arthroscopy. These infections have caused no permanent damage to the knee joint. Nevertheless, it behooves the arthroscopist to take the same precautions as with an arthrotomy.

Vascular Damage

Serious complications have been reported recently involving damage to the popliteal vessels. In patients who have undergone arthroscopy in the presence of a torn capsule, attempts at distending the joint have resulted in escape of the fluid into the popliteal area with transient vascular embarrassment. Much more serious complications, reported anecdotally on several occasions, have involved the loss of a limb following arthroscopic meniscectomy. These complications occurred in patients who had an arthroscopic meniscec-

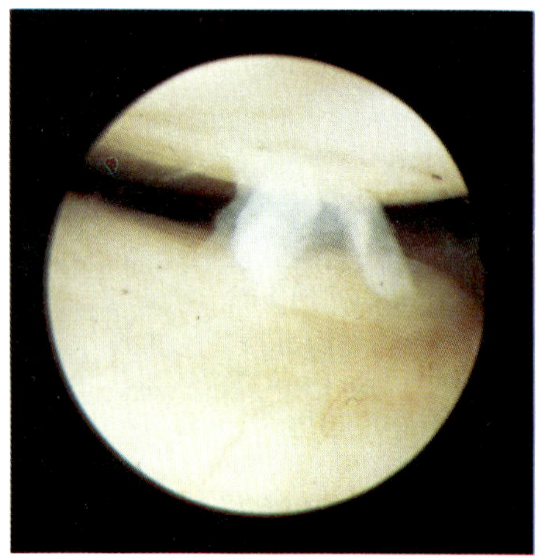
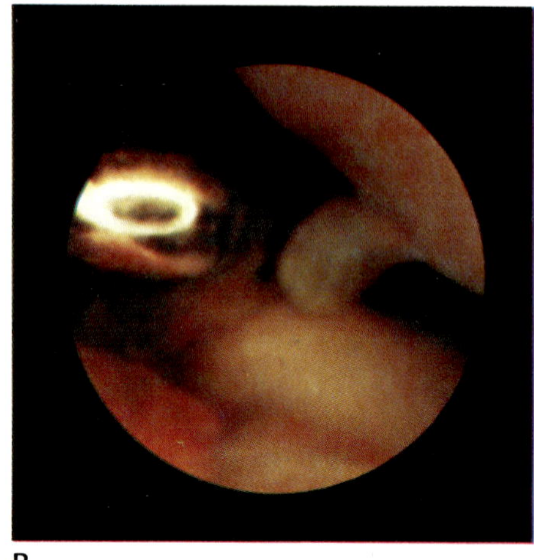

Fig. 10–2. ***A*** **and** ***B,*** **Superficial damage to joint surfaces caused by instruments. More serious damage can occur during arthroscopic surgical procedures.**

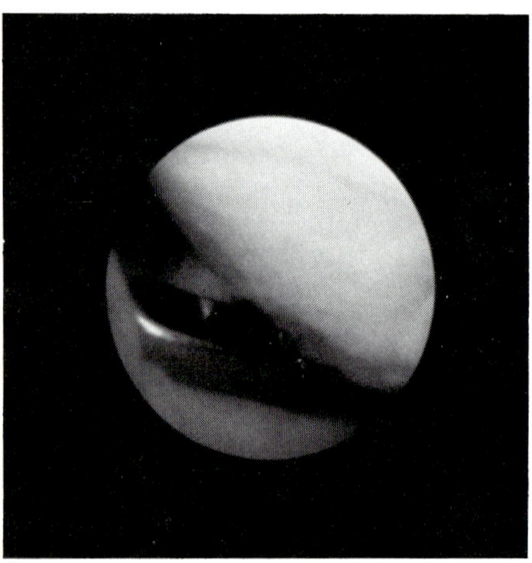

Fig. 10–3. Broken grasping forceps, seen lodged in the tibial femoral joint, were removed arthroscopically.

tomy on an outpatient basis, and the damage to the vascular tree was not recognized at the time. When this damage became apparent, it was too late to save the limb. Vascular damage is possible when one is operating by the posteromedial approach. It is thus extremely important for surgeons to consider this possibility, and if a surgical procedure is attempted in the posteromedial corner of the knee, the patient should be admitted overnight for observation.

Damage to the Articular Cartilage

Of all the complications of diagnostic and especially operative arthroscopy, damage to the articular cartilage is by far the most common. There is no way of knowing how often this complication occurs or how severe it is (Fig. 10–2). Without a doubt, this type of damage has been inflicted by most surgeons who perform operative arthroscopy and by many who restrict themselves to diagnostic arthroscopy. One phrase must be kept constantly in mind: If you cannot see, do not cut. Under such circumstances, an arthrotomy should be performed, to avoid damaging the articular cartilage, thereby possibly promoting the early onset of degenerative arthritis. Although the articular cartilage can be damaged during arthrotomy, the incidence of this complication is certainly much higher during operative arthroscopy.

Instrument Damage

Any instrument can break, and many surgeons have had experience with knife blades and the ends of scissors breaking off in joints (Fig. 10–3). This problem, of course, can be due to faulty equipment, but it is more often the fault of the surgeon. The use of curved, as well as straight, instruments makes it less likely for the surgeon to attempt to force an instrument to perform a task that it is not meant to do. Because of the nature of this task and the confined spaces within which he works, the arthroscopic surgeon must be especially careful not to damage instruments and, more important, the patient himself.

Part II

SURGICAL ARTHROSCOPY

In the past few years, interest in arthroscopic surgery has increased so rapidly that one might well wonder where and how it will end. By its very nature, arthroscopy has appealed not only to patients and orthopedic surgeons, but also to those in the media, and publicity in newspapers and magazines, as well as on television, has been widespread. As a result of this publicity, patients now ask and even demand that, when necessary, their knees be operated arthroscopically and will travel great distances to find a reputed expert. What is unique about this phenomenon is that patients have no fear of this new type of surgery, which they refer to as microsurgery. This confidence is undoubtedly the reason for the sharp increase in the number of surgical procedures performed on the knee. To make arthroscopic surgery available to more patients, it has been necessary to provide more instructional courses. Until recently, this responsibility was borne by a few orthopedic surgeons, but it is now shared by others who also have acquired the necessary expertise.

The need for these courses and the resulting demand for them is the result of the unique nature of arthroscopy. The difficulties in forming a mental image of an object when one is looking through a tiny aperture are considerable, as pointed out in the March, 1981 issue of *Scientific American* entitled "Anorthoscopic Perception." It requires more experience to master this new technique than almost any other orthopedic procedure. Even with experience, some surgeons never become proficient, and those who contemplate learning arthroscopic techniques should know this.

The ability to perform an arthroscopic meniscectomy efficiently and atraumatically is the hallmark of an arthroscopic surgeon. Because so many techniques for arthroscopic meniscectomy are available, this book devotes a considerable amount of space to various techniques. Each chapter on meniscectomy is written by a superb technician and, in many cases, an orthopedic surgeon who devotes all or much of his time to arthroscopic surgery. These techniques are outlined in considerable detail and take the reader step by step through this difficult surgical procedure.

As with any other new operation, the advantages of this procedure are not as great as one might think, and the problems and complications are greater than they appear at first glance. The possibility of an out-patient surgical procedure with little morbidity and the likelihood of return to work or sports in a short time are obvious advantages, especially for highly skilled athletes for whom time is of the essence. The lower morbidity rates and the quick return to work or sports make arthroscopic surgery one of the major advances in our specialty in recent years.

Arthroscopic surgery has several potential disadvantages, however, one of these being that the technique does not lend itself to review by peers, as does an open procedure. As in no other procedure, the surgeon's conscience has to be his guide.

Another inherent disadvantage to arthroscopic surgery is the danger of damaging the articular surface; this danger is much greater than when the same surgical procedure is performed by conventional arthrotomy. In the case of those inexperienced surgeons who spend three or four hours attempting to remove a meniscus, it is almost inevitable that the patient's articular surface will be damaged, and this injury, of course, can result in arthritic changes in later years. As good orthopedic surgeons, we know that the length of the scar in the skin is not as important as the one we may leave behind on the articular surfaces.

The unanswered questions are: who should perform arthroscopic surgical procedures, and on whom should they be performed? Not all surgeons are capable of performing arthroscopic surgery, and not all patients are best handled in this way. In our enthusiasm for arthroscopic surgery, we should not forget that a place still exists for conventional arthrotomy.

Chapter 11

ARTHROSCOPIC SURGERY OF THE ARTICULAR SURFACE OF THE PATELLA

S. Ward Casscells

Although arthroscopic surgery plays an important and well-established role in the treatment of many intra-articular lesions, its role in the treatment of patellofemoral joint disease is limited. The reason for this limitation is that the patients who complain most about anterior knee pain are teenagers who do not, in fact, have chondromalacia, which even when present may not lend itself to patellar shaving. One should question reports that some surgeons have performed hundreds of patellar shavings in a short period of time. Chondromalacia is not so common that anyone can quickly accumulate such a large series; either the reports are untrue or these patients are treated without proper indications.

Most of the current confusion concerning chondromalacia stems from the use of the term by some to designate anyone with pain in the anterior portion of the knee, especially those in their second and third decades. Surgeons who make the diagnosis based on pain may perform unnecessary arthroscopies with the expectation of finding a softening area of patellar cartilage that might lend itself to shaving. The literature does not provide documentation that chondromalacia, especially in the earlier stages, is painful, and my own investigations have led me to the opposite conclusion.

A study of patients whom I evaluated arthroscopically included 163 knees that exhibited either pain or chondromalacia or both, but no other intra-articular disorder. Of this group, 78 patients (48%) had painful knees but no chondromalacia; 44 (27%) had chondromalacia but no pain; and only 41 (25%) had both pain and chondromalacia. From this study, it is obvious that pain and chondromalacia are not synonymous. Hungerford also agrees that knee pain and chondromalacia are not synonymous.[1]

In a review of my first 1000 arthroscopies carried out several years ago, 16% of the patients had no intra-articular disorder whatsoever; most of these patients were teenagers with painful knees.[2] On the basis of this experience, I rarely suggest arthroscopy for young patients who have only anterior knee pain with no clinical or radiologic findings. I find nothing in the literature or in my own experience to explain the suggestion by Sikorski and colleagues that "perhaps there are two types of chondromalacia, one in which there is a lesion and one in which there is not, both of them painful."[3] As in any other surgical procedure, one should have clear-cut indications for operation and at least a reasonable expectation of success and of benefit to the patient.

When treating lesions of the patellar surface by whatever means, it is not currently possible to predict the success of a surgical procedure. The reason is that so little is known about the way human articular cartilage reacts to disease and trauma and, as yet, there have not been even short-term follow-up studies of any sizable group of patients who have had motorized patellar shaving. What we do know is that patellar shaving is a minor surgical procedure that can often be performed on an outpatient basis, and if it does not benefit the patient, at least it does no harm.

Most orthopedic surgeons with the greatest knowledge of the pathophysiology of cartilage believe that little or no benefits accrue to the patient who had his patella shaved.[4] On the other hand, removing loose and damaged articular cartilage may reduce lysosomal enzymes or prostaglandins, which when released into the joint cause further damage to the chondrocytes and produce an inflammatory reaction.

The alternative to patellar shaving is to excise all the damaged articular cartilage including the subchondral bone and to allow the ingrowth of fibroblasts that may be stimulated by joint motion to differentiate into fibrocartilage. If the lesion is in the center of the patella and demands treatment, this is most difficult to do arthroscopically. My own preference is to perform conventional arthrotomy.

PATELLAR SHAVING

Since the development of the motorized shaver by Johnson,[5] patellar shaving has become enormously popular in the orthopedic world. More patellae have probably been shaved since the introduction of the shaver than in all previous years by conventional methods using a knife.

The only patellar lesions that lend themselves to motorized shaving are ones in which the patella has a grass-like or crabmeat appearance (Fig. 11–1). Such lesions are most often found in the younger individuals. Other types of patellar damage such as those in which the patellar cartilage takes on an abraded appearance do not lend themselves to patellar shaving (Figs. 11–2 and 11–3). Such lesions are more often seen in the older individual and are located on the lateral patellar facet.

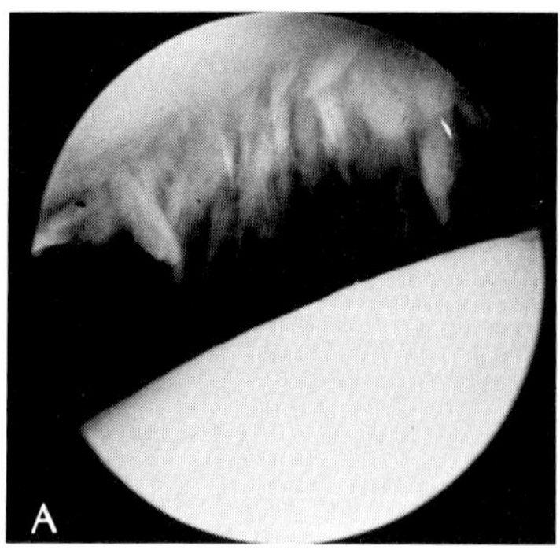

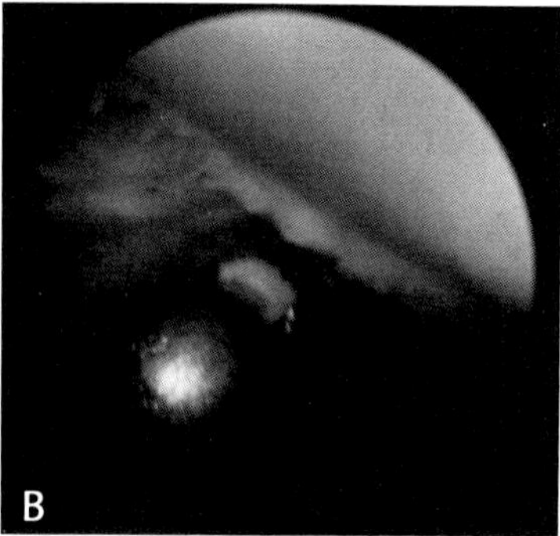

Fig. 11–1. *A,* **A close-up view of the typical crabmeat appearance of chondromalacia patella.** *B,* **Most of the loose and redundant cartilage have been removed by motorized shaver.**

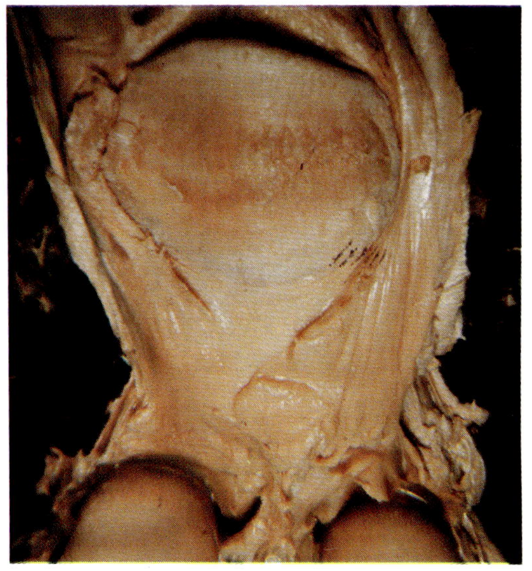

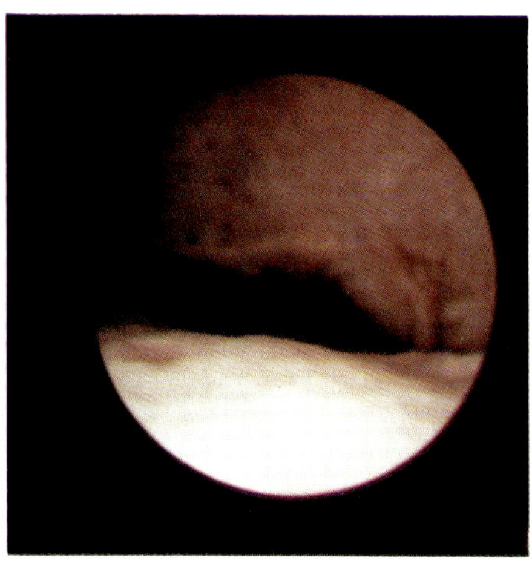

Fig. 11–2. Abraded appearance of the patellar cartilage that does not lend itself to shaving in the cadaver specimen.

Fig. 11–3. Arthroscopic view of patellofemoral joint with abraded appearance that does not lend itself to shaving.

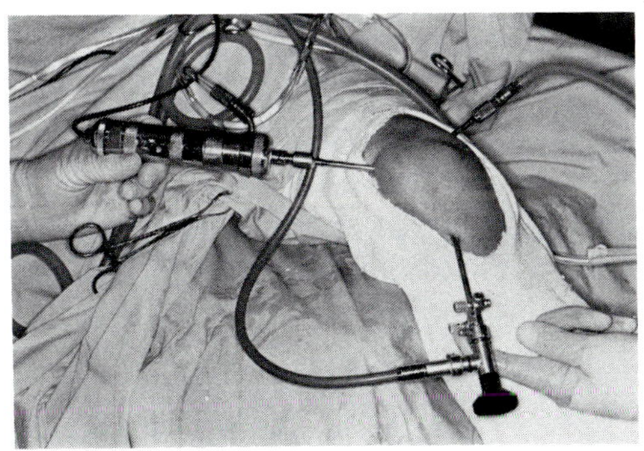

Fig. 11–4. Usual surgical draping of the knee with scope and shaver in place.

Technique

The patient is placed supine on the operating table, and the knee is prepared as for any knee operation (Fig. 11–4). Although some have maintained that patellar shaving can be performed satisfactorily and easily under a local anesthetic, I find this method to be frustrating and generally unsatisfactory. Not many unanesthetized patients can tolerate a thigh tourniquet, and without a tourniquet, puncturing the joint for insertion of the arthroscope and the shaving equipment causes bleeding that may be difficult to control; this complication makes a simple procedure difficult and time-consuming. The technique of using local anesthesia, of course, can be learned, but general anesthesia is better until one has had considerable experience with arthroscopy in general and patellar shaving in particular.

As in all arthroscopic procedures, especially with patellar shaving, maximal distension of the joint is necessary, and a three-liter bag of saline solution is suspended three feet above the patient. The proper portals for introducing the shaver and the inflow tube can be best determined by first examining the patella to see the location of the area to be shaved. It is my practice to introduce the arthroscope through the usual inferolateral portal (Fig. 11–4). Johnson prefers to use this portal for the inflow tube and introduces the arthroscope anteromedially. The site of introduc-

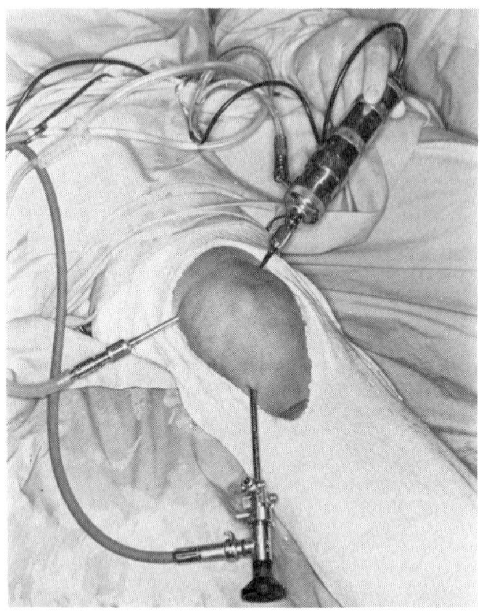

Fig. 11–5. Shaver introduced from the superior medial portal to permit shaving of the medial facet of the patella.

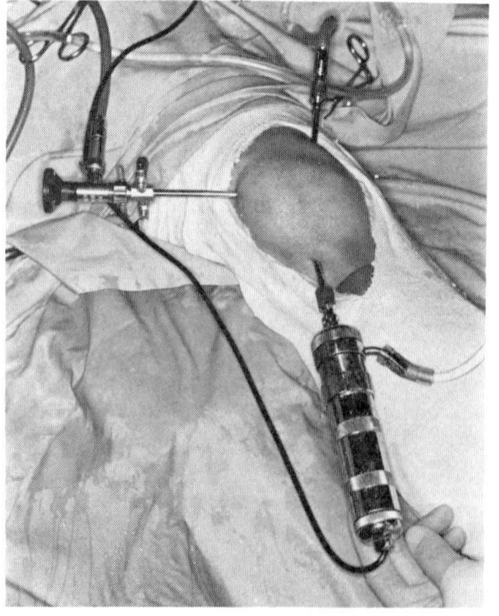

Fig. 11–6. Sometimes the positions are reversed. Lesions of the lower pole of the patella can be best reached from an infrolateral insertion of the shaver with the scope introduced superiorly.

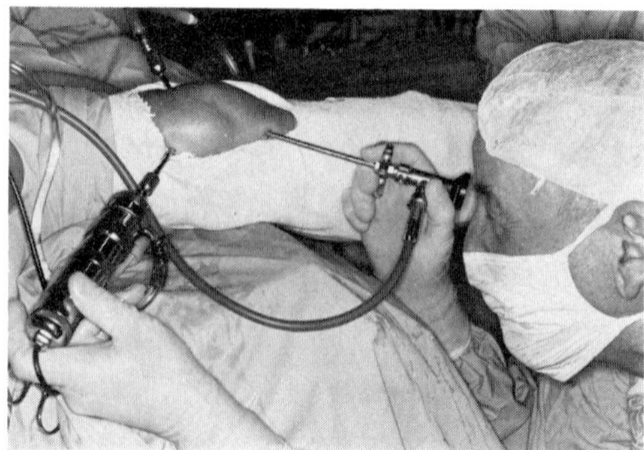

Fig. 11–7. When the arthroscope and the shaver are introduced from the same side, shaving is facilitated because one does not have to reach across the patient. Use of the video camera also makes this procedure easier.

tion of the shaver depends upon the location of the lesion. Because of the convexity of the patellar surface, it is often difficult to shave a lateral lesion when the shaver is introduced medially, and vice versa.

Introducing a Verres or spinal needle first gives the examiner some idea of the accessibility of the lesion. Because the lesions are more commonly found on the medial facet of the patella, the medial portal is usually used for the shaver (Fig. 11–5). The shaver can be introduced from either medially or laterally and from an infrapatellar and a suprapatellar portal (Fig. 11–6). Often, it is necessary to change the shaver from one portal to another in order to remove all the loose cartilage (Fig. 11–7).

During the course of patellar shaving, it may become necessary to tilt the patella to bring the lesion into contact with the shaver, and compressing the patella against the shaver may permit a more thorough debridement of the patellar surface. The shaver may become plugged by the cartilaginous debris sucked through it. Under these circumstances, the shaver must be removed and cleaned. It may be necessary to cut off the outflow through the shaver and wait for a few moments until the patient's joint is again distended with saline solution. It has been my experience that the outflow through the shaver sometimes works more quickly than the inflow, the joint is emptied of fluid, and further shaving becomes impossible until the situation is corrected.

Except for isolated case reports, no one knows what happens to the patella after it has been shaved. Whether shaved or not, many small lesions of the articular surface remain stable for many years, and it is likely that this stability also occurs following shaving. If pain has been a prominent feature, the pain may not be relieved or may return at a later date. If it does, it is unlikely that a repeat shaving will benefit the patient.

REFERENCES

1. Ficat, R.P., and Hungerford, D.S.: Disorders of the Patello-Femoral Joint. Baltimore, Williams & Wilkins, 1977.
2. Casscells, S.W.: The place of arthroscopy in the diagnosis and treatment of internal derangement of the knee—an analysis of 1,000 cases. Clin. Orthop., *151*:135, 1980.
3. Sikorski, J.M., Peters, J., and Watt, I.: The importance of femoral rotation in chondromalacia patellae as shown by serial radiography. J. Bone Joint Surg. (Br.), *61*:442, 1979.
4. Mankin, H.: Personal communication.
5. Johnson, L.L.: Diagnostic and Surgical Arthroscopy: The Knee and Other Joints. St. Louis, C.V. Mosby, 1981.

Chapter 12

SURGERY OF THE SYNOVIAL FOLDS

John J. Joyce, III,
Michael Harty,
John E. Tetzlaff

Synovial folds in the knee have been recognized by a number of observers. *Told's Atlas of Anatomy*, published in 1903, Spalteholtz,[1] and Gray[2] all acknowledged the anatomic presence of these folds, but only in passing. Although these structures were well recognized, their clinical manifestations were largely unknown and were ignored until recent years. Several Japanese observers discussed these structures and their clinical significance.[3–4] Pipkin in 1950[5] and again in 1971[6] mentioned that these plicae could be mistaken for adhesions and suggested that their presence caused symptoms.

Because arthroscopy has assumed a more widespread and popular role in the diagnosis and treatment of joint disorders, the clinical importance of the various plicae has become increasingly evident. The results of excision of these structures have been described by several observers.[7–13]

Despite this extensive background, several problems still exist. First, confusion has arisen over the nomenclature of various bands. Second, the actual existence of suprapatellar and medial plicae as separate entities has been questioned. The incidence of the different types of plicae has varied among observers, and finally the range of clinical symptoms of the synovial folds is still questioned by a number of observers.

A comparison of observations made on cadaver knees with follow-up findings on patients in whom plicae were found and treated has shown that the suprapatellar and medial plicae are distinct structures with distinctive clinical significance.

ANATOMIC OBSERVATIONS

In early fetal life, the knee joint cavity develops from medial, lateral, and suprapatellar compartments, which are separated by synovial septa (Fig. 12–1). During the third month, these membranes are reduced and absorbed, resulting in the commonly accepted anatomic features of the joint. Incomplete resorption of the septa provides the appearance of the various synovial folds.

In the suprapatellar area, complete failure of absorption of the septum is not uncommon and results in a bicompartmental cavity. The suprapatellar pouch remains completely isolated from the remainder of

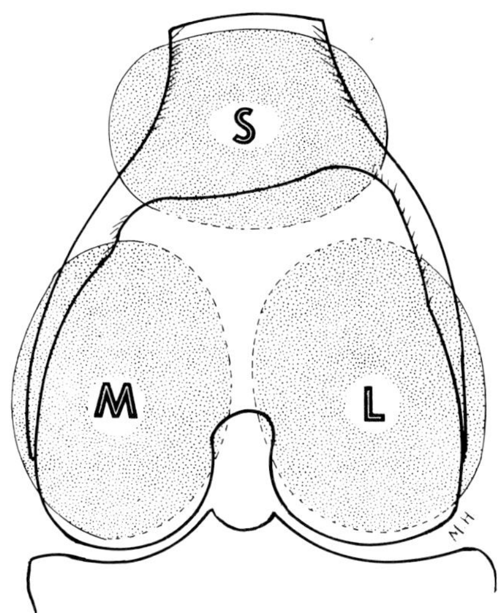

Fig. 12–1. Embryonic loculi of knee joint. The septa indicated by broken lines commonly disappear. S, Suprapatellar; M, medial; L, lateral.

the knee joint (Fig. 12–2). More frequently, partial absorption of the membrane occurs. A so-called "porta" is noted when a small opening occurs between the knee joint and the suprapatellar pouch (Fig. 12–3). More complete absorption results in a suprapatellar fold or plica (Fig. 12–4). All the aforementioned structures are proximal to the patella and extend from the anterior and posterior walls forming the pouch orifice.

The plica synovialis medialis originates in the region of the suprapatellar pouch and may be attached to the plica suprapatellaris. The structure extends distally and obliquely over the medial femoral condyle to insert into the general area of the fat pad. Several observers have referred to this fold as a "shelf" or "band" (Fig. 12–4). The suggestion that the suprapatellar structure be referred to as the plica synovialis suprapatellaris and that the "shelf" or "band" be called the plica synovialis medialis seems sound and should eliminate the confusion.

The plica synovialis infrapatellaris is more commonly called the ligamentum mucosum and lies parallel to the anterior cruciate ligament. Although it is usually small, the fold may be minimally absorbed to leave a septum. The intercondylar area is thus divided into medial and lateral compartments.

ANATOMIC SPECIMENS

The reported incidence and clinical importance of the different plicae varies widely among observers.

We have examined 492 cadaver knees (Table 12–1). A plica suprapatellaris of varying size was found in 89% of the specimens. A total septum was encountered in 7% of the knees. Central absorption of the membrane resulted in the formation of a "porta" in 9% of the specimens, and a residual fold of the medial margin was observed in 73%. Some sort of plica synovialis medialis (shelf or Iino's band) was found in 47% of the cadaver knees. Only 17% of these structures measured more than 1 cm on transverse section and joined with a suprapatellar plica to form the inverted "L" configuration. A fenestration of the distal end of the medial plica was seen in about 1% of the specimens, to form the so-called "chorda synovialis" of Watanabe. A synovial septum that extended between the fat pad and the intercondylar notch was encountered in 2 knees. The structure thus divided the area into medial and lateral halves.

Flexion and extension of the knee joint produced changes in the relationships between the synovial folds and the femoral condyles. With the knee fully extended, the plica suprapatellaris lies transverse to the longitudinal axis of the femur. No pressure was exerted by the synovial fold on any portion of the joint. As flexion of the joint was increased, the suprapatellar plica approached the longitudinal axis of the femur to stretch diagonally across the medial (commonly) femoral condyle. As the joint was flexed to 90° or more, the plica exerted increasing pressure on the articular surface. In several specimens, the inelastic suprapatellar plica fit into a small groove

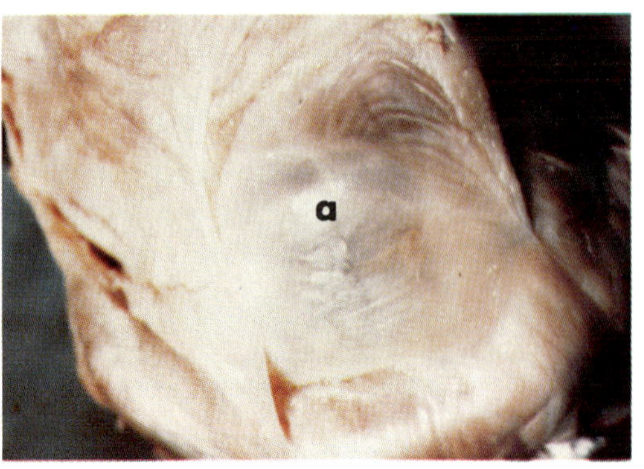

Fig. 12–2.

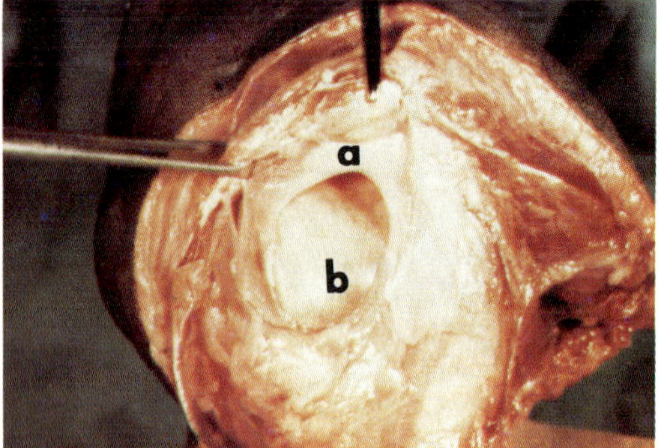

Fig. 12–3.

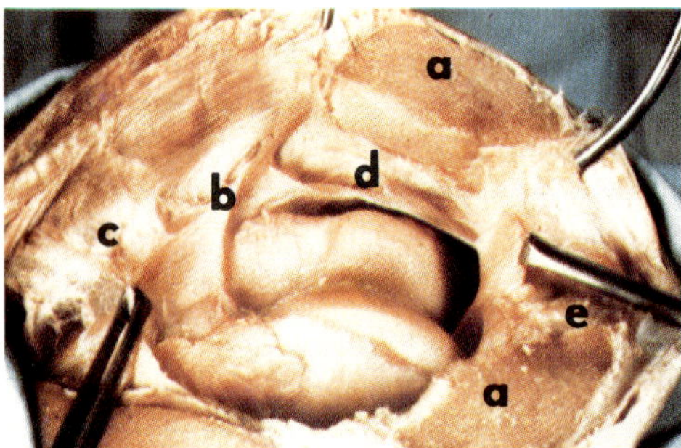

Fig. 12–4.

Fig. 12–5.

Fig. 12–6.

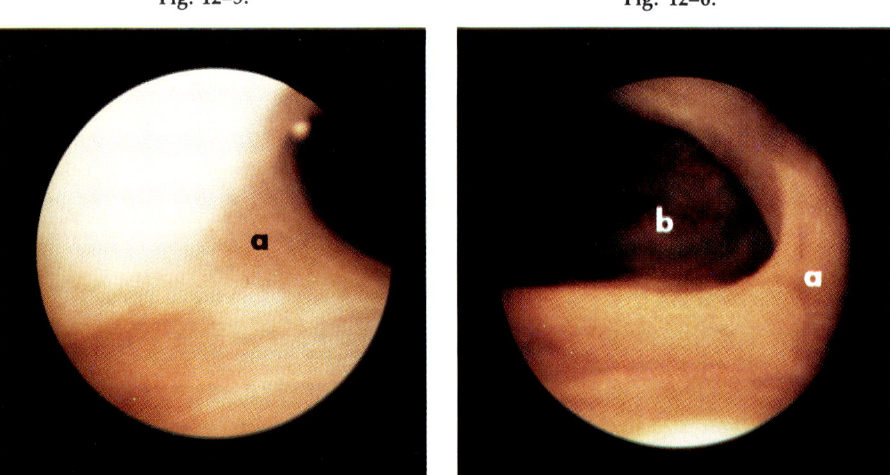

Fig. 12–2. Anatomic specimen. Suprapatellar plica (septum) (a) viewed from the suprapatellar pouch. The latter structure has been opened and spread apart to demonstrate the septum, which is distended by fluid injected into the joint.

Fig. 12–3. Anatomic specimen. Suprapatellar plica (porta) (a) viewed from the suprapatellar pouch, which has been spread open. The femoral condyle (b) can be seen through the small opening.

Fig. 12–4. Anatomic specimen showing suprapatellar and medial synovial plicae: The patella (a) has been split longitudinally. Suprapatellar plica (b); suprapatellar pouch (c). The medial patellar plica (d) forms a typical inverted "L" as it joins the suprapatellar plica superiorly and extends to the fat pad (e) distally.

Fig. 12–5. Arthroscopic view of suprapatellar plica (a) seen from inferiorly. Although the plica is narrow, it is thick and inelastic. Excision relieved the patient's symptoms.

Fig. 12–6. Arthroscopic view of porta seen from inferiorly. (a) Porta; (b) suprapatellar pouch. Resection relieved the patient's symptoms of pain and catching, and unrestricted activities were resumed.

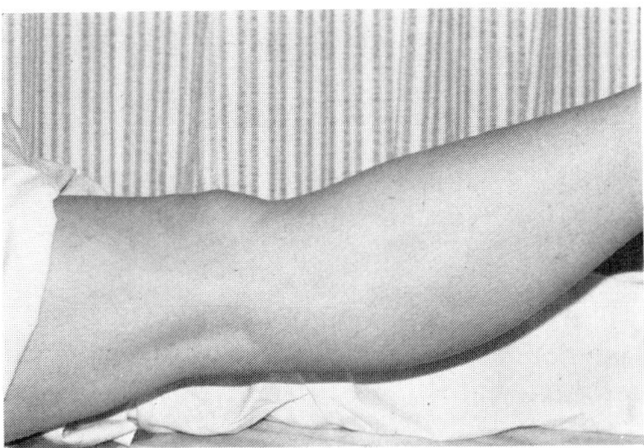

Fig. 13–1. Hyperextension of the knee characteristic of patients with ligamentous laxity.

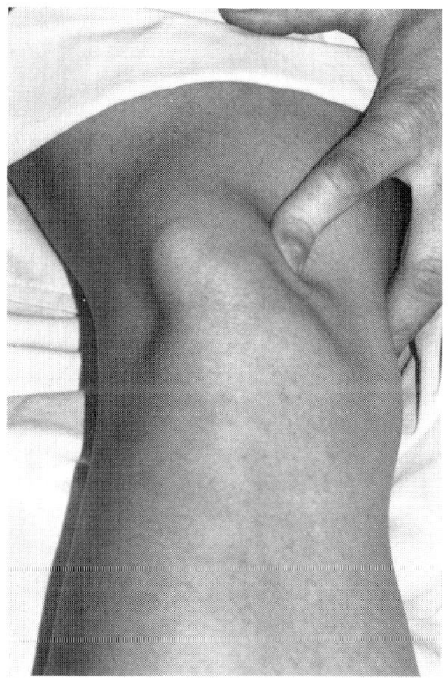

Fig. 13–2. Abnormal lateral mobility of the patella.

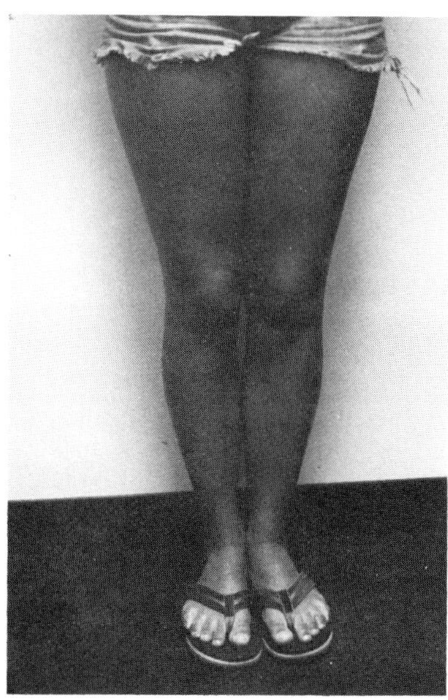

Fig. 13–3. With feet together, patellae point in the direction of each other.

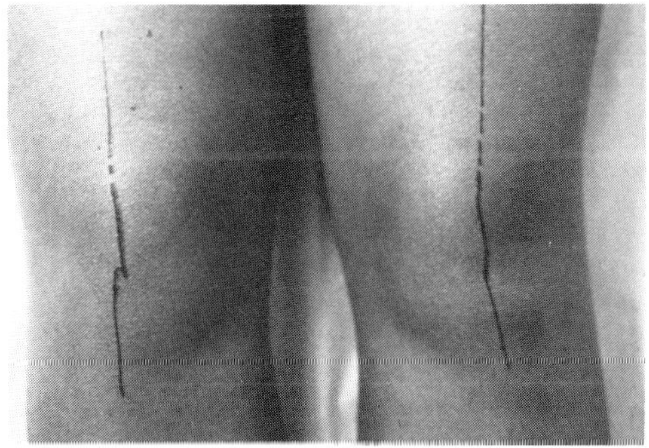

Fig. 13–4. The external position of the tibial tubercle of the left knee effectively creates an increased quadriceps angle.

short-term results of the lateral retinacular release appear favorable, long-term studies are currently unavailable to substantiate the lasting effects of this procedure. A study was initiated to obtain intermediate results of patients who had undergone endoscopic lateral retinacular release previously reported by McGinty and McCarthy, to evaluate any possible change in the previously reported results. The results of this intermediate study follow.

INDICATIONS

Patients in our group were selected for endoscopic lateral release only if symptoms persisted despite a 3-month course of vigorous, documented isometric quadriceps muscle exercise. In addition, each patient demonstrated one or more of the following factors associated with patellofemoral malalignment prior to the surgical procedure: generalized ligamentous laxity (Fig. 13–1), abnormal lateral mobility of the

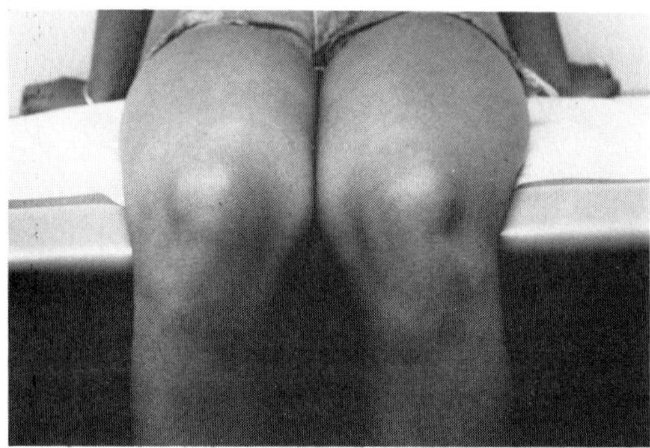

Fig. 13–5. Patellae sit laterally with the knees in 90° of flexion.

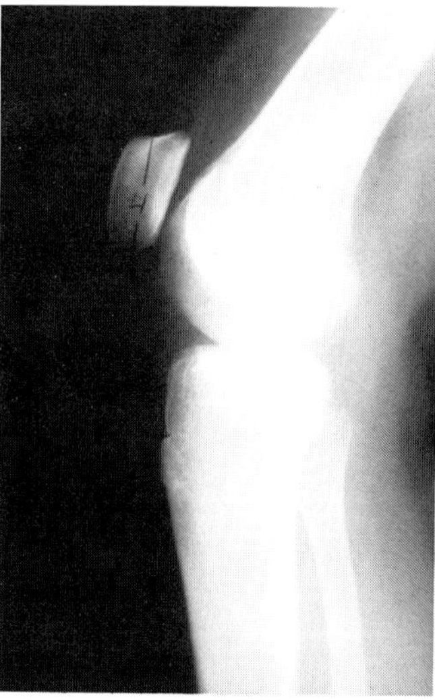

Fig. 13–6. Patella alta. The distance between the tibial tubercle and the inferior pole of the patella is more than 20% greater than the longest diameter of the patella.

patella (Fig. 13–2), a positive patellar apprehension test, medial facet tenderness, exaggerated femoral anteversion (Fig. 13–3), an increased quadriceps muscle angle (Fig. 13–4), lateral tracking of the patella in extension, lateral position of the patella in flexion (Fig. 13–5), or patella alta (Fig. 13–6).

MATERIALS AND METHODS

Endoscopic lateral retinacular release was performed on 45 consecutive knees in 42 patients from October 1977 to December 1978. Thirty-nine knees were evaluated, and the results reported for an average follow-up time of 18 months.[7] Thirty-one (79%) of these knees were evaluated a second time with a mean and median follow-up of 40 months, ranging from 27 to 48 months. Twenty knees were re-evaluated during a formal office examination and interview; for the remaining 11, patients were interviewed by telephone using a standardized questionnaire. Three aspects of knee function were evaluated: objective physical findings, subjective evaluations of pain and activities, and functional evaluation of knee performance. Each knee was then classified into 1 of 3 categories: excellent, improved, or poor, according to the criteria of the previous study as a means of obtaining comparable and longitudinal data.

The study included 22 female and 5 male patients whose average age at follow-up was 22.5 years, ranging from 14 to 35 years. All patients initially had retropatellar pain lasting an average of 3 years (range 4 months to 10 years). Eight patients had documented patellofemoral instability, 6 had recurrent subluxations, and 2 had recurrent dislocations. Three patients had undergone previous surgical procedures, one arthrotomy for a loose body, one tibial tubercle transplant, and one medial meniscectomy. Three patients had realignment procedures performed upon the opposite knee.

Twelve patients were documented to have generalized ligamentous laxity with hyperextensibility of the knees, the elbows, and the metacarpal phalangeal joints of both hands. Twenty-one patients had medial facet tenderness. Twelve patients had a positive apprehension test, including all 8 with a history of patellofemoral instability. Three patients had a preoperative knee effusion. Fourteen knees demonstrated lateral tracking in extension, but only one demonstrated lateral position of the patella in 90° of flexion. Eleven knees were noted to have an exaggerated quad-

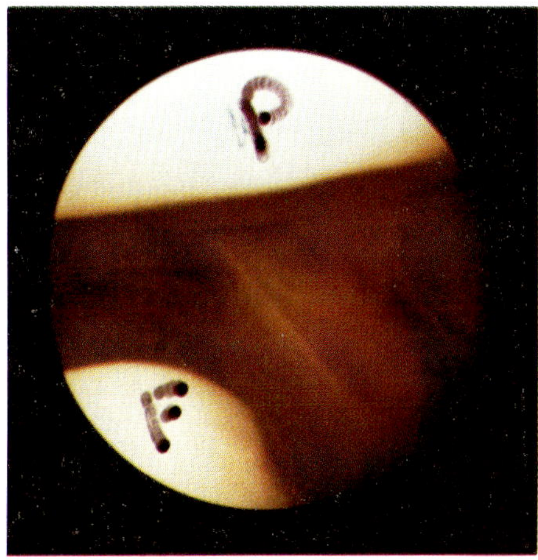

Fig. 13–7. Large percentage of the patella (P) overriding the lateral femoral condyle (F) in 60° of flexion.

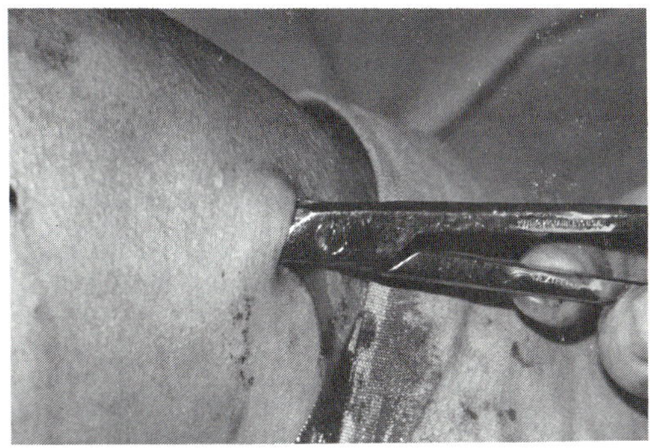

Fig. 13–8. Scissors developing subcutaneous tunnel through anterolateral portal prior to lateral release.

riceps muscle angle, and 16 showed increased femoral anteversion.

Complete arthroscopic evaluation was performed just prior to lateral retinacular release. Lateral patellar overhang (Fig. 13–7), the percentage of the patellar articular surface that protrudes beyond the border of the lateral femoral condyle, was measured through the arthroscope with the knee flexed at 60° and was found to range from 15 to 50%, averaging 30%. Chondromalacia of the patella was observed in 12 knees, moderate in 9 and severe in 3. The severity of the appearance did not correlate with the patient's symptoms. The only additional finding during arthroscopic evaluation was the presence of mild chondromalacia of the medial femoral condyle in 2 knees and the absence of the medial meniscus in one. Patellar shavings were not performed on any of the knees.

PROCEDURE

All procedures are performed in a hospital operating room under spinal or general anesthesia with aseptic technique. A tourniquet is inflated prior to examination in anticipation of bleeding from the lateral geniculate artery. All knees undergo a complete arthroscopic examination through a standard anterolateral portal. At the conclusion of the examination, Mayo scissors are inserted into the anterolateral portal, and a subcutaneous tunnel is bluntly dissected just lateral to the patella up to the junction of the vastus lateralis and the rectus femoris muscles (Fig. 13–8). The subcutaneous dissection is also carried distally toward the margin of the patellar tendon. The scissors are then inserted into the knee through the arthroscopic incision with one blade intra-articularly and the other blade lying in the subcutaneous tunnel previously created. The lateral retinaculum and synovium are then cut blindly to the midpoint of the patella. The retinaculum distal to the anterolateral portal is also cut in a similar manner.

The arthroscope is then reinserted into the knee through the original anterolateral incision. The cut retinaculum is identified (Fig. 13–9*A*) through the arthroscope, and the remainder of the release is completed with the 4- or 5-mm endoscopic scissors inserted either through the same incision (Fig. 13–9*B*) or through a second incision 1 cm proximal to the original anterolateral portal. Under direct observation, one can then extend the release proximally into the junction of the vastus lateralis and the rectus femoris muscles (Fig. 13–10). The lateral overhang of the patella may again be

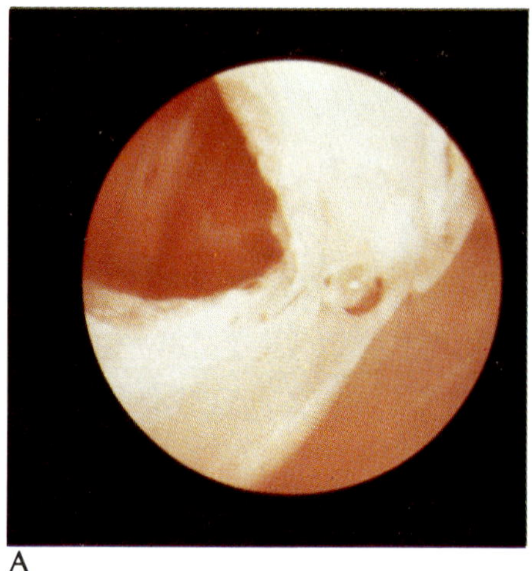

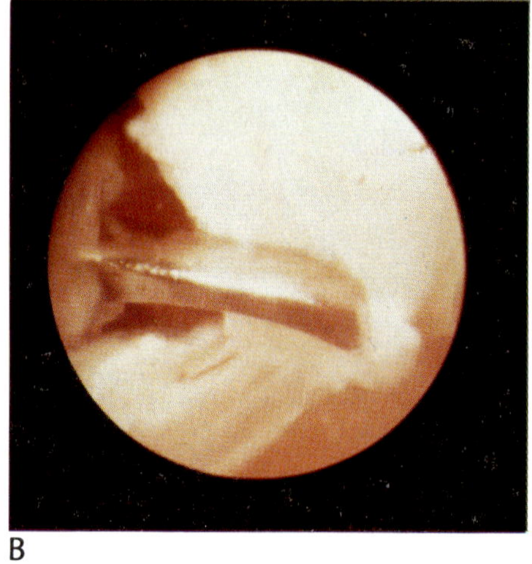

Fig. 13–9. *A*, In right knee, arthroscopic identification of the preliminary "blind" cut in the retinaculum. *B*, Completion of lateral retinacular release with endoscopic scissors.

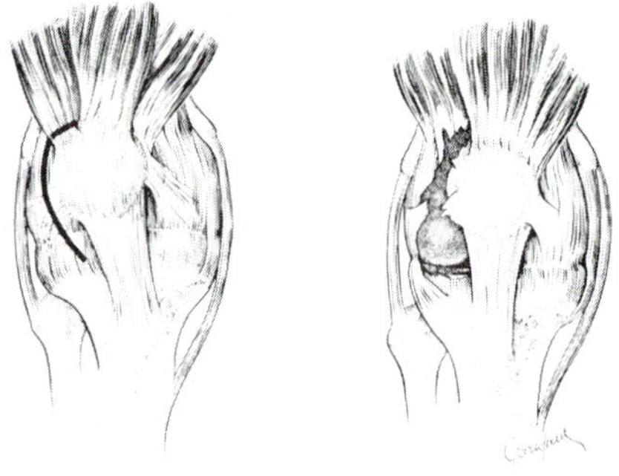

Fig. 13–10. Release must be completed proximally to the junction of the vastus lateralis and rectus femoris muscles.

inspected to confirm correction of the lateral displacement.

Before the tourniquet is released, it is important to place a compressive dressing on the knee. The incisions may be closed with simple interrupted sutures, and the knee may be covered with standard, soft gauze dressings. We prefer using a pressure pad made of inch-thick foam rubber covered with a stockinette measuring 4 by 8 inches. This pad is placed directly over the lateral incision and is held in place with an elastic bandage. The pad is not removed for 48 hours. The patient is then instructed to leave it in place for a total of 10 days except while washing. Isometric quadriceps muscle exercises are started on the first postoperative day, and crutches are generally required for 10 to 14 days. The patient is discharged from the hospital on the first or second postoperative day, depending upon postoperative pain.

POSTOPERATIVE RESULTS

The re-evaluated knees were placed in the 3 categories established in our initial report and modified from Merchant and Mercer.[4] An excellent result constituted total relief of preoperative pain and instability, absence of symptoms, and a complete return to full activity, both occupational and recreational including competitive athletics. An improved knee constituted one in which the symptoms of pain and instability were improved over the preoperative level, but the patient was forced to perform at a reduced level of activity. Poor results constituted no improvement over preoperative function. At the initial follow-up examination, an average of 18 months later, 19 (49%) knees were rated as excellent, 13 (33%) as improved, and 7 (18%) as poor. In the present re-evaluation, 7 (23%) knees were rated as excellent, 13 (42%) of the knees were rated as

TABLE 13–1

POSTOPERATIVE EVALUATION OF PATIENTS UNDERGOING ENDOSCOPIC LATERAL RETINACULAR RELEASE

INITIAL EVALUATION (18 months)	CURRENT EVALUATION (40 Months)	
	Changes by Category	Current Status
19 (49%) Excellent	5 (26%) Excellent 7 (37%) Improved 2 (10%) Poor 5 (27%) Lost	7 (22%) Excellent
13 (33%) Improved	2 (15%) Excellent 6 (47%) Improved 2 (15%) Poor 3 (23%) Lost	13 (42%) Improved
7 (18%) Poor	7 (100%) Poor	11 (35%) Poor 8 (21%) Lost

improved, and 11 (35%) knees were rated as poor.

Table 13–1 demonstrates the change of rating among the 3 groups. Overall, 7 (21%) knees were lost to follow-up. Two (5%) knees demonstrated improved function at the present evaluation. Both patients were re-evaluated as excellent from a previous assessment of improved. Eighteen (46%) knees remained unchanged, including all 7 that were originally rated poor. Three of these patients have subsequently undergone open realignment procedures, but it is too soon to evaluate them further. The remaining 11 (28%) knees functionally deteriorated, as shown in Table 13–1. Thus, of the patients reviewed, 6% showed improved function, 58% remained unchanged, and 35% showed a deterioration in their original evaluation.

Functionally, all three groups of patients could be easily differentiated. Those with excellent function were able to participate in all activities. Patients with improved knees could participate in all normal activities of daily living, but were restricted in their recreational and athletic endeavors, primarily with the onset of pain during strenuous participation. Patients who were rated as poor were restricted from all types of strenuous activities and could participate only in the activities of daily living.

The two patients who showed improved function felt that their knees had gradually improved over a 2-year period. One of these patients now dances professionally. Similarly, the patients who noted deterioration in their knee function reported that at approximately 2 years postoperatively they began to notice a recurrence of their initial symptoms.

Neither of the two patients with documented dislocation preoperatively had sustained a redislocation postoperatively, although both continue to have positive apprehension tests. Similarly, the six patients with preoperative subluxation had no symptoms of subluxation postoperatively, and moreover, only one of the six patients demonstrated a positive apprehension test postoperatively at the follow-up examination.

Subjectively, all patients in the series noted barometric sensitivity in the operated knee. Most complained of a mild, peculiar sensation in cold or damp weather, and six of the seven with a poor rating reported the sensitivity to cold and damp weather to be totally incapacitating. No specific correlations were seen between the final results and the patients' age, ligamentous laxity, Q-angle, or previous history of subluxation or dislocation.

COMPLICATIONS

One patient had a deep thrombophlebitis that responded to rest and anticoagulants. Two patients had significant hemarthrosis, probably the result of premature removal of the pressure pad. Both patients had a poor result. No infections were reported.

DISCUSSION

The number of reports of lateral retinacular release in treating patellofemoral pain and malalignment is increasing. The majority of these reports show favorable results, but have an average follow-up time of less than 18 months. Previously, the longest review for either open or endoscopic lateral retinacular releases was reported by Harwin and Stern.[8] These authors reviewed 25 knees in 15 patients for an average period of 35 months, with a range of 24 to 45 months. Twenty (80%) knees were rated as excellent, 5 (20%) were rated as good, and no poor results were seen in their series. Moreover, they found no change in the patient's functional evaluation for up to 45 months. These authors attribute their overall excellent results to proper selection of patients.

On the contrary, the shorter-term follow-up studies previously noted generally reported poor results in approximately 15 to 20% of operated knees.[1,4-7] This discrepancy does appear to be the result of selection of patients. Earlier studies included a more diversified population representing patients with a variety of patellofemoral disorders and a more widely distributed age range. It is also significant that none of the previously reported series noted any detrimental effects on knee function following lateral retinacular release.

A major distinction in our present review, in comparison to previous reports, is the decrease in the total number of patients who remain asymptomatic. Two patients previously rated as excellent were re-evaluated as poor with a full return of preoperative symptoms. Both patients attributed their regression of knee function to decreased physical activity and an associated weight gain. Furthermore, both noted the recurrence of their symptoms approximately 24 months postoperatively. The remaining 9 patients whose knee function dropped from excellent to improved also noted a change approximately 24 months postoperatively. Most of these patients complained of an insidious onset of retropatellar pain that slowly progressed. Three patients correlated the intensifying symptoms with their own increased athletic participation including long-distance running, crew, and track. These 9 patients were, however, able to participate in most recreational activities, but not at the same level of intensity as over the first 2 postoperative years. All 9 patients had modified their activity to avoid recurrent pain in the knee and were satisfied with their results. Thus, although their overall functional rating fell, their general performance and activity remained improved over preoperative levels.

Factors previously associated with poor results using the isolated retinacular release are patients (1) older than 35 years of age, (2) with significant degenerative joint disease, (3) with generalized ligamentous laxity, (4) with an increased Q-angle and (5) with increased body weight.[1,6] Moreover, Micheli and Stanitski noted a predominance of females in the poor-results category. Our present review cannot confirm that any of the factors previously noted are related to a poor result. In fact, 4 of 5 males in our study group were rated as poor, in contradistinction to the reports of Micheli and Stanitski.[1] In addition, of the 5 patients 30 years of age or older, 4 were rated as improved postoperatively, and only one retained poor knee function. Finally, no significant relationship was seen between a poor result and ligamentous laxity or an increased Q-angle, although, as previously noted, both patients who dropped from an excellent to a poor rating did undergo a substantial weight gain.

Micheli and Stanitski also emphasize the role of muscle rehabilitation and a closely supervised physical therapy regimen as essential for maximizing the effects of the surgical release, particularly in the first 6 months. They find the overall rating of each knee directly proportional to rehabilitative effort. Patients in our present series were instructed in an isometric quadriceps muscle strengthening program, which began the first day postoperatively and continued throughout the initial 3 months of postoperative office visits. All patients regained good quadriceps muscle tone with this schedule. Among the 11 patients who subsequently developed increasing symptoms, however, the resumption of quadriceps muscle strengthening exercises following the operation failed to improve the recurrent complaints. The effect of an intense physical therapy rehabilitation program, therefore, appears to be confined to the immediate postoperative period.

Although open lateral retinacular releases have been used in the past, the development of an endoscopic approach has facilitated the ability to perform a complete endoscopic evaluation of the knee and a controlled retinacular release by directly observing, and therefore controlling, the full extent of the release. In addition, the endoscopic technique results in minimum morbidity, provides a better cosmetic appearance, generally requires a shorter hospitalization and thereby costs less, does not interfere with subsequent reconstruction procedures, and produces results comparable to those of open procedures. The current reports on the use of endoscopic surgical procedures and the population of patients available for study are limited, so that significant factors influencing the results of endoscopic lateral retinacular release cannot be specifically defined. It remains for a larger review of patients and long-term studies to define the limits of the procedure further. The present intermediate results are again favorable. Although the number of patients who are completely asymptomatic has declined, most remain improved over preoperative levels, and the role of endoscopic lateral retinacular release remains an initial surgical technique in the treatment of patellofemoral pain in malalignment syndromes.

In summary, endoscopic lateral retinacular release is as effective as open retinacular release in the treatment of lateral malalignment syndromes of the patella. In addition, the technique provides specific advantages over an open procedure. Short-term follow-up results of this technique in treating patellofemoral disorders have been favorable. Long-term results have not been reported, however. This intermediate evaluation continues to support the use of lateral retinacular release as an initial procedure in patients unresponsive to conservative measures. Although asymptomatic knees apparently deteriorate approximately 2 years postoperatively, the overall function of the patient remains improved over preoperative levels. The simplicity and efficacy of the procedure make it useful as an initial treatment in lateral malalignment problems of the patella.

REFERENCES

1. Micheli, L.J., and Stanitski, C.L.: Lateral patellar retinacular release. Am. J. Sports Med., *9*:330, 1981.
2. DeHaven, K.E., Dolan, W.A., and Mayer, P.J.: Chondromalacia patella in athletes—clinical presentation and conservative management. Am. J. Sports Med., *7*:1, 1979.
3. Corta, H.: Zur Therapie der habituellen patellaren Luxation. Arch. Orthop. Unfallchir., *51*:256, 1959.
4. Merchant, A.C., and Mercer, R.L.: Lateral release of the patella: a preliminary report. Clin. Orthop., *103*:40, 1974.
5. Larson, R.L., et al.: The patellar compression syndrome. Clin. Orthop., *134*:158, 1978.
6. Betz, R.R., et al.: The percutaneous lateral retinacular release. Orthopedics, *5*:57, 1982.
7. McGinty, J.B., and McCarthy, J.C.: Endoscopic lateral retinacular release. Clin. Orthop., *158*:120, 1981.
8. Harwin, S.F., and Stern, R.E.: Subcutaneous lateral retinacular release for chondromalacia patellae: a preliminary report. Clin. Orthop., *156*:207, 1981.

Chapter 14

SURGERY OF LOOSE BODIES IN THE KNEE JOINT

John J. Joyce, III

ETIOLOGIC FACTORS

Loose bodies arise from several conditions. Although trauma is one of the most frequent causes, metabolic disorders, arthritis, synovial disorders, growth disturbances, and meniscal problems are all important etiologic factors. Foreign bodies within the joint are also of significance and frequently are loose within its confines.

Direct external injury, such as produced by a blow on the knee, may result in a chondral or an osteochondral fragment that floats about in the joint. Symptoms arise shortly after such an episode. Purely cartilaginous tissue is not seen on regular roentgenograms. On the other hand, a fragment containing a small piece of bone may appear to be deceptively small. Finally, an isolated flap of bony or cartilaginous tissue may be located in such a position that it causes intermittent disturbance of motion (Fig. 14–1). The femoral condyles, the patella, and the menisci are the areas from which loose bodies most commonly arise (Fig. 14–2).

Metabolic disorders such as gout or diabetes often produce changes that cause osteochondral material to float freely within the joint. Loose bodies may arise early in the course of such an ailment. Although rheumatoid disease may be the source of loose fragments, the detached osteophytes of osteoarthritis are encountered more frequently. The latter fragments vary in size and consistency.

Synovial osteochondromatosis is a common source of multiple "rice bodies" within the joint. Although their presence is usually evident, early diagnosis may be a problem. Not only is radiolucency of the material deceptive, but also the number of fragments may be small in the early stages of the condition. Only in its later stages may the disorder be accurately recognized.

The presence of osteocartilaginous bodies in both knees is not often associated with injury. A "constitutional factor," as well as a growth disturbance, has been suggested.

Foreign bodies assume many forms and present many problems. Pieces of wire suture, fragments of broken operating instruments, broken glass, and even bullets have all challenged and frustrated the surgeon (Fig. 14–3). Although most of the offending objects can be extracted with an ar-

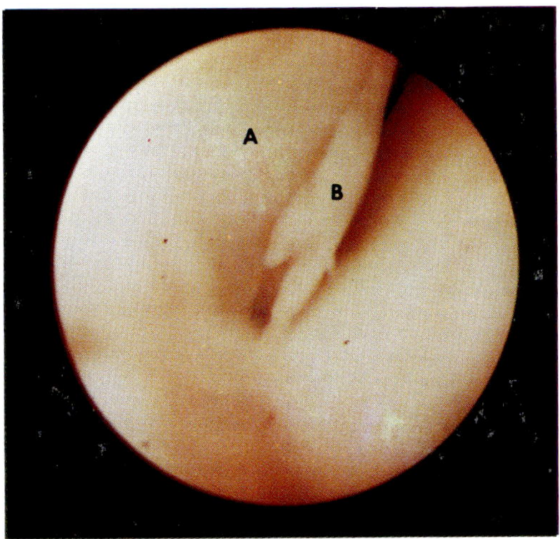

Fig. 14–1. Arthroscopic view of medial femoral condyle (A) with an attached fragment (B) that caused "catching" and swelling. Because the patient was 30 years old and the appearance of the remaining articular cartilage was good, excision was performed. Two years later, patient was engaging in sports without handicap.

throscope, arthrotomy is sometimes necessary.

DIAGNOSIS

Recognition of the presence of a loose body within the knee joint is usually straightforward. A history of an injury is followed by episodes of transitory "catching" or "locking" of the extremity. The patient usually can feel something moving about within the articular cavity.

Physical examination usually reveals a swollen knee with a demonstrable effusion. The swelling is often accompanied by limitation of motion. Local tenderness may be present in the region of the femoral condyles. A palpable mass is sometimes felt within the suprapatellar pouch.

Roentgenographic examination demonstrates the presence of a radiopaque osteochondral fragment (Fig. 14–4). An osseous defect is often noted in the patella or the femoral condyle (Fig. 14–5). An arthrogram may be helpful to demonstrate a radiolucent fragment. Although metallic or bony materials are usually observed roentgenographically, overlying bone may interfere with visualization. Anteroposterior, notch, oblique, and tangential views offer a solution to the problem of recognition and localization of the loose body.

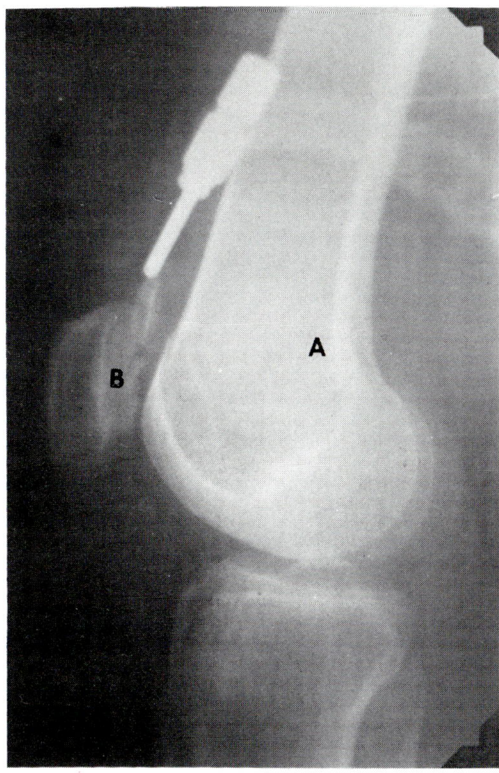

Fig. 14–2. Although this loose body may appear free in the suprapatellar pouch, it was so firmly attached to the patella that a small incision directly over it was necessary for removal. The subsequent patellar defect healed with minimal residua at 18 months. *A,* medial femoral condyle; *B,* attached fragment.

TREATMENT

Although excision of the loose body is the usual treatment, drilling and pin fixation of the partially detached fragment is desirable in younger patients. A large loose body may also be replaced, and bone may be grafted in a condylar defect. The adjoining surfaces of condyle and fragment require debridement. The incidence of success is greatest in younger patients. A bub-

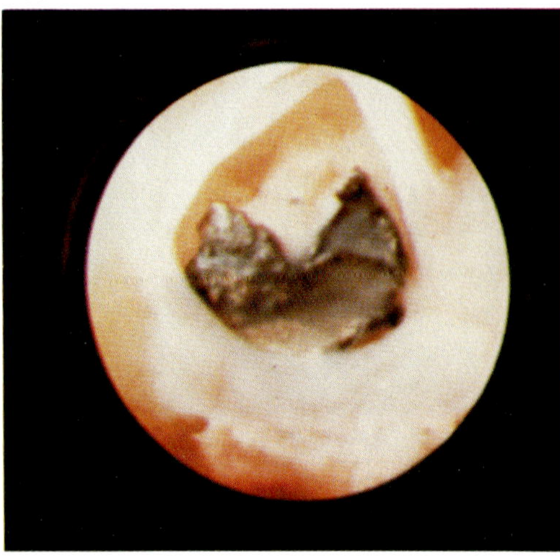

Fig. 14–3. This 22-caliber bullet is an example of a foreign body deeply embedded in the articular surface of the femoral condyle. Arthroscopic removal was followed by good function.

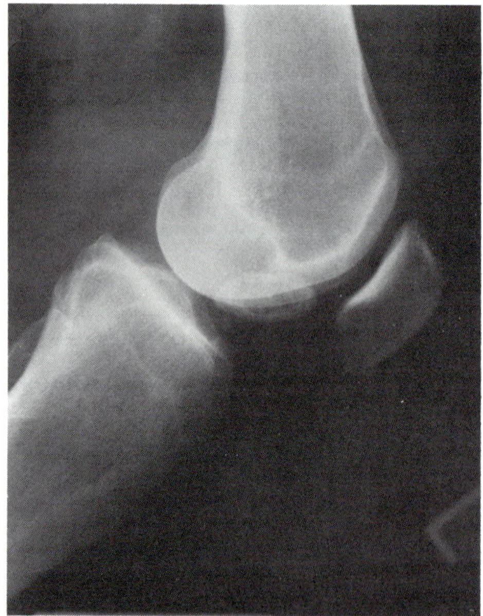

Fig. 14–4. A large osteochondral fragment is easily seen roentgenographically. Pure cartilaginous bodies can sometimes be shown by arthrogram, but often must be located arthroscopically. The size and location of this fragment facilitated its arthroscopic removal.

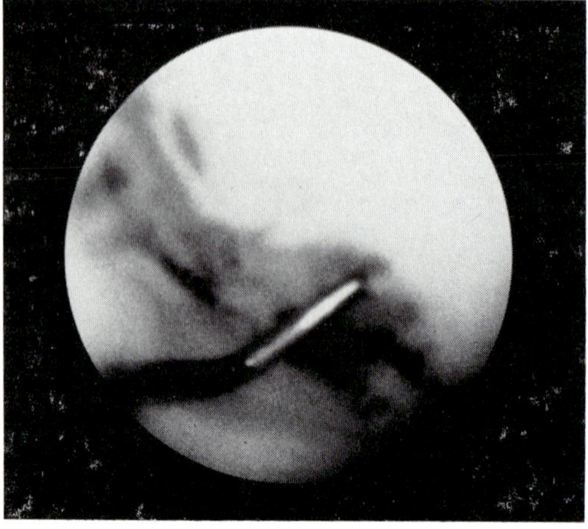

Fig. 14–5. The tip of the probe rests in an osseous defect of the medial femoral condyle. An osteochondral loose body had been removed by an open procedure elsewhere.

ble-like lesion with an intact articular surface usually heals by drilling alone.

A magnet is helpful in removing steel foreign bodies. Nonmagnetic materials must be visualized and extracted by means of a grasping device. If the object is too large to grasp with the available instruments or if multiple fragments are present, an open procedure may be advisable.

Evacuation of the multiple rice bodies found in synovial osteochondromatosis usually affords temporary relief. Synovectomy, either by arthroscope or by an open procedure, is required for a more permanent cure.

Arthroscopic Technique

Although loose bodies can be removed arthroscopically, an open procedure is occasionally necessary. A roentgenogram taken with the patient on the operating table is helpful. After surgical preparation and draping of the patient's knee, the surgeon inserts the arthroscope through the anterolateral portal. Gentle manipulation of the instrument and of the extremity is essential to avoid displacement of the fragment.

The suprapatellar pouch is a common lodging place for extraneous masses. In this

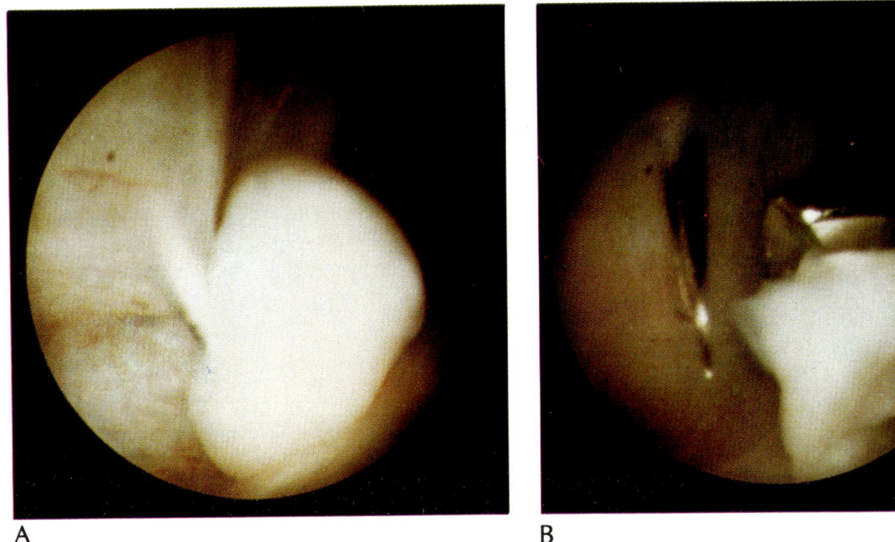

Fig. 14–6. *A,* Following an exasperating pursuit through the joint cavity, the loose body was coaxed into the suprapatellar pouch, where a gently inserted needle was used to transfix it. *B,* The fragment was then grasped and was gently removed through a slightly enlarged stab wound.

locale, the loose body can usually be seen and palpated. Unfortunately, the fragment is mobile and frequently hides in the recesses of the area. Interruption of the inflow and outflow of the distending fluid helps to stabilize the position of the loose body. The suction created by a needle carefully inserted over the mass lures it into an area where it may be impaled. Grasping forceps are then inserted, and the loose body is drawn to the periphery of the pouch under direct vision (Fig. 14–6). At this point, one must be careful not to use excessive force in withdrawing the mass and thereby losing it. While the loose body is held against the periphery of the pouch, the incision is sufficiently widened to permit gentle extraction of the mass.

The posterior compartment, the popliteal recess, the medial or lateral gutters, and the intercondylar notch provide favorite hiding places for inaccessible fragments. Loose bodies may be dislodged from the popliteal recess by manipulation with a nerve hook inserted posteromedially, by grasping the mass with small forceps through the same route, by extra-articular digital manipulation, by a suction device, or finally, by direct incision over the fragment. Figure 14–7 illustrates several instruments useful in removing loose bodies. A 70 or 120° arthroscope may be useful in

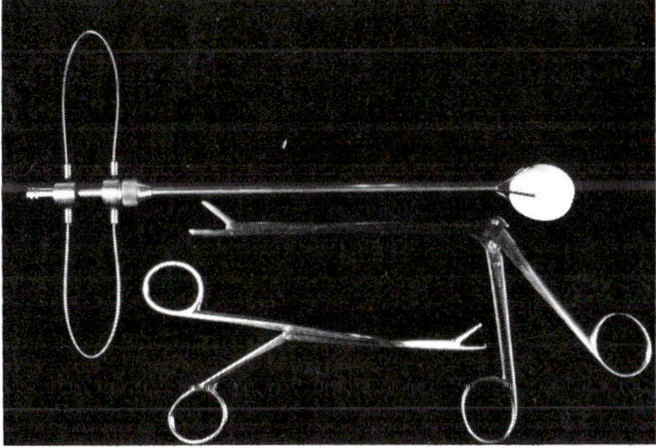

Fig. 14–7. Instruments used in the removal of loose bodies. Top: This device has metallic fingers activated by a spring mechanism. Suction can be applied. Middle: Pituitary grasping forceps. Bottom: Tendon passing forceps.

visualizing unusual areas. A roentgenogram is essential.

Although gas distension of the knee joint is used in other countries, its advantages are just now being appreciated in the United States. Surgeons who have used this method find that the area visualized is clearer and wider than with fluid distension. Further, the loose fragment does not migrate.

The removal of foreign bodies presents problems similar to those mentioned in the preceding discussion. Open removal is sometimes required to dislodge fragments imbedded in bone or soft tissue. It is essential that the arthroscopist set a time limit of an hour and a half for the procedure, beyond which he either performs an open arthrotomy or abandons an unsuccessful search.

Following replacement and pinning of a loose osteochondral fragment, the patient's knee should be immobilized until roentgenographic evidence of healing is present. Previous investigation has shown that repair is more likely to occur in younger patients. Laminograms are often helpful in demonstrating union of the fragments.

Although the arthroscope affords an excellent view of the knee joint, localization of loose bodies and their extraction may present a challenge to the surgeon. As in attempts at open removal, the offending material can elude the most experienced operator. The surgeon must have a variety of arthroscopes and instruments available to him. Furthermore, he must be able to use the various portals. Replacement of loose bodies by one of several techniques should be considered, especially in younger patients. Significant defects in the articular surfaces can result from the loss of a fragment, and early degenerative joint changes may then follow (see Fig. 14–5).

Arthroscopic removal of loose bodies is potentially one of the most frustrating procedures the surgeon undertakes. As seen from the foregoing discussion, a number of therapeutic possibilities exist. The treatment selected must comply with the condition dictated by the individual's needs.

SUGGESTED READINGS

Dandy, D.J.: Arthroscopic Surgery of the Knee. Edinburgh, Churchill Livingstone, 1981.

Guhl, J.F.: Arthroscopic treatment of osteochondritis dissecans: preliminary report. Orthop. Clin. North Am., *10*:671, 1979.

Milgram, J.E.: Osteochondral fractures of the articular surfaces of the knee. *In* Disorders of the Knee Joint. Edited by A. Helfet. Philadelphia, J.B. Lippincott, 1974.

O'Connor, R.L.: Arthroscopic surgery of the knee. *In* American Academy of Orthopaedic Surgeons Symposium on Arthroscopy and Arthrography of the Knee. St. Louis, C.V. Mosby, 1978.

O'Connor, R.L.: Arthroscopy. A Scope Publication. Kalamazoo, MI, Upjohn, 1977.

Smillie, I.S.: Injuries of the Knee Joint. 2nd Ed. Baltimore, Williams & Wilkins, 1951.

Watanabe, M., Takeda, S., and Ikeuchi, H.: Atlas of Arthroscopy. 3rd Ed. Tokyo, Igakushoin, 1978.

Watanabe, M.: Arthroscopy of the knee joint. *In* Disorders of the Knee Joint. Edited by A. Helfet. Philadelphia, J.B. Lippincott, 1974.

Chapter 15

OSTEOCHONDRITIS DISSECANS

James Guhl

HISTORY OF TREATMENT

The treatment of osteochondritis dissecans has been controversial for the past half century. Conservative measures such as restricted activity and immobilization for those 12 years of age and under have been successful according to Green,[1] Green and Banks,[2] Helfet,[3] Campbell and Ranawat,[4] and others. Smillie,[5] however, has pointed out that many of these lesions probably were anomalies of ossification and disappeared without treatment.

In the 12- to 14-year age group, the lesions were often intact and were treated by immobilization or drilling by open arthrotomy. The success rate was not as high as in younger patients. The success rate in patients 15 years and older was much less predictable, whether treated by immobilization or some other means, and the lesion frequently separated from its bed. As a result, Smillie in 1957 advocated fixing these loose fragments,[6] using a small nail that was later removed. Aichroth,[7] on the other hand, removed loose and separated fragments and expressed the opinion that fixation with wires and nails was of little value. Other methods of fixation by bone pegs were used by Scott and Stevenson[8] and also by Lindholm and Pylkkanen.[9] Lipscomb and associates[10] obtained success in a few cases by curetting the base of the crater, filling it in with cancellous bone, and then replacing the fragment, maintaining it with Kirschner wires that were later removed.

ARTHROSCOPIC TREATMENT

With the advent of arthroscopy in the early 1970s, accurate evaluation of these lesions became possible. In my early experience with 50 patients, all of whom were evaluated arthroscopically, I was able to classify the lesions accurately and to establish a protocol for treatment. All patients over the age of 12 years with lesions more than 1 cm in diameter and located in the weight-bearing area of the joint were promptly examined arthroscopically and were treated.

The majority of the lesions of the medial femoral condyle were mediolateral, involving part of the weight-bearing area but close to the intercondylar notch. In the lateral view, most lesions appeared in an area bounded by two lines: one projecting distally from the posterior femoral shaft, and the other projecting anteriorly from the femoral groove. Lesions of the lateral femoral condyle were usually inferomedial and more posterior than those on the medial condyle.

The position of the lesion on the condyle often determined treatment. Lesions too far posterior were usually inaccessible and could not be pinned or drilled. In some cases, the lesion, though clearly visible roentgenographically, was difficult to see arthroscopically, and special techniques were needed to identify it. Palpation with a probe for a softened area is of value in locating the lesion, and light-dimming techniques and the use of methylene blue dye are also helpful.

In our clinic, the type of treatment depends on the age of the patient and also on the physical appearance of the lesion. In children under 12, treatment is nonsurgical without arthroscopy. In this group, the prognosis for healing is good. In the intact lesion in the patient over 12 years of age, drilling is done routinely, and the success rate is over 90%. Drilling appears to be the preferred treatment because good results are achieved, and the morbidity, such as joint stiffness and muscle atrophy, is avoided.

In the third group, in which early separation or a crack in the articular cartilage is seen, the fibrous tissue under the lesion is curetted or removed with a power-driven bur, and the lesion is pinned.

In the fourth group, the older teenager and adults, bone grafting is added to the curettage and pinning technique.

Contraindications

In the following situations, open arthrotomy is preferred to closed arthroscopic techniques:

1. Large lesions 3 to 4 cm in diameter with a displaced loose body. These lesions require shaping, trimming, and replacement by open methods.
2. Lesions in which multiple, small, loose fragments are present.
3. Large craters with a hard sclerotic base.
4. Lesions that are arthroscopically inaccessible, such as those in the posterior portion of the lateral femoral condyle.
5. Failure in previous attempts at treatment by arthroscopic means.

In all instances, one's experience with arthroscopy should be taken into consideration before attempting to treat these lesions arthroscopically. The technique is difficult and demanding, and one should not attempt something beyond one's capabilities.

Techniques

Arthroscopic surgical procedures are performed in a hospital operating room with the patient under general anesthesia or, in some cases, local anesthesia. Sterile technique is required. The patient's knee should be flexed as much as possible with the aid of a triangular-shaped knee pad. An image intensifier or a roetgenogram is rarely indicated except for inexperienced surgeons.

Drilling. Drilling is done with a plain or smooth .062 Kirschner wire by the method

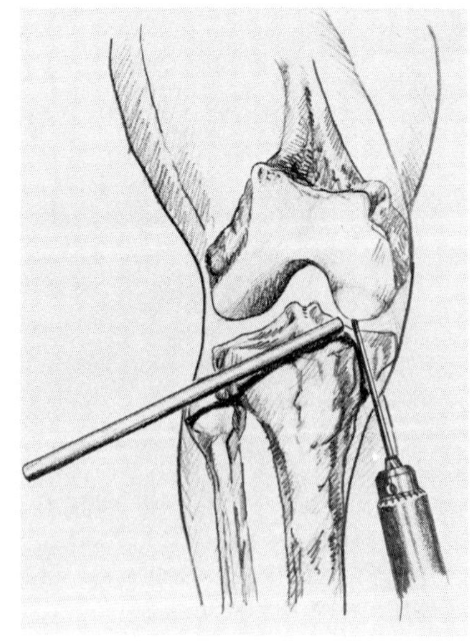

Fig. 15–1. Drilling by triangulation.

of triangulation (Fig. 15–1). A large wire, a Steinman pin, or a drill can be used if one is reconstructing a defect with an unsalvageable fragment. A needlescope cannula or a similar device is neccesary to avoid damage to the soft tissues when using a Kirschner wire. The anteromedial or anterolateral approaches can be alternated as necessary for the arthroscope and pin, depending upon the position of the lesion. If necessary, the proximal approach, as described by Patel, can also be used. If the lesion is located far posteriorly, the needlescope cannula for drilling must often be inserted as inferiorly as possible, just adjacent to the patellar tendon.

When the lesion is located in the lateral femoral condyle, as it is occasionally, drilling can be done with a needlescope cannula through the posterolateral approach. When the lesion has been sighted, the cannula is held firm, and the needlescope is replaced by the .062 Kirschner wire for drilling.

The purpose of each approach is to obtain a perpendicular approach to the lesion. The best technique is to use one or two entry points into the articular cartilage of the non-weight-bearing portion and to drill in several different directions down to bleeding bone. Little damage is done to the articular cartilage, if multiple punctures are required, when one uses nothing larger than an .062 Kirschner wire.

Pinning. Pinning is best done with a 9-inch, .062 Kirschner wire with a raised thread on the distal end or trailing 3 inches (Fig. 15–2). Completely threaded wires are far too difficult to insert, to direct, and to remove, and they often break. Two or more smooth Kirschner wires may suffice if inserted at divergent angles, but fixation may not be as secure.

Once the boundaries of the lesion are established, the wire should be placed under arthroscopic visualization and tapped in a few millimeters beneath the articular cartilage. A 25 to 70° oblique arthroscope is helpful for this method of

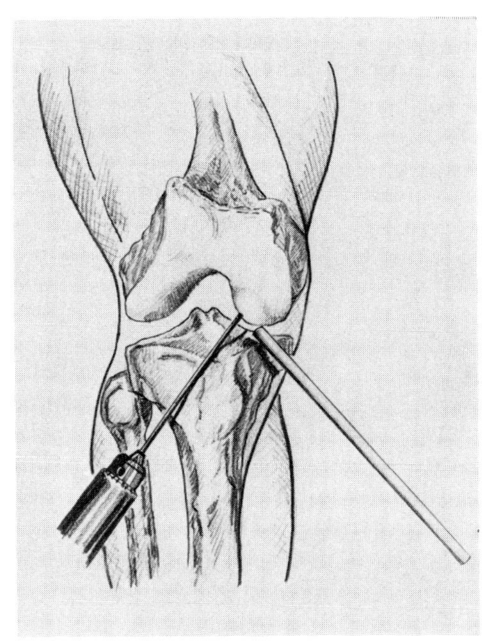

Fig. 15–2. Wire driven by a power drill.

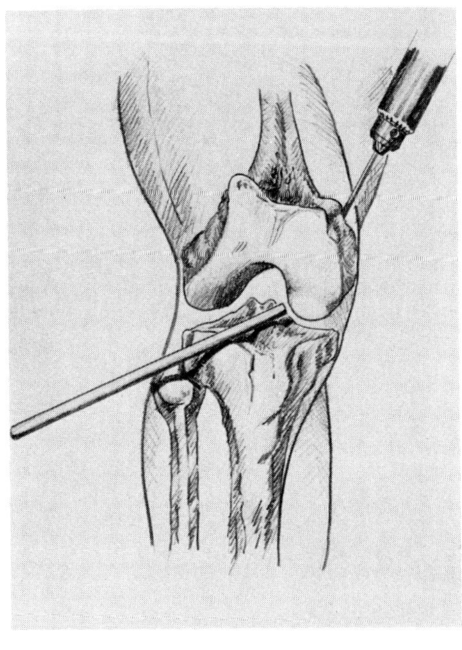

Fig. 15–3. Wire withdrawn in a retrograde manner.

triangulation. The wire is aimed for the posterosuperior flare of the medial femoral condyle. When the wire is placed, it is driven as far as possible with a powered instrument in a proximal direction; the wire is then withdrawn in a retrograde manner until it disappears into the joint and is barely palpable by the double-gloved thumb (Fig. 15–3). The joint is then redistended, and the arthroscope is reinserted with care to avoid scratching the lens. The remainder of the threaded portion of the wire is withdrawn fully until it is flush with or just slightly inferior to the articular cartilage. Several wires may be necessary (Fig. 15–4). The proximal end is then cut off just beneath the skin.

The wire is removed in 4 to 6 weeks as an outpatient procedure, with the patient under local anesthesia.

Pinning partially separated fragments should be accompanied by adequate debridement of fibrous tissue from the boundary, as already described, as well as by drilling the base.

Reduction and Fixation. Partially detached lesions held by a hinge of articular cartilage require complete debridement of all fibrous tissue from the undersurface of the detached fragment as well as from the crater of the lesion. The loose piece can be hinged away, usually held against the femoral condyle, and the undersurface is then debrided with small rongeurs inserted through another portal. Accurate reduction must be obtained. Further debridement of the fragment or crater may be necessary, or bone may be packed down through a channel superiorly, as described in the next paragraphs. When adequate reduction has been obtained, fixation by multiple wires is then done. It is sometimes possible to replace and reduce a completely detached fragment by this technique.

Bone Grafting. Local cancellous bone, iliac cancellous or cortical cancellous bone pegs, matchstick grafts, allografts, and freeze-dried grafts supplemented by local bone have all been used. These grafts can be obtained by a small stab incision over

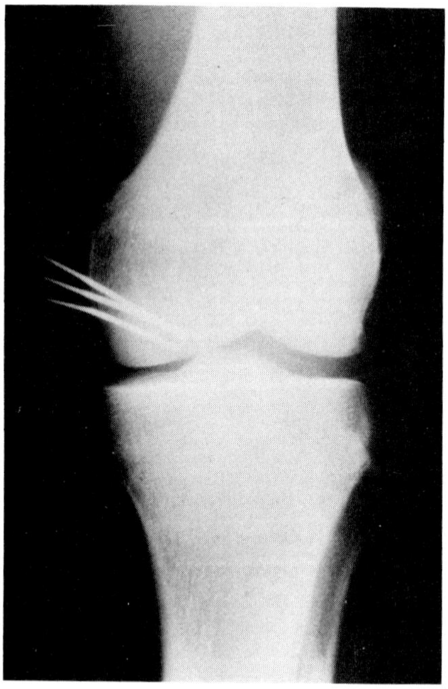

Fig. 15–4. Anteroposterior roentgenographic view showing lesion after debridement, hairline reduction, and fixation with three pins.

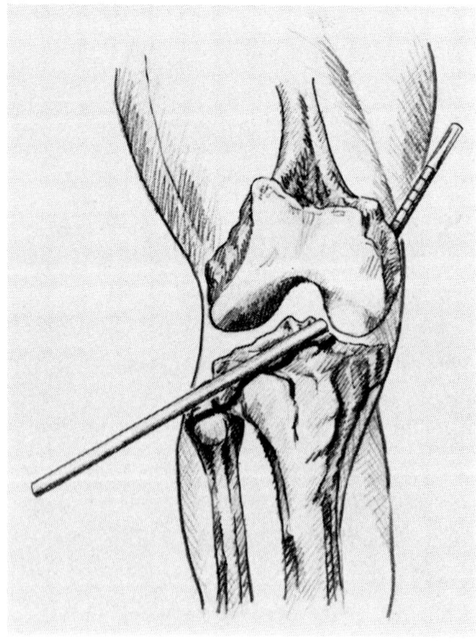

Fig. 15–5. Bone grafting by the first method from the proximal position.

the iliac crest or proximal condyle and taken with a trephine. Two methods of grafting exist, with some variations.

The first method establishes a channel, and grafting is accomplished from a proximal position. First, one places a .062 Kirschner wire, as described for pinning, as a guide. A 5-mm or larger cannulated reamer, which should be calibrated, is driven distally over the wire by an assistant arthroscopically (Fig. 15–5). This maneuver can be accomplished without passing through the articular cartilage. If a larger reamer is chosen, 8 to 10 mm in diameter, penetration can be avoided by taking accurate measurements and by observing the articular cartilage carefully as it is approached slowly by the reamer. If penetration occurs with a small 5-mm reamer, particularly in the intercondylar notch, where no weight bearing takes place, little damage is done. Two or 3 small channels or a single large channel can be constructed. The pegs, struts, cancellous bone, or any combinations of these are packed distally down to the lesion to complete the graft. A firm fit is mandatory.

The second method involves creating the channel from the distal position for placement of smaller, 3- to 4-mm matchstick grafts. The channels are formed by driving the reamer over a guide wire from the distal position by the triangulation method (Fig. 15–6). It is important to construct the channel perpendicular to the articular surface. The wire and reamer are subsequently withdrawn and are replaced by a second arthroscopic cannula (Fig. 15–7). The graft is passed through the cannula and into the channel. As experience is gained, the surgeon may no longer require the cannula. A loose graft in the joint can be retrieved by the experienced arthroscopist.

This second method of grafting is preferable when used for the combined purpose of fixing the lesion and acting as a graft. The first method is preferable for larger lesions and for packing bone at the

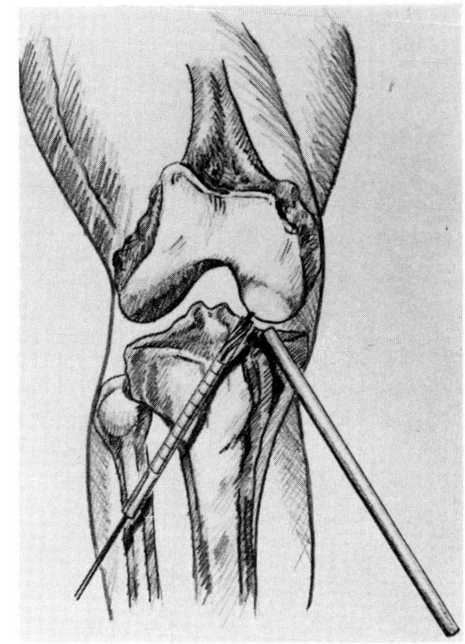

Fig. 15–6. Bone grafting by the second method from the distal approach.

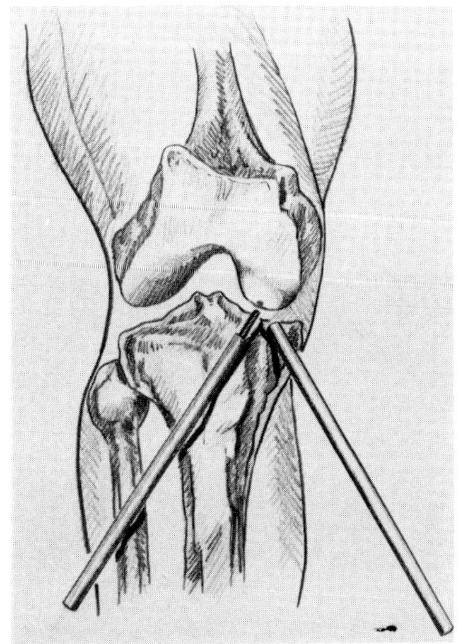

Fig. 15–7. Cannula replacing a reamer for placement of the graft.

site of the lesion to correct an incongruity or an irregularity of the articular cartilage. When grafting, it is imperative that all fibrous tissue be removed, as described, and that the base be drilled.

Reconstruction and Loose Body Removal. Reconstruction means trimming the rim of the crater of the lesion and trephining to form a sharp, perpendicular margin. This operation is performed with basket forceps, knives, dental chisels, curettes, and dental burs. The reason for the sharp margin is that fibrocartilage replacement forms in a perpendicular manner from the base. The tissue in the lesion's crater must be thoroughly debrided and then abraded several millimeters with a dental bur or drilled to freshly bleeding bone. This maneuver results in a smooth, continuous surface of fibrocartilage and hyaline cartilage for the best possible articular surface. All unsalvageable loose bodies are removed.

OPEN SURGICAL PROCEDURES

When open procedures are indicated, pinning and drilling are done in essentially the same manner. Bone grafting can be accomplished by three methods. Cancellous bone can be packed into the bed of the lesion directly to fill space before replacing the fragment, as described by Lipscomb and associates.[10] Multiple pegs taken from an area immediately adjacent to the tibial spine are excellent for fixation (Fig. 15–8), as well as grafting. A third method is to use a large hip trephine. A 10- to 12-cm plug of bone is taken from the femoral condyle proximally and is broken and detached a few millimeters before the articular cartilage and bone junction are reached. The break is created by making several fine drill holes with a small Kirschner wire perpendicular to the end point of the plug. When the plug has been carefully removed, it is reversed so that fresh bone at the proximal end is used to replace the necrotic bone of the lesion. Additional drill holes through the lesion and parallel to the graft may be made with an .062 Kirschner wire when indicated.

For lesions that are unusually large and unsalvageable, one may have to consider cancellous-cartilaginous allograft replacement, and one may choose to refer such patients to centers in Toronto, Boston, or Dallas.

POSTOPERATIVE CARE

Intact lesions that are drilled require minimal immobilization, as judged by the

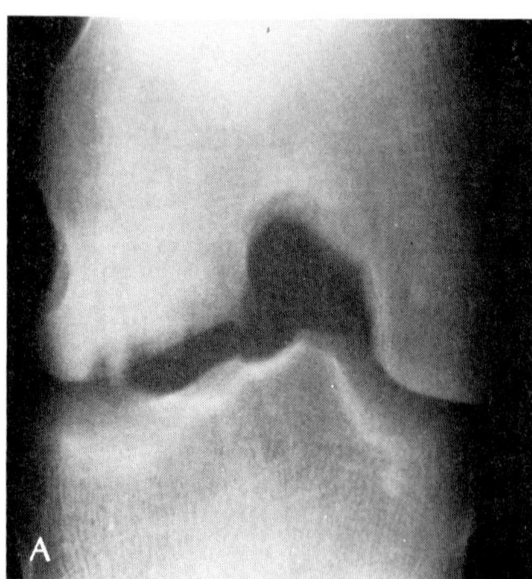

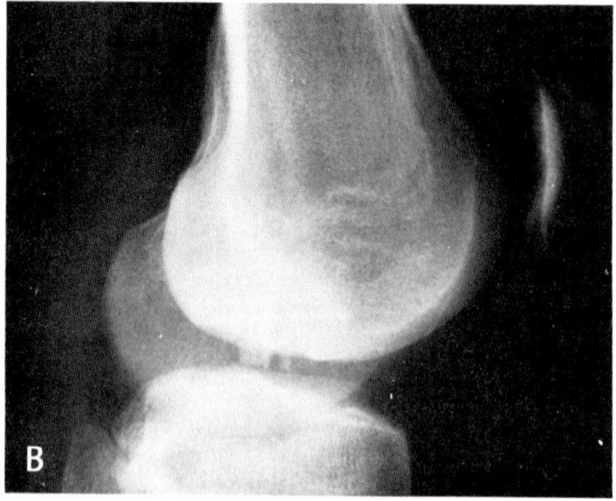

Fig. 15–8. ***A,*** **Anteroposterior roentgenographic view of an inferocentral lesion of the lateral femoral condyle treated with multiple cortical pegs by an open surgical procedure.** ***B,*** **Lateral view showing the same lesion. Note the posterior location.**

size of the lesion and the individual patient. I feel that it is best in some cases to restrict the patient's activity, with partial or full weight bearing, particularly in the younger patient. If a rare lesion does not heal, treatment can be repeated in these younger individuals without the penalty of long-term immobilization. I learned this through experience with several of my patients whose activities were difficult or impossible to control, as is common in this age group.

Lesions that are pinned or grafted should be immobilized until the pins are removed and early trabeculae are seen to cross the margin of the lesion and the graft bed. Early motion can then be started either with no weight bearing or with protected weight bearing, as judged best for each patient. Full weight bearing should be prohibited until healing is sufficient, as shown by adequate trabecular formation. In most cases, sports should be restricted for at least a year, and in some cases, indefinitely.

Reconstructed lesions require early or immediate motion, as soon as the patient is comfortable. I advise full weight bearing based on my experience in this series with arthroscopic follow-up and the results of Tippet's experience[11] with abrasion chondroplasties. The price of a 2- or 3-month period on crutches seems too high when one considers the size of the lesion and the minimal morbidity associated with a repeat of treatment, if the rare lesion should not heal.

In a few of my patients, in whom lesions were drilled, pinned, or grafted, and from roentgenograms sent to me by others in similar cases, I have noted that often 6 months or more may transpire without evidence of full or adequate progressive healing. In most cases, the patients became active on their own due to impatience. When roentgenograms were repeated in these patients 6 months to a year later, further healing had occurred with activity, and the patients were asymptomatic. Further follow-up will have to bear out these observations.

Bone scarring does persist in all adults and in most adolescents, although it is of little significance as long as the articular surface is congruous and smooth.

COMPLICATIONS

Broken pins were left buried in place in two patients.[8] The bone grafts loosened in two cases, but were retrieved and replaced. Early in my experience, two patients developed iatrogenic chondromalacia, most likely due to prolonged immobilization. This evidence again speaks in favor of early motion. Quadriceps muscle atrophy and limited motion were also kept to a minimum for this reason in the patients that followed. Aspirations were rarely necessary, and no joint infections occurred.

When bone grafting is employed, greater precautions should be taken than in other arthroscopic procedures. I routinely use intravenous antibiotics during the procedure and soak the bone grafts in antibiotics while the procedure is in progress. Final irrigation is done with plain saline solution. If the procedure is to be documented, these extra precautions must be taken into consideration because contamination is of much greater significance than in routine arthroscopic procedures.

RESULTS

The results of arthroscopic treatment of osteochondritis dissecans have been extensively analyzed and reported in *Clinical Orthopedics and Related Research.* In general, the rate of healing appeared far more promising when the treatment methods previously outlined had been followed carefully. These reports include patients treated by nonoperative means as well as those in whom arthrotomy was performed. The rate of healing was 90%, both in patients treated nonsurgically and those treated arthroscopically. The patients who underwent arthrotomy are also doing well, so far, although some additional failures will probably be reported in the next 6 years. Improved techniques and equipment have resulted in a better rate of healing of these osteochondritic lesions than in the past.

Benefits to the patient from arthroscopic surgical procedures, are evidenced by shorter hospitalization, decreased costs, less morbidity and fewer complications, and decreased scar formation.

In some cases, repeated arthroscopic evaluations, when necessary, can be performed with the patient under local anesthesia, and additional loose fragments can be drilled or removed. Outpatient operations under local anesthesia are obviously much more acceptable to patients than arthrotomy.

Total treatment time has been reduced by early arthroscopic evaluation and early treatment of these lesions, in contradistinction to following them radiologically and starting treatment after a period of months or years. Based on the first 6 years' experience, long-term results in the future should be superior to those in the past.

REFERENCES

1. Green, J.: Osteochondritis dissecans of the knee. J. Bone Joint Surg. (Br.), *48*:82, 1966.
2. Green, W., and Banks, H.: Osteochondritis dissecans in children. J. Bone Joint Surg., *14*:26, 1953.
3. Helfet, A.: Disorders of the Knee. Philadelphia, J.B. Lippincott, 1974.
4. Campbell, C., and Ranawat, C.: Osteochondritis dissecans: the question of etiology. J. Trauma, *6*:201, 1966.
5. Smillie, I.: Injuries of the Knee Joint. Edinburgh, Churchill Livingstone, 1970.
6. Smillie, I.: Treatment of osteochondritis dissecans. J. Bone Joint Surg. (Br.), *39*:248, 1957.
7. Aichroth, P.: Osteochondritis dissecans of the knee: a clinical study. J. Bone Joint Surg., *53*:440, 1971.
8. Scott, D., and Stevenson, C.: Osteochondritis dissecans of the knee in adults. Clin. Orthop., *76*:82, 1971.
9. Lindholm, S., and Pylkkanen, P.: Internal fixation of the fragments of osteochondritis dissecans of the knee by means of a bone pin. Acta Chir. Scand., *140*:626, 1974.
10. Lipscomb, P.R., Jr., Lipscomb, P.R.S., and Byron, R.: Osteochondritis dissecans of the knee with loose fragments: treatment by replacement and fixation with readily removed pins. J. Bone Joint Surg. (Am), *60*:235, 1978.
11. Tippet, J.W.: Unpublished data.

Chapter 16

MENISCECTOMY AND OTHER SURGICAL TECHNIQUES USING THE OPERATING ARTHROSCOPES

Robert W. Carson

OPERATING ARTHROSCOPES

Operative arthroscopy is a natural outgrowth of diagnostic arthroscopy, and the basic techniques of both originated with the Japanese. In 1918, Dr. Kenji Takagi of Tokyo was the first to examine with a cystoscope the knee joint of a corpse; by 1920, he had developed the first arthroscope.[1] In 1962, his pupil, Dr. Masaki Watanabe, performed the first *partial* meniscectomy under arthroscopic control.[1] Dr. Hiroshi Ikeuchi, Dr. Watanabe's pupil, was the first to perform a total arthroscopic meniscectomy in 1968.[2] These historic cases notwithstanding, from 1962 to 1978 only 48 arthroscopic meniscectomies were performed by the Tokyo group.[2]

It was another disciple of the Japanese, the late Dr. Richard O'Connor of West Covina, California, who finally established and popularized meniscectomy as a routine operation in the late 1970s. This procedure then became the cornerstone for a new surgical discipline, operative arthroscopy. The major hindrance to O'Connor's early meniscectomies was the lack of suitable instruments. His laparoscopic scissors and forceps were long and awkward. They seemed too fragile for meniscal tissue or else too large in diameter for the joint spaces. His frustration with triangulating these long instruments through a second portal and crowding a grasping instrument into the knee through a third portal led O'Connor to develop the first operating arthroscope in 1976.[3]

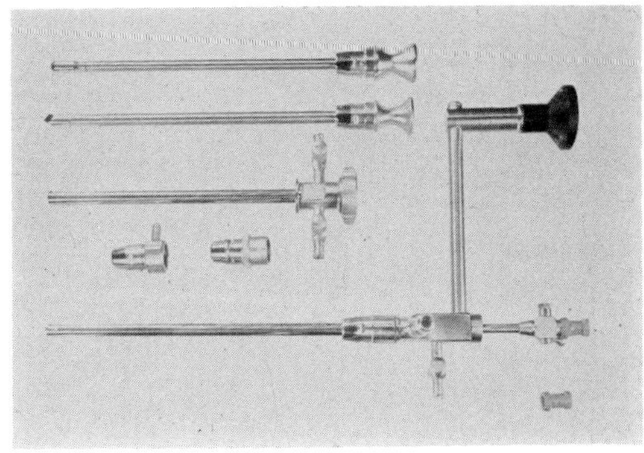

Fig. 16–1. The original Wolf-O'Connor operating arthroscope system with an adaptor for 5-mm diagnostic arthroscopes.

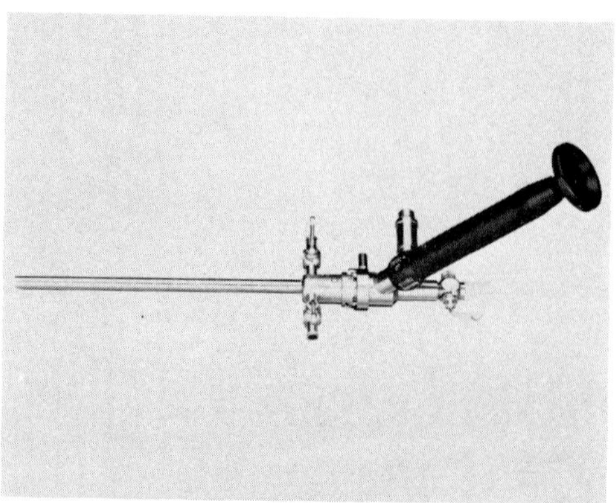

Fig. 16–2. The Storz operating arthroscope with an angled eyepiece. This has a 6.5-mm water sheath that also accepts 4-mm diagnostic arthroscopes.

Wolf-O'Connor Arthroscope

With the Richard Wolf Company of Germany, O'Connor modified a Palmer-Jacobs laparoscope. The size was reduced, and it was optically changed for the knee joint. The instrument has an offset eyepiece with a long barrel and a 7.2-mm (outside diameter) sheath. Because of the small optics in the operating instrument, the sheath has an adaptor that accepts a diagnostic telescope with an outer diameter of 5 mm for better viewing and photography. The instrument was designed for the right eye and the right hand with a 3-mm instrument channel lying directly beneath the lens system. The operating instruments have 12-inch shafts (Fig. 16–1).

Other Round Arthroscopes

Storz, Eder, and Stryker marketed copies of Wolf's original arthroscope with minor modifications. Storz also introduced a model with an angled eyepiece (Fig. 16–2). In 1980, Wolf modified their original instrument to a shorter barrel, a longer eyepiece, and better optics. The new model carries shorter instruments and is less awkward to use than the original. It has a 3.4-mm instrument channel and a correspondingly larger outside diameter (7.5 mm) (Fig. 16–3).

Stryker-Carson Arthroscope

Most endoscopy is performed in soft tissue body cavities that are anatomically appropriate for conventional round endoscopes. Joint spaces, on the other hand, are

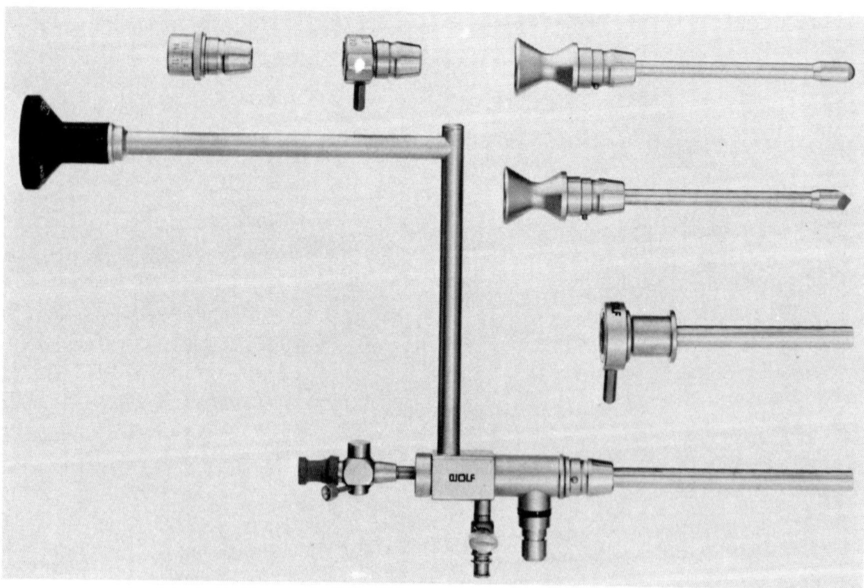

Fig. 16–3. The Wolf-O'Connor operating arthroscope II. This has a 7.5-mm sheath and accepts working instruments of 3.4-mm diameter.

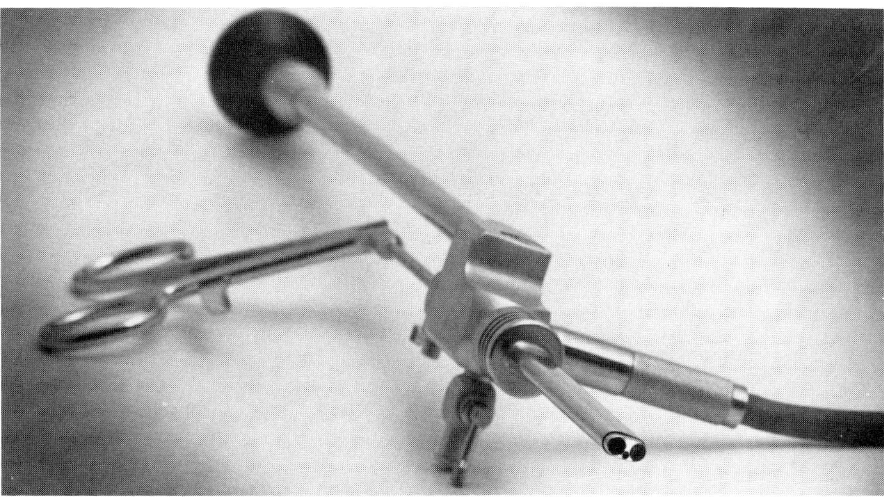

Fig. 16–4. The Stryker-Carson flat, in-line operating arthroscope, showing its thin profile (4.2-mm barrel that fits a 4.5-mm sheath) and the separated and canted lens for enhancing depth perception.

thin and wide and therefore are more suited to thin, wide endoscopes. Having made this simple assumption, I designed a new operating arthroscope in 1977, with a flat barrel to fit the narrow, rigid confines of the knee. This instrument was given an *in-line* configuration, to allow a comfortable, straight-ahead working position for the surgeon (Fig. 16–4).

Flat Design. The distal end of the instrument has the minimum length (80 mm) that accommodates a large knee joint, and its thinness (4.2 mm) is determined by the diameter of its largest element (the 3-mm instrument channel). A round operating arthroscope can be no smaller in diameter than the sum of its two largest elements (the lens system and the instrument channel). This factor sharply constrains the diameters of both elements. No such relationship compromises the flat design, and therefore a full-size lens is installed, identical to that of the largest (5-mm) diagnostic arthroscope.

Depth Perception. A round operating arthroscope, because of the juxtaposition of its lens and instrument channel, has an inherent lack of depth perception. This problem is solved in the flat design by separating these elements and by angling the lens 15° toward the instrument channel. This design gives the arthroscopist a side view of the tip of the working instruments and the monocular clues to depth perception that one observes with the triangulation technique. The 15° lens also enlarges the visual cone (30°) and permits oblique viewing and alternate cutting angles.

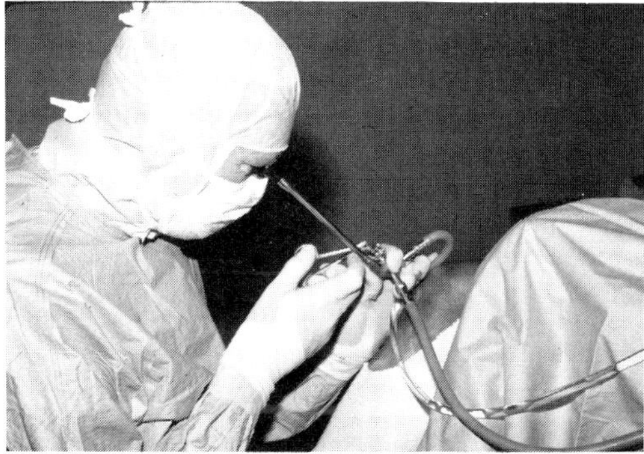

Fig. 16–5. With the Stryker in-line operating arthroscope, the surgeon has a comfortable working position, using either eye or either hand.

In-line Configuration. Offset and angled operating arthroscopes do not conform to human engineering standards for a "normal work area."[4] Working with one's hand beside one's ear is awkward and fatiguing. The most significant experimental work on instrument design was sponsored by the United States Army Air Force in World War II. Its objective was the optimal positioning of cockpit controls and instruments in the first-generation jet fighter planes. This study concluded that the most comfortable, efficient, and accurate working area for blind positioning movements is below shoulder height and in the dead-ahead position.[5] These experimental findings validate my intuitive choice for an in-line configuration (Fig. 16–5).

The in-line arrangement offers one additional advantage. Strongly left-eyed or left-handed surgeons cannot adapt to the offset arthroscope, which was designed for use with the right eye and right hand. By contrast, the in-line configuration is equally convenient for either eye or either hand in any combination.

INSTRUMENTS FOR OPERATING ARTHROSCOPE

More than a dozen different types of instruments are available for operating arthroscopes; however, only scissors, basket forceps, grasping forceps, and front-cutting knives are essential for a versatile system. Beyond this basic set, one should have a specific need before cluttering the instrument cabinet (Fig. 16–6).

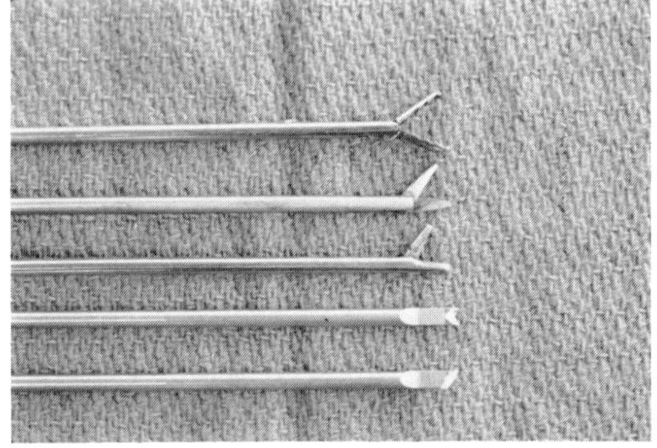

Fig. 16–6. Basic working instruments for an operating arthroscope include grasping forceps, basket forceps, scissors, a Smillie-type knife, and a full front-cutting knife.

ALTERNATIVES TO OPERATING ARTHROSCOPES

Arthroscopic meniscectomies can be performed without an operating arthroscope, as originally demonstrated by Watanabe and Ikeuchi.[1–2] O'Connor, at first, removed menisci piecemeal with basket forceps. He also used a 15-gauge intravenous needle and a Kocher clamp through a third puncture to provide traction as he made his scissor cuts.[3] I made do without an operating arthroscope by passing 4-inch scissors and a small arthroscope through the same puncture.[6] In Sweden, Oretorp and Gillquist developed the transpatellar tendon (triple-puncture) technique.[7] Patel has popularized the midpatellar lateral (triple-puncture) approach to relieve the congestion of instruments along the joint line,[8] and Sprague preserves intact bridges of tissue as he makes his cuts. These bridges provide counter traction without a grasping instrument and prevent the loss of fragments. Eventually, however, the final threads must be either avulsed or cut through.[9] Johnson developed, and others have copied, a powered meniscal cutter that he uses in conjunction with hand instruments for excising the meniscus.[10]

Every arthroscopist should be familiar with all of the foregoing techniques. A difficult meniscectomy or an instrument failure may force one to try different approaches. Routine triple-puncture methods, however, usually require an extra assistant and a television system, and no method has eliminated the need to view, grasp, and cut simultaneously.

GENERAL INDICATIONS FOR OPERATING ARTHROSCOPES

Operating arthroscopes permit the surgeon both to view and to operate through a single puncture. This facility enables one to perform the three functions of viewing, grasping, and cutting through only two anterior punctures—the basis for O'Connor's original two-puncture meniscectomy techniques.

The best use for an operating arthroscope is *viewing* and *cutting* through one puncture while applying traction to a meniscal fragment through another. The best example of this use is the posterior detachment of a displaced bucket-handle tear. Conversely, the operating arthroscope can be used for *viewing* and *applying traction* while cutting through a separate portal. Occasional meniscal flaps and most medial patellar plicae lend themselves to this approach.

Apart from being able to perform two functions through a single portal, the capability to view and to operate straight ahead through a single puncture gives the surgeon advantageous cutting and grasping angles. Some of these angles are difficult or impossible to achieve by triangulation because of crowding and interference with multiple instruments in a single compartment. Cutting entries into the thin rim of a contralateral meniscus and the removal of fragments through the intercondylar notch are examples.

DISADVANTAGES OF OPERATING ARTHROSCOPES

Some surgeons abandoned their original Wolf operating arthroscopes for various reasons and changed to other methods. Undoubtedly, the tiny optics, lack of depth perception, and awkwardness were contributing factors. The second generation of operating arthroscopes have overcome most of these shortcomings. Wolf's second operating arthroscope is less awkward and has better optics, but it also has a 3.5-mm instrument channel, a dubious advantage. The outside diameter of the new instrument is even larger (7.5 mm), and the 3.4-mm instruments, although stronger, must be handled with great care to avoid damaging the articular cartilage, especially in the medial compartment.

The Stryker operating arthroscope has the largest optics, but its photographic advantage is partially offset by its having fewer light fibers. This instrument also has a slower flow rate for saline solution, a deliberate design compromise made with full consideration of the instrument's limited purpose. The only occasion for a continuous flow of saline solution during arthroscopy is to maintain joint distension for powered instruments. For this purpose, any operating arthroscope delivers saline solution much faster than any diagnostic arthroscope by simply transferring inflow to the instrument channel.

Finally, the advantage of using any instrument *through* an arthroscope is coupled with the disadvantage of restricting that instrument to in-and-out and rotary motions in the *alignment* of the arthroscope. This attribute must be taken into account in planning puncture sites, in positioning the patient's knee, and in rotating the arthroscope for better cutting angles.

SURGICAL TECHNIQUES

Arthroscopy attracted widespread interest only when O'Connor had developed and had promoted his techniques for meniscectomy. Many of the maneuvers described here originated with him; they are not published except as syllabus material for his seminars in operative arthroscopy, which began in 1978 at the University of California, Los Angeles.

Meniscectomies

An operating arthroscope, in the course of a particular meniscectomy, may be used for the entire excision, for one or two cuts, or not at all. Meniscal tears are either longitudinal (vertical) to the body of a meniscus, horizontal, radial, or a combination of these. An operating arthroscope is most suited to the management of *longitudinal* tears, but the focus here is on the instrument, and the emphasis is on specific cuts rather than on tear patterns.

Anterior Cuts. The best cutting and viewing angles sometimes coincide, as when entering the thin edge of the medial meniscus to begin a well-blended cut from the opposite portal. An anterior horn can

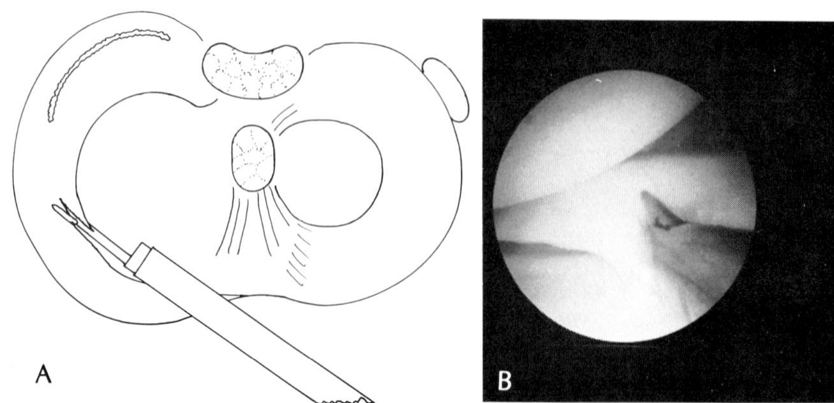

Fig. 16–7. *A* **and** *B,* **The best viewing or cutting approach to the anterior half of a meniscus is from the opposite portal. An operating arthroscope makes the most consistent "blended" rim entries in this area.**

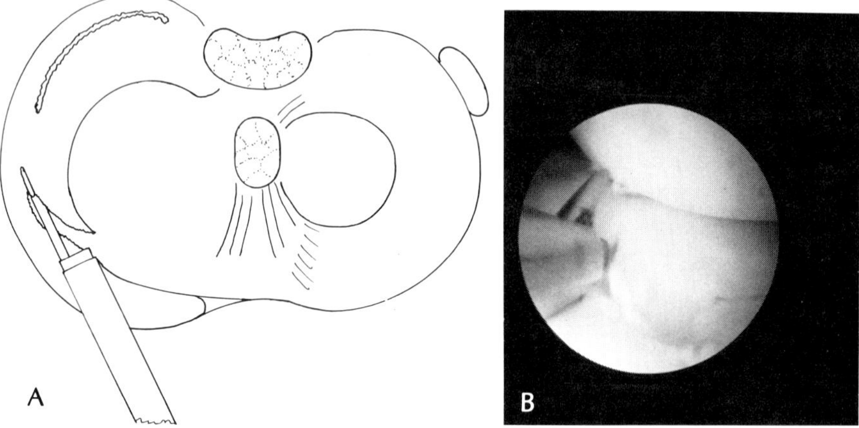

Fig. 16–8. *A* **and** *B,* **Moving a** ***flat*** **operating arthroscope to the medial portal permits continuing the cut straight posteriorly. (Note that straight scissors make curved cuts if side pressure is applied.)**

be seen from the ipsilateral portal, preferably with an angled arthroscope, but the view is always better from the opposite portal, and so is the cutting angle (Fig. 16–7).

With the flat design, the operating arthroscope and scissors can be switched to the ipsilateral portal for cutting straight back through the middle third of the meniscus (Fig. 16–8). One can than enter a short longitudinal tear by retracting it with a probe from the opposite portal (Fig. 16–9).

The anterior attachment of a locked bucket-handle tear of either meniscus can be managed with an operating arthroscope from the opposite portal. Traction or probing from the ipsilateral portal keeps the axilla in view to avoid leaving a stump on the remaining rim (Fig. 16–10).

Posterior Cuts. The operating arthroscope is particularly helpful in the posterior detachment of a locked bucket-handle tear of either meniscus. From an ipsilateral portal, the operating arthroscope is used to cut as closely as possible to the posterior attachment while the fragment is retracted by a clamp from the opposite portal. Rotation of the fragment from time to time, as cutting progresses, defines the remaining fibers. The flat arthroscope can be rotated to great advantage to change the angle of view and the position of the cutting instruments (Fig. 16–11).

Either knives or scissors can be used for

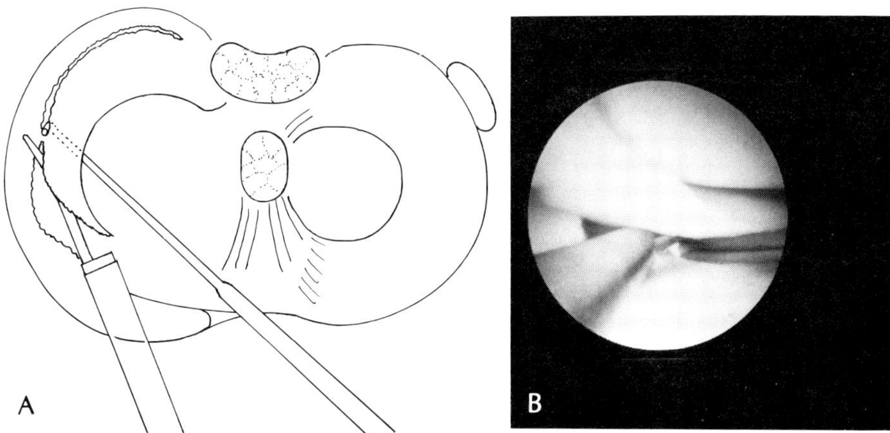

Fig. 16–9. *A* **and** *B,* **By shifting the operating arthroscope to cut along the middle third of the meniscus, it is possible to probe or retract a short hidden tear from the opposite portal. This technique permits an accurate entry into the tear.**

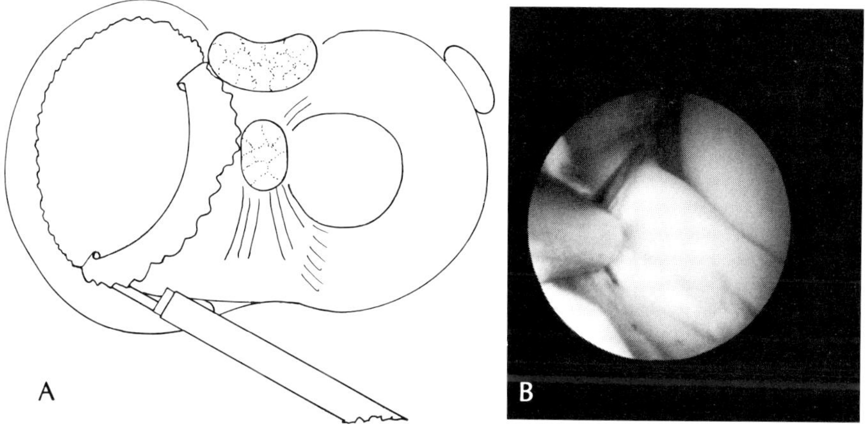

Fig. 16–10. *A* **and** *B,* **Cutting the anterior attachment of a locked bucket-handle tear with the** ***flat*** **operating arthroscope permits one to rotate the angled lens and check the position of the axilla or probe it from the ipsilateral portal.**

this particular cut. Knives have certain advantages over scissors; they are thin, cheap, and easily sharpened. They are also less likely to scuff articular cartilage than scissors (especially hook scissors), which require a space more than twice their diameter for their jaws to open. Scissors are also expensive and fragile, but breakage can be minimized by taking small bites and by avoiding bending forces on their shafts.

Detached longitudinal tears (broken bucket-handle tears) can be managed in the same manner as locked bucket-handle tears, by anterior or posterior stump releases under traction. If a stump is hopelessly trapped in the posteromedial space, the flat operating arthroscope will pass easily through a posteromedial puncture to release this fragment as traction is applied through the notch.

Sprague finds the operating arthroscope helpful for removing oblique (horizontal or radial) flap tears of the posterior horn of the medial meniscus, in which traction helps him to define the anterior attachment[7] (Fig. 16–12).

For any lateral tear, the operating arthroscope can be used to release the entire

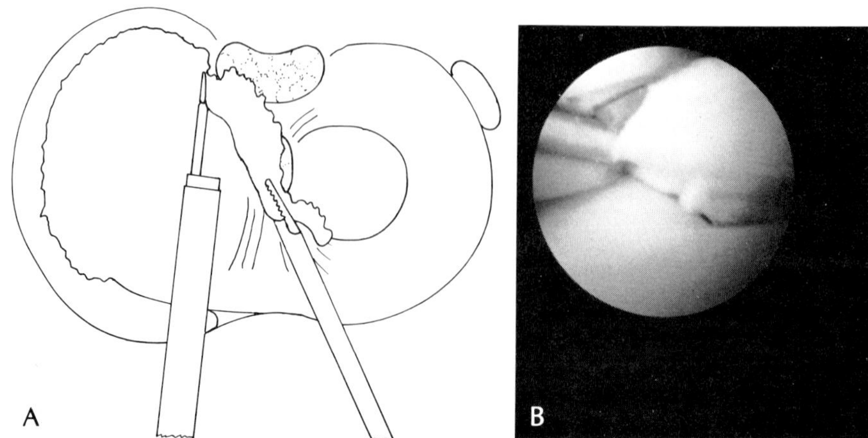

Fig. 16–11. *A* **and** *B,* **Releasing a posterior attachment can be a particularly tight situation in which, again, the ability to switch viewing angles 30° with the flat operating arthroscope is helpful. Strong lateral traction on the tibia with the patient's knee flexed 90° gives the best exposure.**

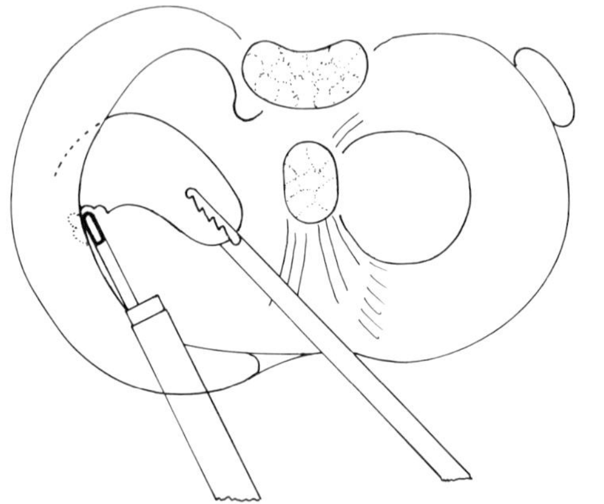

Fig. 16–12. Separating a torn horizontal leaf from an intact rim is easiest when the fragment is under traction.

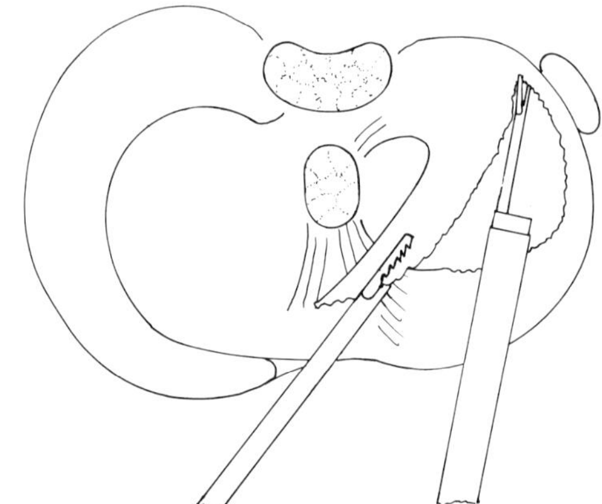

Fig. 16–13. For a torn lateral meniscus with intact fibers in the posterior horn, this technique is a good alternative to piecemeal removal. This procedure requires small nibbles with the scissor tips. One should avoid extending a tear into the popliteus sulcus.

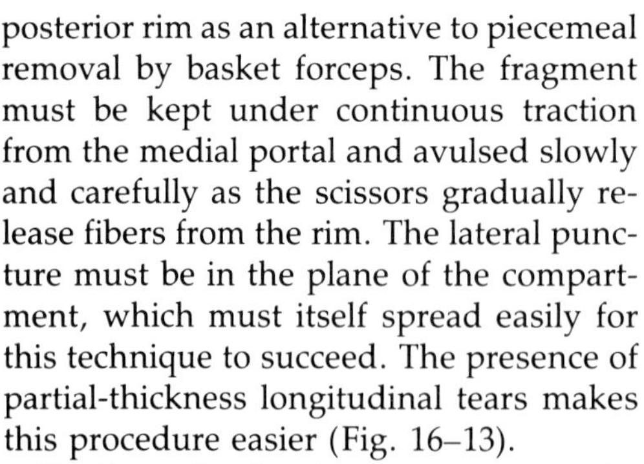

posterior rim as an alternative to piecemeal removal by basket forceps. The fragment must be kept under continuous traction from the medial portal and avulsed slowly and carefully as the scissors gradually release fibers from the rim. The lateral puncture must be in the plane of the compartment, which must itself spread easily for this technique to succeed. The presence of partial-thickness longitudinal tears makes this procedure easier (Fig. 16–13).

Caution. Cutting instruments must be meticulously controlled in the posterolateral compartment. Laceration of the popliteal artery, which lies only 1 cm behind the joint capsule, can lead to amputation of the patient's leg.

Loose Body Removal

Loose bodies are usually easy to retrieve by viewing from one puncture and removing from another. This method is preferable because meniscus clamps, alligator forceps, or Kocher hemostats are stronger than any grasping instrument that can be passed

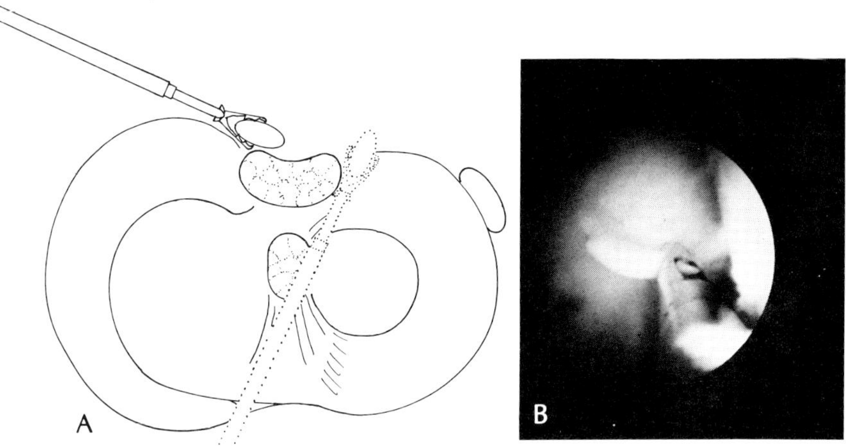

Fig. 16–14. ***A*** **and** ***B,*** **The operating arthroscope can be used for loose bodies if they are not too large. A posteromedial puncture is shown here, but the posterolateral space can be reached easily from an anteromedial puncture (*A*, dotted lines).**

through an operating arthroscope. This technique may fail, however, in two particular areas of the knee to which one has limited access.

Posteromedial Space. Ordinarily, loose bodies in the medial popliteal space can be grasped and removed from a posteromedial puncture while the surgeon views through the intercondylar notch, or vice versa. On occasion, it is best to divide a large loose body before removal and then simply flush the fragments through a large sheath. When a loose body is particularly elusive, prolonged fumbling can be avoided by using the grasping forceps of the operating arthroscope through the posteromedial puncture. With the patient's knee in a figure 4 position, gravity assists one to pin the loose body directly against the posterior cruciate ligament (Fig. 16–14). The grasping instrument is fragile, however, and it cannot be withdrawn through the channel with any object in its mouth. The sheath, arthroscope, instrument, and fragment must all be removed together (Fig. 16–15). An ample puncture tract is essential to avoid leaving the loose body in the subcutaneous tissue.

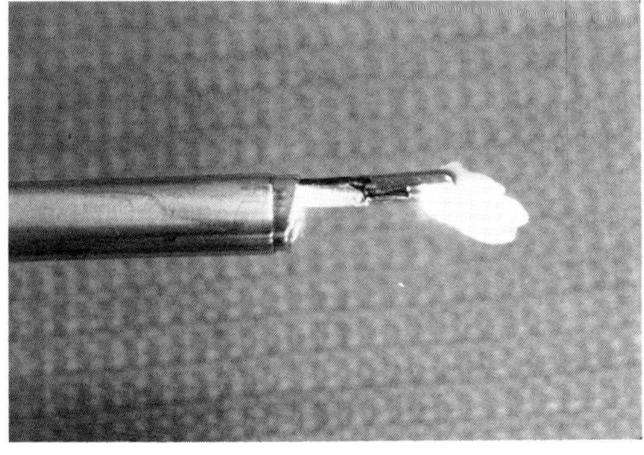

Fig. 16–15. In using grasping forceps, the entire system, including the sheath, must be removed as a unit to avoid losing the object.

Posterolateral Space. The lateral popliteal compartment is approachable posteriorly as is the medial, but repeated instrumentation is unsafe on the lateral side because of the crowded anatomic structures. Furthermore, posterolateral loose bodies can be impossible to retrieve by triangulation from the anterior side because of collision of the arthroscope with the grasping instrument. Grasping forceps through an operating arthroscope in the medial portal remove these loose bodies easily (Fig. 16–14*A*, dotted lines).

Medial Patellar Plica

If a surgical procedure is indicated for a medial patellar plica, excision rather than

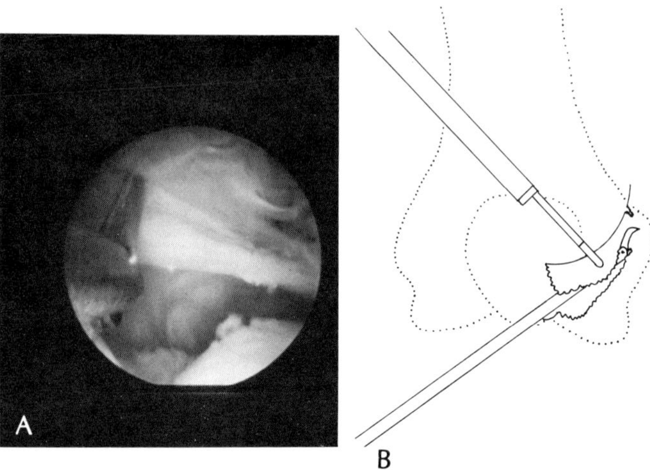

Fig. 16–16. ***A* and *B*, A medial patellar shelf can be approached superiorly or inferiorly with an operating arthroscope. The best view is superiorly. After releasing each end with scissors, the surgeon retracts the fragment with grasping forceps *(A)*, and large hook scissors finish the excision by triangulation from the anterolateral puncture *(B)*.**

incision is preferred to avoid a contracted scar. Viewing from a superolateral portal and cutting with hand and powered instruments from an anterolateral portal, one can quickly excise a plica, including a large area of adjacent synovium. For a *controlled* excision, an operating arthroscope is placed through a superolateral portal and the extremities of the plica are released with scissors. Then, one can remove the plica by triangulation with *large* scissors from an anterolateral portal while it is retracted with grasping forceps through the operating arthroscope (Fig. 16–16).

Miscellaneous Procedures

These uses represent my experience with a new instrument in a new field of surgery; this list is not comprehensive. Additional uses of the operating arthroscope include: lysis of adhesions, biopsies, foreign body removals, bone drilling for osteochondritis dissecans,[11] and lateral retinacular releases.[12] If, in any other situation, the ability to view and to operate straight ahead through a single puncture seems preferable, the operating arthroscope should be kept in mind.

REFERENCES

1. Watanabe, M., Takeda, S., and Ikeuchi, H.: Atlas of Arthroscopy. 2nd Ed. Tokyo, Igaku-Shoin, 1969.
2. Ikeuchi, H.: Meniscus surgery using the Watanabe arthroscope. Orthop. Clin. North Am., *10*:629, 1979.
3. O'Connor, R.: Arthroscopy. Philadelphia, J.B. Lippincott, 1977.
4. McCormick, E.J.: Human Factors Engineering. 3rd Ed. New York, McGraw-Hill, 1970.
5. Fitts, P.M.: A study of location discrimination ability, psychological research on equipment and design. Army Air Force Aviation Psychology Program, Research Report No. 19, 1947.
6. Carson, R.W.: Arthroscopic meniscectomy. Orthop. Clin. North Am., *10*:619, 1979.
7. Oretorp, N., and Gillquist, J.: Transcutaneous meniscectomy under arthroscopic control. Int. Orthop., *3*:19, 1979.
8. Patel, D.: Personal communication, 1980.
9. Sprague, N.: Personal communication, 1981.
10. Johnson, L.L.: Diagnostic and Surgical Arthroscopy. St. Louis, C.V. Mosby, 1981.
11. Guhl, J.: Arthroscopic treatment of osteochondritis dissecans. Orthop. Clin. North Am., *10*:671, 1979.
12. Metcalf, R.: Personal communication, 1977.

Chapter 17

MENISCECTOMY BY TRIANGULATION THROUGH MEDIAL AND LATERAL PORTALS

Robert W. Metcalf

The purpose of this chapter is to describe a two-portal "triangulation" technique for arthroscopic meniscectomy that uses mainly anteromedial and anterolateral incisions for the viewing arthroscope and resecting instrument. A skilled arthroscopic surgeon should be familiar with all the other techniques described in this book, however.

Sometimes, changing from one approach to another enables one to finish a meniscal resection. For example, a mediolateral two-portal approach may not allow proper progress and may be abandoned in favor of the use of an operating arthroscope, or a superior approach may be used to see the anterior meniscal horn better. I find that no single method of endoscopic meniscal surgery works best in every case. On the other hand, surgeons who are just beginning to learn arthroscopic surgical techniques should start with one basic approach or another and become proficient with it. Then, other approaches can be added until one is familiar with all the available techniques. The goals of arthroscopic partial meniscectomy should be the same, no matter which approach is used. These goals are:

1. Resection of the torn portion of the meniscus that is catching or sliding into the central tibial femoral interface with weight bearing.
2. Trimming of the remaining meniscal rim to prevent further tearing.
3. Preservation, if at all possible, of the capsular rim of the meniscus, to help retain knee-joint stability.

Sometimes, the meniscal tear is so extensive and fragmented that a partial meniscectomy cannot be performed. In such a case, total meniscectomy may be needed; this procedure can also be performed with arthroscopic techniques. The objective of this new technique, however, is to perform a partial meniscectomy whenever possible.

Long-term studies[1–5] of open total meniscectomy show a significant percentage of knees with progressive degenerative changes and recurring knee symptoms. Properly performed, arthroscopic partial meniscectomy can reduce these known problems.

My results at a 5-year minimum follow-up show that 86% of knees following arthroscopic partial meniscectomy have a good or excellent objective result, with minimal Fairbank's changes noted on weight-bearing roentgenograms.[6] Although this follow-up time is not yet long enough to state categorically that partial meniscectomy is better than total meniscectomy, the results are encouraging with regard to the goals that have been mentioned.

The main advantage to endoscopic technique[7,8] is the ability to approach the meniscus from inside the joint, at the inner margin, where most tears begin. The magnification afforded by modern fiberoptic and lens technology enables the surgeon accurately to visualize even minute tears in the meniscus.[9] A probe can be inserted to palpate tears and to determine their exact extent and location. Most often, the tear does not extend out into the capsular rim, and this stabilizing structure can be preserved. An arthrotomy, which comes from outside the joint, cuts through this capsular ring, and the meniscal resection is usually total because of the larger instruments and less-refined technique.

PORTALS

The first incision (portal) made for arthroscopic examination of the knee is anterolateral,[10] just adjacent to the lateral border of the patellar tendon and superior to the edge of the tibia (Fig. 17–1). It is important to make this incision at least 1.5 cm superior to the palpable tibia so as to avoid injury to the anterior horn of the meniscus. If the portal hugs the tibia too closely, it will be difficult to move an arthroscope or an instrument freely over the tibial and meniscal edge, and meniscal resection will be thereby rendered difficult. Moreover, the slightly more superior incision, almost to the inferior border of the patella, allows the viewing arthroscope to enter the joint *over* the fat pad, rather than through it, thus avoiding the entanglement of hypertrophied strands of synovium that can so easily block the surgeon's view.

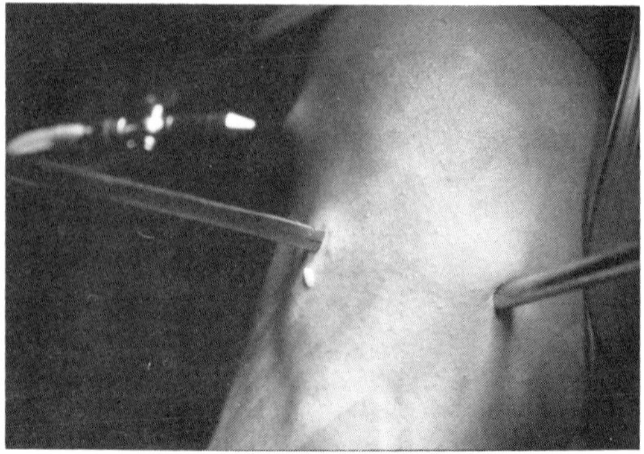

Fig. 17–1. Viewing arthroscope is anteromedial and grasping clamp is anterolateral.

The anteromedial portal, used initially for insertion of the probe in diagnostic arthroscopy, is in a location that mirrors the lateral portal, that is, superior to the joint line and adjacent to the patellar tendon. When the surgeon makes these two anterior portals through which the majority of meniscal surgical procedures are performed, the patient's knee should be at about 30° of flexion. The skin is cut either transversely or longitudinally with a scalpel. The joint capsule is then pierced with a sharp trocar; then this trocar is replaced in the sleeve of the arthroscope with a blunt obturator. The final entry into the joint is *always* made with a blunt obturator to avoid scratching the joint surfaces.

Once the joint is entered, the blunt obturator is used to "stretch" the incision by moving the obturator 360° a few times. This action loosens the portal and makes it much easier to maneuver instruments later because the fascial layers are less resistant to fine movements. One other point about these incisions is that one can always return the patient's knee to its original position of flexion, such as 30°, to line up the tracts through the skin, capsule, and synovium if re-entry through a portal becomes difficult. Other portals that I use are, in order of frequency, posteromedial, superolateral, accessory joint line, superomedial, posterolateral, and rarely, patellar ligament or central.

Posteromedial Portal

The posteromedial puncture allows direct viewing of the posteromedial compartment and shows meniscal capsular tears better than any other approach. This portal is used routinely in all meniscal cases with tears of the posterior horn or any question of loose bodies. The range of lesions visible from this posteromedial corner is often surprising and includes tears of the posterior cruciate ligament, tags and flaps of meniscus folded back and hidden from anterior view, loose bodies, especially those imbedded near the posterior cruciate ligament, and capsular tears. It is also possible to see the remaining rim after meniscal resection, if the knee is flexed to 90° and the tibia is internally rotated. One should not hesitate to make the posteromedial puncture; and even using it routinely during diagnostic arthroscopy helps the surgeon to become familiar with the normal posterior compartment's anatomic features.

To make this posteromedial puncture, one should flex the patient's knee to 90° and palpate the posteromedial edge of the femur and tibia (Fig. 17–2). A small triangular soft spot lies just posterior to this corner. An incision is made over this space through the skin only. A smooth cannula, such as that used for outflow, is then inserted through one of the anterior joint line portals and is passed through the intercondylar notch to the posterior compartment. Then, 30 to 60 ml saline solution is injected to distend the posterior compartment, thus making entry easier. The sleeve of the arthroscope (I use a 5-mm scope for this) is then inserted, using a sharp trocar. One directs the trocar and sleeve slightly anteriorly, aiming toward the intercondylar notch. This puncture is made right at the moment of maximum distension of the knee joint with saline solution. One should not direct the trocar posteriorly because of the danger of piercing the popliteal artery or vein.

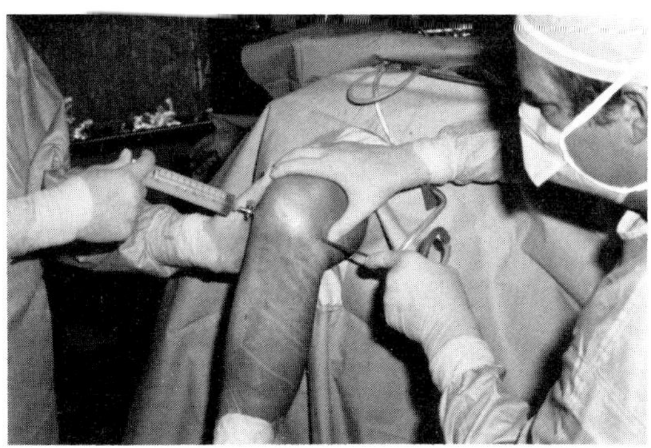

Fig. 17–2. With the knee flexed at 90°, a posteromedial puncture is made after first injecting saline solution to distend the posteromedial capsule.

Posterolateral punctures are not used as often as posteromedial, because the posterolateral compartment can be seen so well from an anterolateral approach. The landmarks and technique are identical to that just described, only they are lateral instead of medial.

Superior portals are used as necessary to view the patellofemoral joint, the medial or lateral synovial walls, or to look inferiorly onto the anterior horns of the menisci.

It is important to shift the viewing arthroscope from one portal to another as indicated by the need of the particular case; this concept helps one to become skillful at triangulation technique. Often, it is tempting to persist for a long time with an approach that does not allow the best view of the meniscus. Changing the arthroscope to another portal,[11] to give a different angle of view and perspective, usually solves the problem, and valuable time is thereby saved.

TRIANGULATION

Angles of Triangulation

The further apart the entry portals are for insertion of instrument and arthroscope, the easier it is to bring the instruments' tips together to a desired placement inside the joint. Incisions that closely parallel each other are more difficult to manage with triangulation technique. For this reason, I prefer the mediolateral two-puncture method most of the time. When additional portals are added around the joint line, it is best to keep them as far apart as possible. A needle can be inserted percutaneously to test the desired angle and location of a new portal.[12]

Once the surgeon is satisfied that the needle shows the proper angle, it is removed and an incision is made at that site. I usually insert a knife, scissors, or basket forceps directly into the joint, without using a cannula, once I have established the entry tract with a blunt obturator. A cannula system can be used, but I find that it often is in the way, slides into the joint, and has to be pulled back or adjusted. One exception, however, is a posteromedial portal, in which I always use a cannula to keep the entry tract established; it can be most difficult to find these posterior tracts for repeated insertion of an instrument. For anterior punctures, however, no cannula (sleeve) is usually used for inserting resecting instruments.

Developing Triangulation Skills

The word "triangulation" as used in arthroscopic surgery describes the positioning of an instrument inside of the knee joint from one angle while the surgeon looks through an arthroscope from another angle. Triangulation implies an exact science, much as a mathematician talks about geometry. In actual practice, the ability to position instruments to a desired location within the knee joint is an inexact skill at first. It takes time to develop this skill, and it is a matter of trial and practice as it is learned. Eventually, this skill becomes almost automatic, and when an instrument, such as a probe or scissors, is placed into the knee from one angle, the surgeon knows that this angle is proper and that the tip of the scissors is guided to the exact location desired on the meniscal rim.

Using a blunt probe in all diagnostic arthroscopic examinations is a good way to develop this skill. By looking from one side of the knee and probing from the other, the surgeon soon learns the "feel" of triangulation. The blunt probe does not damage the knee joint surfaces and increases diagnostic accuracy. Probing is the first step in endoscopic surgical techniques and should be performed routinely in all diagnostic examinations (Fig. 17–3).

I highly recommend knee models that accurately simulate conditions of arthro-

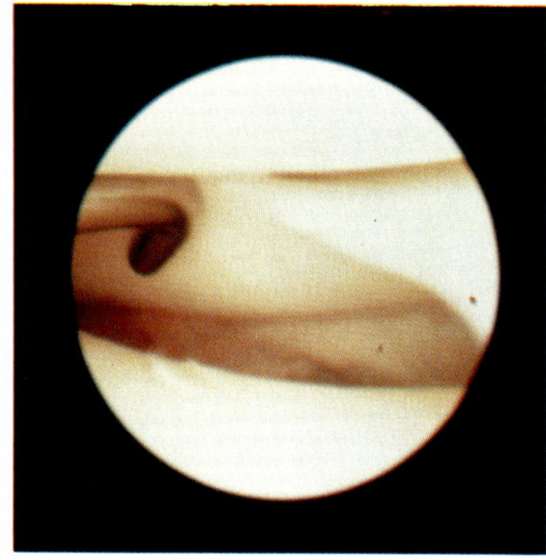

Fig. 17–3. Arthroscopic view showing the posterior horn of the lateral meniscus being lifted with a probe.

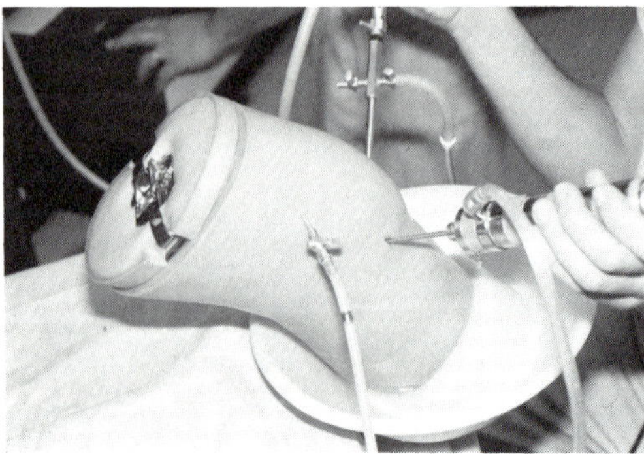

Fig. 17–4. Surgery Simulator designed by H. Sweeney, M.D. The continuous irrigation system allows practice of the triangulation technique, here using a motorized cutting device.

scopic meniscectomy and allow an "in vitro" practice of triangulation. Such practice speeds up the learning process and also avoids the risk of scratching normal articular surfaces during an actual surgical procedure. Knives, scissors, cutting forceps, grasping instruments, and motorized devices can all be used in these models. The model developed by Dr. H. Sweeney adds the important dimension of having a fluid medium, so one learns to operate with an irrigation system flowing (Fig. 17–4).

Depth perception in arthroscopy must be learned by experience and observation. Because a monocular lens system is used, everything is seen in two dimensions, and no real depth perception exists. This factor alone accounts for much of the problem in learning to "triangulate." As orthopedic surgeons, we are used to bringing two instruments together in front of us in an open operation, relying on our stereoscopic vision, which gives true depth perception. To change to endoscopic methods, in which this depth perception is lost, takes time and is the cause of some frustration. With practice, however, this disadvantage is soon overcome.

Triangulation and the Use of Television

Having a television camera attached to the viewing arthroscope enables the surgeon to view the interior of the knee from a monitor, enhancing the ability to teach others and to involve the operating room personnel in the procedure. The question arises, however, about whether television enhances or detracts from the skill of triangulation.

The use of television is definitely an additional skill that must be learned. The beginning arthroscopist finds that it is generally easier to learn triangulation techniques without television. By looking directly through the arthroscope, the surgeon can see the interior of the patient's knee joint in crystal clear detail and natural color. Everything looks much as it does during an arthrotomy, and therefore it is easier to make a correlation with the arthroscopic view.

Television cameras, even at their best, give a picture that is not nearly as detailed or clear as the direct view. For this reason, depth perception is harder to master. I recommend that a surgeon first become proficient with triangulation and probing while looking directly through the arthroscope before a television camera is introduced. Hand-eye coordination is thus easier, and one learns to appreciate the minute details of meniscal tears that might be missed on a television monitor. When using television, it is true that the surgeon can assume a more comfortable body position, but his hands are moving in one area while he is looking in another—almost a "remote control" operation.

When the surgeon views directly through the arthroscope, his head position and vision are all directed right to the spatial location to which an instrument is passed with triangulation. Once the skill of triangulation is mastered by this direct-viewing technique, then the transition to television is much easier.

INSTRUMENTS

Single-Jaw Forceps

I use this instrument most often in resecting torn meniscal fragments. We often call this instrument "basket forceps" because of the small bar that used to be placed across the lower jaw to catch each small fragment of meniscus as it was cut. This bar has been removed on most current cutting forceps, however, because it was time consuming to remove each meniscal fragment as it was cut, and the instrument also frequently became jammed, causing breakage of the upper jaw. The term "basket forceps" is still used commonly.

This instrument has several advantages. First, it cuts right at the end of the tip (Fig. 17–5). This feature makes it possible to advance the instrument inferior to the fem-

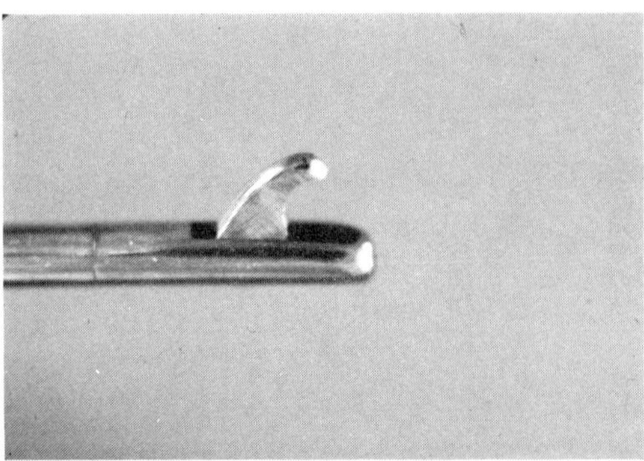

Fig. 17–5. Tip of a single-jaw cutting forceps. The upper jaw has a curved, "hook" design that has a crisp, accurate cutting action. This instrument is used extensively in meniscal trimming.

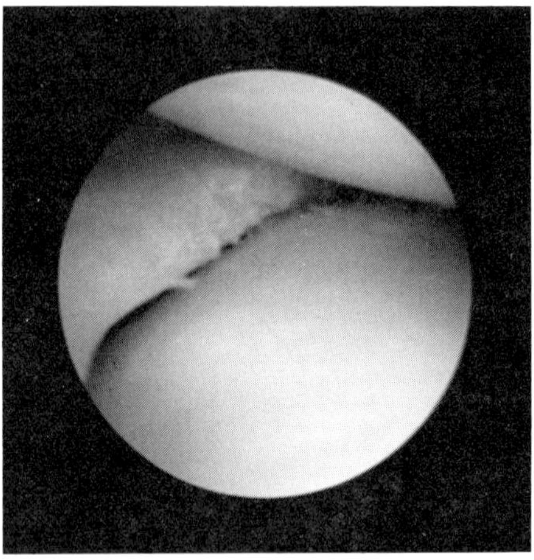

Fig. 17–6. Remaining rim after resection of a medial meniscal tear. Single-jaw forceps are used to trim away only the damaged portion.

oral condyle and accurately trim away, bit by bit, torn fragments from the posterior horn of the meniscus. No other instrument does this. Knives are difficult to position posteriorly at the proper cutting angle. Scissors cut at their tips, but the angle of approach when passed from anterior to posterior favors cutting transversely across the body of the meniscus, rather than cutting longitudinally or paralleling the normal meniscal curve.

Another advantage to basket forceps is their ability to control the depth of cut. When trimming the meniscal rim, one can remove an even amount of meniscus with multiple bites of the forceps. A proper contour can thus be developed in the remaining rim (Fig. 17–6). Much as in sculpturing, the meniscal rim is shaped little by little, to protect the capsule that rings the joint.

This type of cutting forceps gives tactile feedback that is transmitted through the instrument to the surgeon's hand as meniscal tissue is cut. Often, degenerative meniscus cartilage has a characteristic texture, as opposed to normal, firm, more fibrous meniscal cartilage. The surgeon soon learns to differentiate the normal from the abnormal as the meniscus is trimmed away, to avoid excising normal meniscus. Arthroscopic meniscal resection is not performed blindly. The tips of the cutting instrument are *always* kept in view, but this differentiation of cartilage texture is helpful as the trimming process continues.

Cutting forceps must be sharp; otherwise, they have a chewing action on meniscal cartilage. The instrument should be returned to the manufacturer for sharpening. The microscopic sharpening process that is required must be done in a laboratory by properly trained technicians.

Numerous shapes and sizes of single-jaw cutting forceps are now available. Curved shafts and angled tips can facilitate reaching various areas of the meniscal rim from a particular portal. These curved and angled forceps are making the 2-portal triangulation technique much easier. A basic set of instruments should include basket forceps 3 to 3.5 mm in diameter with a straight, right-, and left-curved set of shafts. A 90° tip-angle basket forceps is also helpful for resecting anterior meniscal horn tears.

Knives

Although a knife can make a clean incision around the rim of the meniscus in its medial and anterior portions, such a cut is much more difficult in the posteromedial meniscal horn because the femoral condyle obstructs the proper angle of approach.

Therefore, knives are most often used in resecting a portion of the anterior rim or cutting across the base of a meniscal tag. Occasionally, the anterior attachment of a bucket-handle fragment can be more readily cut with a retrograde knife.

I use three basic configurations of knife tips. The first has a curve at the tip with cutting action on both sides of the blade. The second type is shaped like a Smillie meniscotome, and the third is a retrograde knife.

Knives can easily scratch the articular surfaces of the femur or tibia and should always be kept in view when using within the knee joint. Knives are not introduced through an incision unless the surgeon positions the viewing arthroscope to see the entry of the knife into the joint. Disposable knife blades are the sharpest but they also break more readily, sometimes within the knee joint. The nondisposable knife blades have more resiliency to breakage, but dull with use and must be resharpened. A dull knife blade is dangerous because more force has to be used in cutting, and an inadvertent slip of the knife can cause a cut across the meniscal capsule or into articular cartilage.

Scissors

Arthroscopic scissors can be helpful to cut across the base of a meniscal tag or flap or to resect anterior and posterior ends of a bucket-handle fragment. Scissors have the advantage of being smooth when introduced into the joint and therefore the chance of damage to the articular cartilage is less. Care should still be taken, however, to keep the tip of the scissors in direct view at all times within the knee joint.

Scissors come in a variety of shapes and shaft configurations. Right- and left-curved shafts are helpful in addition to straight scissors. Angled tips can also facilitate resection in the posterior meniscal horn area. Scissors do not dull as readily as knives and basket forceps. The "hook" design at the scissor tip grasps the meniscal fragment and keeps it from being pushed way from the scissors during cutting (Fig. 17–7).

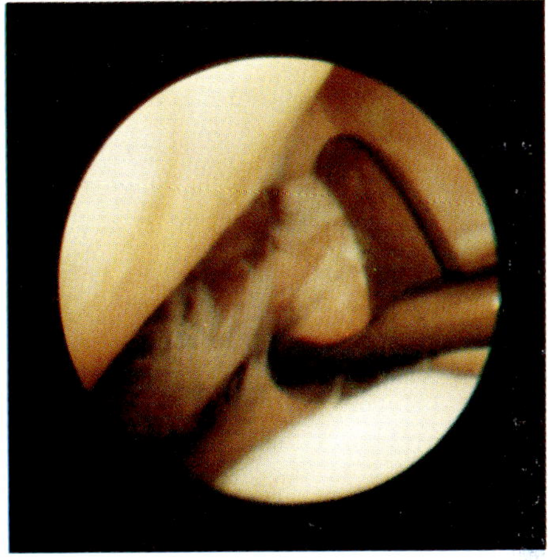

Fig. 17–7. Tip of a 3-mm "hook" designed scissor positioned in the posterior knee compartment. This type of scissor grasps tissue as it cuts.

Motorized Meniscal Cutters

Motorized instruments are most often used with a 2-portal triangulation technique. The viewing arthroscope may be contralateral, with the motorized cutting tip introduced on the ipsilateral side of the meniscal tear, or vice versa, depending on the particular situation. An adequate flow of saline solution into the joint must be present to operate these cutters properly. If a 5-mm arthroscope is used, the sleeve is of a diameter sufficiently large to admit an adequate flow. With a 4-mm-diameter arthroscope, which has a smaller sleeve diameter and reduced flow rates, an accessory inflow cannula should be inserted into the suprapatellar pouch. None of the currently available motorized meniscal cutters (Dyonics, Storz, Stryker, Wolf) aggressively cut into normal meniscal tissue. This safety feature is inherent in the design of an inner blade rotating against the outer blade, but it means that motorized cutters are limited when trimming torn meniscal fragments. The fragments have to be small enough to fit into the window opening of the device and also soft enough to be readily cut. Therefore, these motorized instruments are used mainly for trimming, alternating with either a knife or basket forceps to accomplish the final desired contour of the meniscal rim.

The motorized cutter is also useful for suctioning away small pieces of meniscus that might be floating free in the joint. Motorized devices can damage normal articular cartilage, and the cutting edge of the tip must always be kept in view or positioned so that the surgeon knows the window is facing away from normal articular cartilage. The advantage to suction down the center of these instruments is that meniscal tissue to be cut is drawn into the window rather than being pushed away, as often occurs with a hand-operated instrument. This feature can be a great help when one trims difficult-to-reach areas of the posterior meniscus. Motorized cutters are often used to trim away synovium in the anterior part of the knee joint that may be blocking the view of the entire meniscal rim. This excision of hypertrophied synovium allows better visualization.

REMAINING MENISCAL RIM

It is difficult to give strict criteria for how much meniscus to leave after partial meniscectomy. It is a matter of judgment in each particular case, Experience has taught, however, that some general guidelines are helpful to those just learning to perform this type of surgical procedure.

The underlying principle in all meniscal operations now is to "save the meniscus" as much as possible. We have come to realize that the meniscus has many important functions for the knee joint, including load transmission, space-filling capacity to add to joint congruence, lubrication, prevention of synovial intrusion into the joint, shock absorption, and most important, knee stabilization.[13,14]

Resection

Removal of the Mobile Fragment. One must resect any torn part of the meniscus that could protrude beyond what would be the inner margin of the normal meniscus (Fig. 17–8). If an imaginary line were drawn to show the normal inner margin of the meniscus, that line would represent a boundary beyond which a meniscal fragment must not go without becoming caught between the interface of the femur and the tibia during weight bearing. If a tag of meniscus can be pulled in beyond this imaginary line with a blunt probe, then that tag will likely become caught during knee flexion and weight bearing, and either a further tearing of the meniscal rim or a pull on the joint capsule and adjacent synovium will result, causing localized symptoms of pain and catching (Fig. 17–9). Therefore, the surgeon knows that this fragment should be resected.

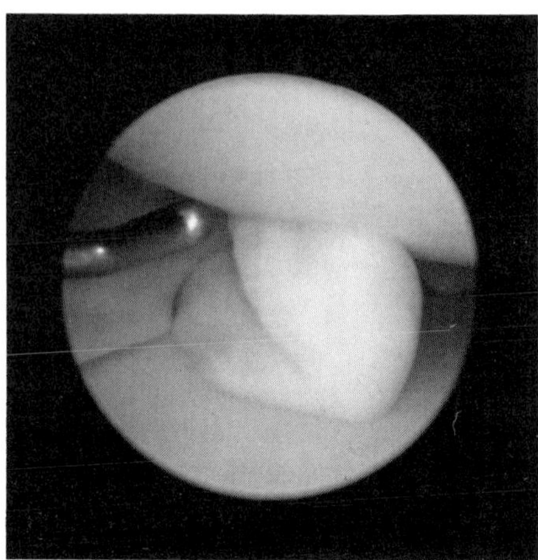

Fig. 17–8. Arthroscopic view of a torn mobile "flap" of the medial meniscus. Probe is at the junction of the middle and posterior thirds of the meniscus.

Importance of Not Leaving Sudden Changes in the Contour of the Remaining Rim. If a segmental resection is performed, such as in resecting a transverse type of meniscal tear, the remaining corners should be tapered (Fig. 17–10). It is not necessary to leave a rim that is exactly even in width from anterior to posterior, however. More of the anterior rim can be left because this area of the meniscus does not come under the same shearing stresses as the posterior

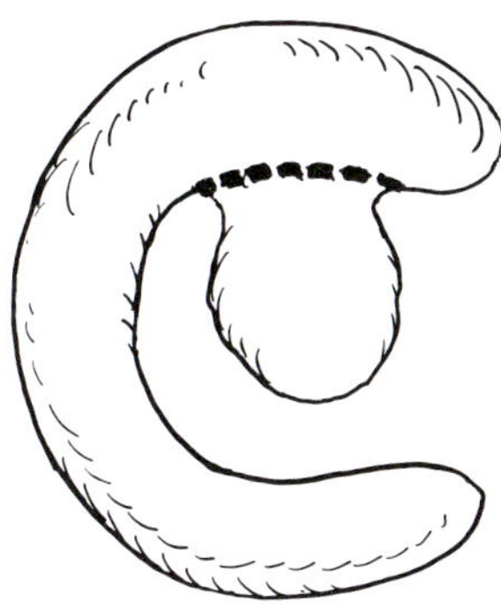

Fig. 17–9. Flap tear of a posterior meniscus that extends into the center of the joint beyond what would normally be the inner margin of the meniscus (dotted line). Any fragment that can be pulled beyond this imaginary line with a probe should be resected.

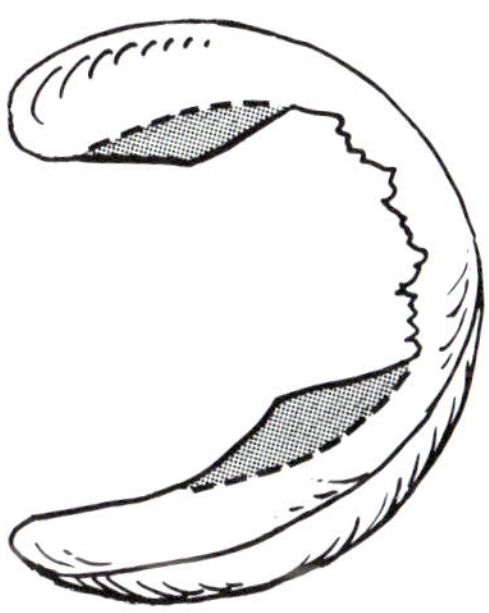

Fig. 17–10. If a segmental resection of a torn meniscal fragment is performed, the triangular corners that are left should be trimmed to give a more even contour to the remaining rim.

horn. I routinely leave the anterior meniscal horn completely intact, even when most of the posterior horn has been removed, and I taper the resection gradually from anterior to posterior. To date, none of my patients have had a further tear or other problem from such a remaining anterior rim. The reverse is not true, however. If a tear exists in the anterior horn alone (rare), then the line of resection must include an equal amount of posterior horn to leave an even contour to the remaining meniscal rim. If this procedure is not done, the remaining posterior horn will likely tear further because it has been rendered less stable by the removal of its anterior attachments.

Contraindications to Obtaining a Perfectly Smooth Meniscal Rim. It is impossible to obtain such a meniscal rim anyway, and much time is wasted trying to trim every last little irregularity (Fig. 17–11). The remaining meniscus rim heals with time. I have seen this healing whenever a second arthroscopic look is possible (Fig. 17–12). Of course, the meniscal rim should

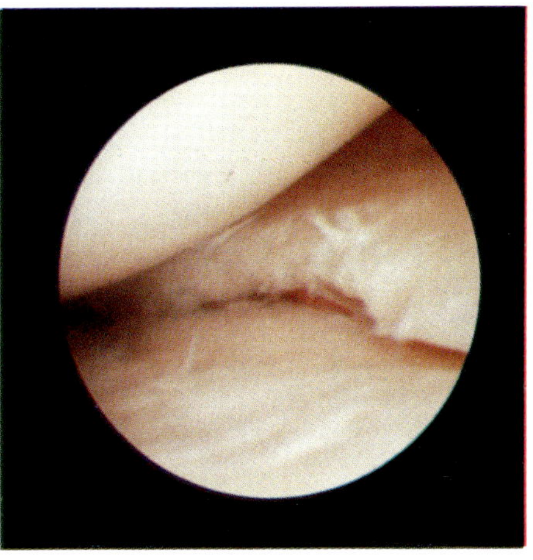

Fig. 17–11. Meniscal rim remaining after arthroscopic resection. Note that some roughening of both the meniscus and the tibia are still present from the resection.

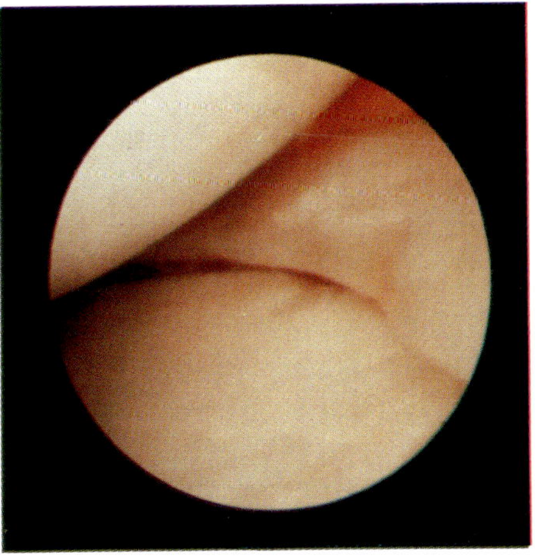

Fig. 17–12. Meniscal rim viewed 9 months after arthroscopic resection. This meniscus has an almost normal appearance, and the articular surfaces also look healthy.

not be left in a haphazardly trimmed or extremely ragged state—the surgeon's judgment must prevail—but the trimming process should be reasonable, and excessive time should not be spent in trying to excise every last cutting mark from the rim. The remaining meniscal rim will be smooth and will retriangulate with the normal walking action of the patient.

Probing of the Meniscal Rim. Resect, then probe; resect some more, then probe again. It is similar to sculpturing in that one must back away frequently to obtain a perspective. The probe allows evaluation of texture, stability, and mobility.

Protection of the Meniscocapsular Junction. Once this junction is divided, the meniscus is rendered unstable. One must avoid cutting too deeply into the meniscus in any one area. It is better to trim an even amount from the entire posterior horn, for example, then to advance the resection a little deeper toward the capsular border, taking an equal amount off the entire area. By advancing little by little in this manner, an error can be avoided. If the first cut with a knife or basket forceps is made too deeply toward the capsule, placement of the next cut is then much more difficult to judge. If the capsular junction is transected, then the meniscus on either side will be unstable, and a "total" arthroscopic meniscectomy must be performed.

Leaving More Rim Rather Than Less. It is much better to leave the meniscal rim intact, with its capsular attachment, rather than to risk cutting through it and ending up with a total meniscectomy. This advice is especially applicable to the lateral meniscus in which a small rim left anterior to the popliteal tendon heals and provides better stability. It is always possible to repeat an arthroscopic procedure at a later date and to resect more meniscus. In actual practice, this repetition is rarely necessary, but if doubt exists about the first resection, it should be explained carefully to the patient, and the surgeon should state that it is better to leave the meniscal rim for stability of the joint. If "catching" continues, then a second operation can easily be performed to resect more (or all) of the meniscal rim. Such a secondary tear in the remaining meniscal rim is rare—the incidence is under 1% in my experience over the past 6 years.

Visualization of the Posterior Horn

During arthroscopic partial meniscectomy, the lateral joint usually opens up 4 to 5 mm when a varus internal rotational stress is applied to allow satisfactory access to the posterior horn of the lateral meniscus. The medial joint is not so easily opened. Many knees are so "tight" that no more space than 3 or 4 mm can be gained, even with maximal stress. This problem affects both visualization and the passage of instruments to the posterior meniscal horn.

General anesthesia gives the best muscle relaxation, which is important for proper manipulation of the joint. With a local anesthetic, the thigh muscles involuntarily tighten, especially if a tourniquet is used, and this tightening seriously restricts the surgeon's ability to stress open the joint. Spinal anesthesia provides adequate muscle relaxation, but the patient cannot start active quadriceps muscle exercises for several hours, and this is a major disadvantage. Spinal anesthetics also have some increased risk. We routinely use general anesthesia for all meniscal surgical procedures at the Salt Lake Surgical Center. A

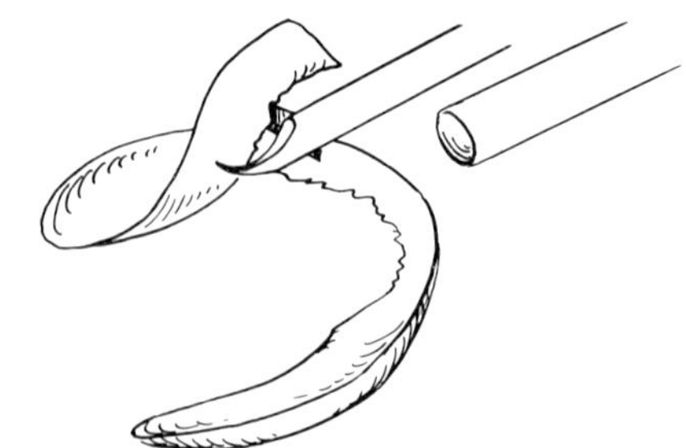

Fig. 17–13. Drawing shows how two instruments can be inserted posteromedially for a triangulation technique to resect a piece of meniscus that is folded into the posterior compartment.

thigh-holding device is a great help in applying the proper stress to the joint. I prefer a holder that encircles the thigh and controls rotation as well as providing a fulcrum for varus and valgus stress.

To best see the medial meniscus, one should flex the patient's knee 20 to 30° and apply a valgus external rotational stress. For the lateral meniscus, the knee is again moderately flexed and a varus internal rotational stress opens the joint. Often, a slight change in position and stress makes the difference in proper joint exposure.

Changing from a 5-mm to a 2.7-mm-diameter arthroscope sometimes allows a better view of the posterior meniscus because the smaller scope can slide under the condyle for a direct look. Then, 3-mm basket forceps can triangulate from an accessory portal just anterior to the collateral ligament and may be used to trim away what is needed to obtain a satisfactory contour of the remaining rim. This triangulation technique can be varied by interchanging the arthroscope and basket forceps as needed to obtain the right angle of approach. Curved instruments can also be helpful.

Sometimes, the patient's knee joint is just so tight that, in spite of all the preceding measures, it is still not possible to resect a posterior meniscal horn tear. In this situation, a posterior puncture should be done (Fig. 17–13). The arthroscope is inserted either directly posteromedially or through the intercondylar notch, and then a resecting instrument is brought in from another direction. An operating arthroscope can also be inserted directly from a posteromedial approach.

Indications for Arthrotomy

In some situations, visualization is so limited and the meniscus is so fragmented that it is better to abandon the arthroscopic procedure and proceed with an arthrotomy. It is much preferable to perform an arthrotomy, especially if the surgeon is not experienced in arthroscopic technique, than to spend an excessive amount of time (over 90 minutes) trying to accomplish the procedure with the arthroscope. The patient's limb should always be reprepared and redraped if an arthrotomy is performed. As the surgeon becomes more experienced with arthroscopic meniscectomy, the need for arthrotomy diminishes proportionately, but arthrotomy should always be an available option.

TRIANGULATION TECHNIQUES FOR SPECIFIC MENISCAL TEARS

Bucket-Handle Tear

The anterior attachment of the bucket-handle fragment is usually divided first, then it is grasped and pulled into the intercondylar notch, and the posterior attachment is divided. This sequence is easier than any other technique because the posterior attachment can be placed under tension before it is cut, thus reducing the chance of leaving a posterior horn tag (Fig. 17–14). The anterior attachment is divided with scissors or a retrograde knife. The viewing arthroscope is usually on the con-

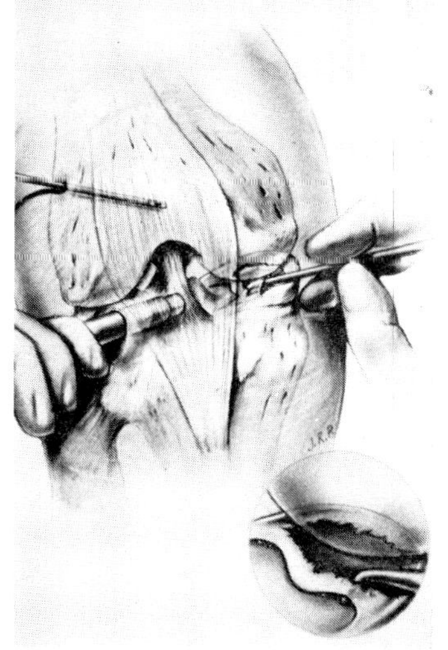

Fig. 17–14. Two-portal technique with a viewing arthroscope anterolateral and a probe anteromedial. The probe is used to palpate the anterior attachment of a bucket-handle tear prior to arthroscopic resection.

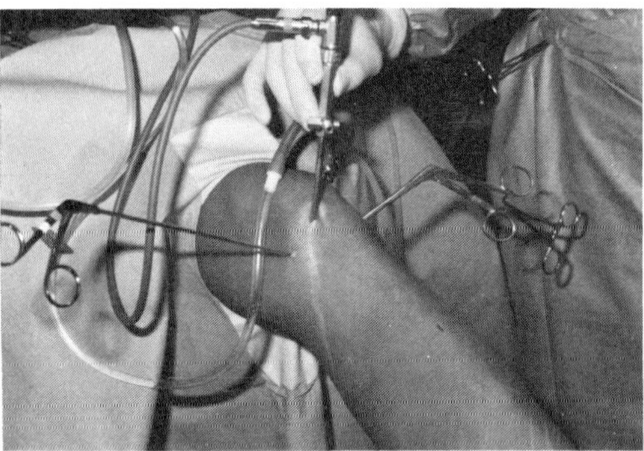

Fig. 17–15. Three-portal triangulation technique. The viewing arthroscope is in the standard anteromedial portal, and a grasping forceps is anterolateral. A third portal has been made just anterior to the medial collateral ligament for insertion of a resecting instrument.

tralateral side and the cutting instrument on the ipsilateral side of the meniscal tear.

Although I usually prefer to make the posterior cut of the bucket-handle fragment using an operating arthroscope, a triangulation technique can be also used by making a third portal anteriorly on the ipsilateral side of the meniscal tear, just anterior to the collateral ligament (Fig. 17–15). The viewing arthroscope is then inserted into the ipsilateral portal, just adjacent to the patellar tendon, and a grasping clamp is brought across the intercondylar notch from the contralateral portal to place the bucket-handle fragment under tension. One may insert scissors or a small meniscotome through the accessory portal, inferior to and beneath the femoral condyle, and one may thereby transect the posterior attachment under direct vision.

The two-portal technique is used for the most important step in resecting a bucket-handle tear—trimming of the remaining meniscal rim. For this step, the basket forceps, either curved or straight, are used to nibble away at the meniscus while the surgeon views with the arthroscope inserted from an opposite portal. A motorized cutter is used alternately. On finishing these steps and feeling satisfied that the remaining meniscal rim is stable, I still routinely perform a posteromedial puncture as a double check of the posterior horn. Sometimes, one finds additional tear that was neither seen nor probed from the anterior portals. Occasionally, one discovers and removes a loose body that might otherwise have been left. A posteromedial puncture should be part of the surgeon's routine.

Oblique ("Flap") Tears

Oblique tears are the most common and account for at least 50% of all meniscal tears. The oblique tear occurs at the junction of the middle and posterior third of the meniscus and produces a mobile segment that can become caught in the joint interface. This "flap" or tag can become larger as the tear extends and may eventually become rounded and firm, producing symptoms of localized joint-line pain and catching.

It is sometimes possible to perform the entire resection by means of a motorized meniscal cutter, without any need for hand instruments. Such is the case if the meniscal tag is small or fragmented and if the tear is degenerative. The two-portal triangulation technique allows the window of the meniscal cutter to be positioned against the flap; the cutting action then proceeds as the surgeon frequently reverses the direction of rotation of the inner cutting blade with a hand or foot switch, depending on the type of cutter. Chondromalacia of the adjacent femoral condyle and tibia may be

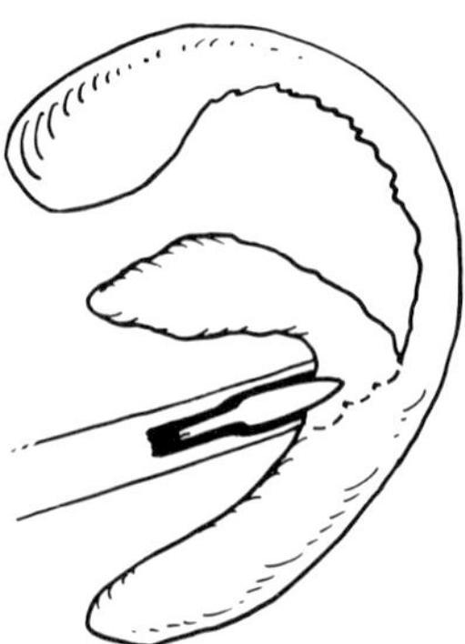

Fig. 17–16. Drawing shows how the base of a flap tear is cut using single-jaw cutting forceps.

present and may exactly match the area of excursion of the torn flap.

If the flap of torn meniscus is too large to be resected with a motorized cutter, it can be cut into several sections using scissors or basket forceps. The pieces of the flap can then be fed into the meniscal cutter. Another triangulation method is to cut across the base of the flap with basket forceps, scissors or a knife (Fig. 17–16). A small attachment can be left at the base of the flap; then, a cutting instrument may be replaced by grasping forceps, and the flap of meniscus may be avulsed from its base.

If the flap is completely transected by the two-portal technique, it becomes a loose body that can be elusive in the joint. If this situation occurs, the irrigation flow should be stopped immediately to prevent washing of the free fragment into some other part of the joint. The fragment is kept carefully under view, grasping forceps are inserted into the joints and the fragment is removed.

As with the bucket-handle tear, the most important part of this arthroscopic resection is the inspection and trimming of the remaining meniscal rim. Fragmentation is usually seen in the posterior horn where the piece of meniscus was torn away. In the knees of patients over age 40, this remaining rim is often especially fibrillated and fragmented. The motorized meniscal cutter is used alternately with the basket forceps to smooth and trim away all fragments that might catch in the joint. A posteromedial puncture may be needed to finish the resection.

Transverse Tears

The transverse or so-called "radial" tear is easily resected by the two-portal technique. This tear usually occurs in the lateral meniscus at the junction of the middle and posterior thirds, but it also may occur medially or laterally at the posterior base of the meniscus as it attaches to the tibia (Fig. 17–17). The viewing arthroscope is placed on the ipsilateral side of the tear, curved or straight basket forceps are passed from the contralateral portal, and the two sides of the tear are trimmed until an even contour is obtained in the remaining rim.

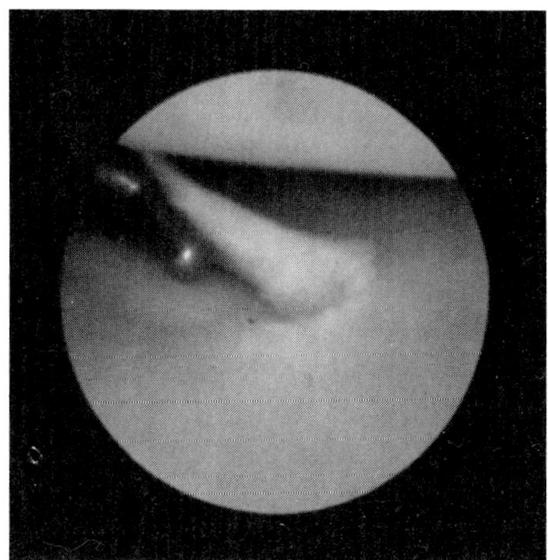

Fig. 17–17. Arthroscopic view of a vertical transverse (radial) tear of the lateral meniscus. The probe lifts up one corner of this tear, which becomes caught in the joint during weight bearing much like a flap tear.

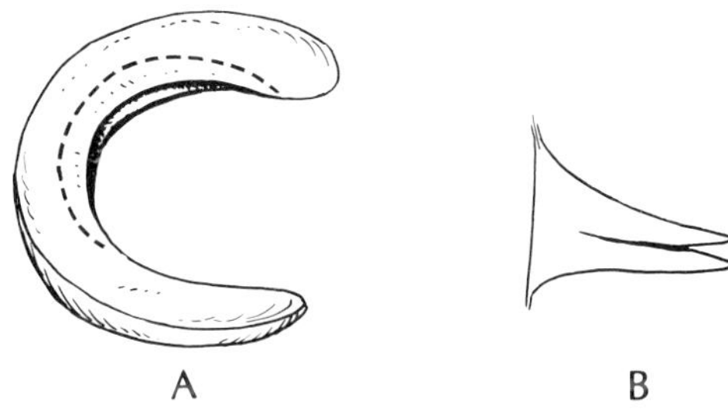

Fig. 17–18. *A,* Horizontal tear of the meniscus can extend deep toward the capsular edge of the meniscus. Dotted line indicates how the tear extends further than its "fishmouth" opening. *B,* Lateral view.

This type of tear is especially difficult to resect with a knife because the two triangular sides of the tear are floppy and the knife may stray across the capsular border.

Horizontal Longitudinal Tears

This "fishmouth" type of tear can present a difficult situation for arthroscopic resection because the tear extends posteriorly into the joint capsule and creates a superior and an inferior leaf. Fortunately, this tear pattern is not common.

The triangulation technique involves a piecemeal resection with basket forceps, cutting progressively deeper toward the depth of the tear (Fig. 17–18). The probe is used frequently to test stability, and once most of the cleft left in the meniscus has been resected and the remaining rim feels stable, then the procedure is ended, even if a small horizontal cleft still remains in the meniscal rim.

This type of tear is often seen in the remaining rim of an old bucket-handle tear and, as such, is usually stable and needs no further resection. Occasionally, only one of the "leaves" of the tear is resected. The remaining leaf, either superior or inferior, can function as a normal meniscus. Thorough probing is the key to determining what must be resected, as judged by the mobility of the portion of the meniscus probed.

Discoid Meniscus

The central part of a discoid meniscus can be excised using an arthroscopic knife or basket forceps (Fig. 17–19). The remaining rim has a thick inner margin that eventually becomes triangular in shape. The width of rim left depends on the type of tear, but usually what remains is about the width of a normal meniscus.

Only those discoid menisci that cause symptoms are excised. The incidental finding of a discoid meniscus at arthroscopy is not an indication for resection. Tears do occur, however, especially transverse (radial) tears and even bucket-handle tears.

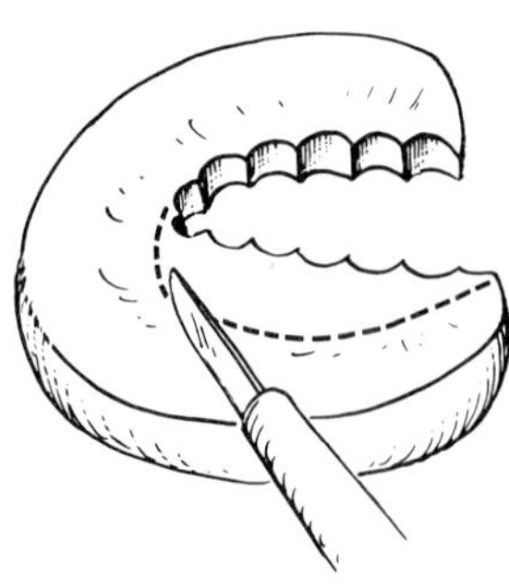

Fig. 17–19. The center portion of a discoid meniscus is resected, leaving a rim about the width of a normal meniscus.

Young children can develop a limp and flexed knee because of the block of terminal extension from a discoid meniscus. Central resection from the thick discoid meniscus is uniformly successful in these children. The youngest patient I have seen was 7 years old. The arthroscopic resection is not difficult because a child's knee is supple and excellent joint exposure can be obtained. By leaving a rim of meniscus of normal width, albeit thicker, the knee has a much better prognosis. Within 3 to 6 months, the child's knee has normal range of motion and normal gait returns, indicating that it takes time for the remaining thick rim to retriangulate.

POSTOPERATIVE MANAGEMENT

All arthroscopic meniscal surgical procedures can be performed in an outpatient surgical facility, either hospital-based or independent. If an arthrotomy should become necessary to repair a capsular tear or to complete a meniscectomy, the patient can be admitted to a hospital for postoperative care. Most patients do not have an arthrotomy, however, and their postoperative care is simple.

At the completion of the operation, the joint is thoroughly irrigated with a bulb syringe, to remove any loose pieces of meniscus that may not have been removed with the motorized meniscal cutter. These pieces can be flushed out of the joint through the arthroscope sleeve inserted into the suprapatellar pouch. Adhesive tapes rather than stitches are used to close incisions.

A few sterile gauze pads are placed over each puncture site, and an elastic bandage is used for mild compression. If the meniscal resection has been extensive or if a total meniscectomy has been necessary, a padded cotton dressing is applied from midthigh to ankle to give more compression and hemostasis for 24 to 48 hours. This dressing is then replaced with an elastic bandage until swelling subsides. The elastic bandage is rewrapped by the patient as needed, with a caution to loosen it if ankle swelling occurs. The patient is permitted to shower the next day but should not soak in a tub until the wounds are sealed. Antibiotics are not used before, during, or after the operation.

Isometric quadriceps muscle exercises are started as soon as the patient is awake. Full weight bearing is allowed the day of the procedure and, in fact, is encouraged as soon as possible. Crutches are seldom used, unless an area of chondral fracture has been found or an abrasion chondroplasty has been performed in a weight-bearing area. An early active range of motion is encouraged in all patients. At least 90° of knee flexion should be present at the first postoperative examination a week later. Arthroscopic meniscectomy patients often have full knee motion at that time.

Moderate swelling is normal following this procedure. Rarely, an aspiration is performed 48 to 72 hours postoperatively for excessive bleeding. Swelling usually subsides in proportion to return of quadriceps muscle strength.

At one week, muscle rehabilitation is further encouraged with the help of a physical therapist if necessary, using isometric and isotonic exercises. If chondromalacia of the patella or femoral condyles is significant, only isometric exercises are allowed. Chronic meniscal tears usually produce gradual and significant quadriceps muscle atrophy, often unrecognized by the patient, and a return to full activities following arthroscopic meniscectomy should not be allowed until the knee muscles are strong again. The postoperative criteria for arthrotomy also apply following arthroscopic surgical procedures; namely, adequate quadriceps muscle strength, full range of motion, and absence of swelling and pain.

Most patients are able to return to an office or other sedentary type of work within 2 or 3 days. Athletes in training who had minimal muscle weakness initially can usually return to competitive sports within 2 or 3 weeks, although this return to actvity is not encouraged until the foregoing criteria have been achieved.

If the remaining meniscal rim is thin and if some question exists about its integrity, then the knee is protected from running and jumping stress for a mandatory 6 to 8 weeks. Patients with significant tibial or femoral chondromalacia are discouraged from any running for 6 months or even permanently. Swimming or the use of a bicycle is substituted for running in these patients for a general exercise program.

Persistent swelling following arthroscopic meniscectomy is usually due to overactivity coupled with weak thigh muscles. Both must be corrected. Anti-inflammatory medications may be prescribed for a short time to reduce synovitis.

Patients are routinely seen postoperatively at 1 week, 6 weeks, 3 months, and if possible, at 1 year. Weight-bearing anteroposterior roentgenograms are obtained preoperatively and again at 1 year for comparison.

REFERENCES

1. Appel, H.: Late results after meniscectomy in the knee joint: a clinical and roentgenologic followup investigation. Acta Orthop. Scand., *133 (Suppl.),* 1, 1970.
2. Johnson, R.J., et al.: Factors affecting late results after meniscectomy. J. Bone Joint Surg. (Am.), *56*:719, 1974.
3. Jones, R.E., Smith, E.C., and Reisch, J.S.: Effects of medial meniscectomy in patients older than forty years. J. Bone Joint Surg. (Am.), *60*:783, 1978.
4. Tapper, E.M., and Hoover, N.W.: Late results after meniscectomy. J. Bone Joint Surg. (Am.), *51*:517, 1969.
5. Vahvanen, V., and Aalto, K.: Meniscectomy in children. Acta Orthop. Scand., *50*:791, 1979.
6. Fairbank, T.J.: Knee joint changes after meniscectomy. J. Bone Joint Surg. (Br.), *30*:664, 1948.
7. Dandy, D.J., and Jackson, R.W.: The impact of arthroscopy on the management of disorders of the knee. J. Bone Joint Surg. (Br.), *57*:346, 1975.
8. Jackson, R.W., and Abe, I.: The role of arthroscopy in the management of disorders of the knee: an analysis of 200 consecutive cases. J. Bone Joint Surg. (Br.), *54*:310, 1972.
9. Casscells, S.W.: Arthroscopy of the knee joint. J. Bone Joint Surg. (Am.), *53*:287, 1971.

10. Metcalf, R.W.: Operative arthroscopy of the knee. Instruct. Course Lect., *30*:357, 1981.
11. Whipple, T.L., and Bassett, F.H.: Arthroscopic examination of the knee: polypuncture technique with percutaneous intra-articular manipulation. J. Bone Joint Surg. (Am.), *60*:444, 1978.
12. Johnson, L.L.: Arthroscopic Surgery of the Knee and Other Joints. St. Louis, C.V. Mosby, 1981.
13. Krause, W.R., et al.: Mechanical changes in the knee after meniscectomy. J. Bone Joint Surg. (Am.), *58*:599, 1976.
14. Walker, P.S., and Erkman, M.J.: The role of the menisci in force transmission across the knee. Clin. Orthop., *109*:184, 1975.

Chapter 18

ANTERIOR MIDLINE OR CENTRAL APPROACH FOR ARTHROSCOPIC MENISCECTOMY

Nils Oretorp

In diagnostic and surgical arthrosopy, the process of selecting portals for arthroscopic and operating instruments is of utmost importance for best results. Unfortunately, portals selected for viewing through the telescope are not necessarily the best for operating instruments, whether straight, angled, or curved. The reverse also applies. After learning diagnostic arthroscopy through anteromedial and anterolateral portals, many surgeons begin an operation by inserting instruments through the portal not occupied at the time by the telescope. When difficulties are met, the portals for viewing and operating are switched, sometimes repeatedly. Not infrequently, the surgical procedure is facilitated once a new entry point is selected only for the operating instrument. The advantage of using a midline point of entry for viewing is that access to all areas of the knee, both anterior and posterior, is possible from this single portal.[1] The surgeon can carefully select any other site for the insertion of operating instruments with no need to compromise. This choice leaves him a wide opportunity to triangulate with either the right or left hand, or with both for bimanual operations either medially or laterally.

TREATMENT PLANNING

Although the two semilunar cartilages are not identical, their form and fibrous structure are much the same. Most often, therefore, the same principles for surgical treatment can be applied medially, and laterally for identical tears. When planning the resection, the surgeon should keep in mind the fine fiber structure of the two menisci.[2,3] Not only should torn or degenerated tissue be removed, but also parts that, because another segment was cut, have been deprived of their functional role. After operation, the remaining parts of the meniscus are not stronger than the weakest part anywhere along its course. Consequently, resections should be tangential to the direction of the meniscal fiber to attain a well-controlled meniscal rim instead of a functionless remnant, which risks residual or recurrent symptoms.

TELESCOPE PORTAL

The two cruciate ligaments and the tibial spine constitute roughly a symmetrical center in the knee, with the femoral walls nearly parallel in the intercondylar fossa. A telescope entering this space in the midline anteriorly can be advanced along both medial and lateral walls of the femur and can be passed lateral and inferior to the posterior and anterior cruciate ligaments, respectively. From positions close to the popliteal capsule, a 30 or 70° telescope can be rotated to view the condyle medially or laterally. When the telescope is inserted obliquely, only the opposite posterior compartment can be seen, because the nearest femoral condyle blocks the route to the posterior aspect of the same side. Consequently, for full visual control over both anterior and posterior operations, the entry point for the telescope must be located in the midline anteriorly ±0.5 cm and about 1 cm proximal to the palpated tibial condylar plane.

In practice, one therefore enters either through the patellar tendon[4] or close medially or laterally to it. It is important to avoid damage to tendon fibers when incising the skin. The sharp obturator should be inserted when the patient's knee is flexed to a right angle separating the fibers longitudinally. The blunt trocar is then directed proximally inferior to the patella while the patient's knee is laid flat on the table. When properly placed, the arthroscope enters the joint superior to instead of through the fat pad.

OPERATING PORTALS

A less well trained surgeon may need 4 to 5 portals to cut accurately along the meniscus in all directions. Correctly placed, only 2 portals are needed. They should be located 2 to 3 cm on either side of the telescope and, most importantly, at different levels. The portal ipsilateral to the tear should be just proximal to the tibial plateau and the anterior segment of the meniscus. This portal is needed for the dissection of the medial and posterior segments. Through the second portal, located on the contralateral side of the tear, the operating instruments should reach both the anterior segment and, across the intercondylar notch, the central posterior attachment. Therefore, this portal must be placed higher than the ipsilateral portal, with the correct site 2 to 3 cm superior to the palpated tibial plateau (Fig. 18–1).

Bimanual Surgical Technique

A midline approach for the telescope affords the possibility for the surgeon to work bimanually and to view through the optics between his two hands. An assistant keeps the telescope in position with his lower arm comfortably resting on the patient's thigh and out of the surgeon's way. As in an open surgical procedure cutting by hand is more precise when the other hand stabilizes the structure (Fig. 18–2).

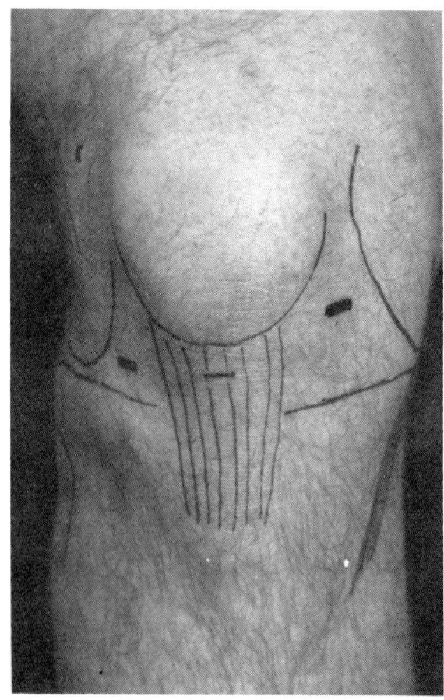

Fig. 18–1. Location of portals for radical excision of a torn lateral meniscus. Lateral to the patella, the site for an outflow cannula is indicated.

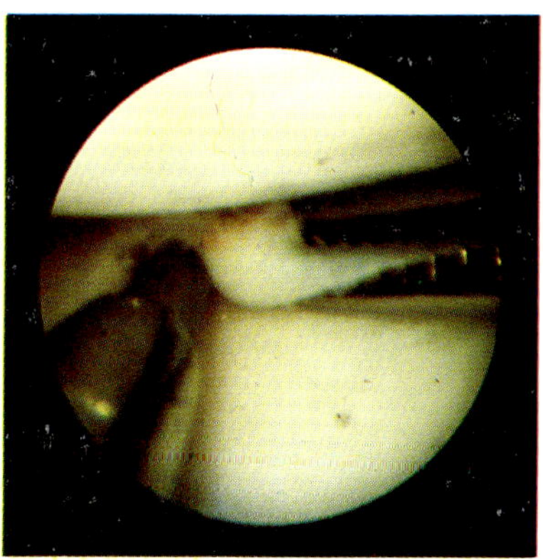

Fig. 18–2. A torn meniscus remnant is excised bimanually using a knife with a retractable protective sheath and grasping forceps.

FLUID FLOW AND PRESSURE CONTROL

The importance of joint distension during arthroscopy is often emphasized.[5,6] The telescope can be retracted more, thus increasing the field of vision. Moreover, the risk of condylar scuffing with the tip is much less. Furthermore, distension stretches the joint capsule and folds back the synovium anteriorly over the menisci. Visual control over anterior segment operations is therefore easily achieved using a midline foreoblique telescope only if the knee is distended enough.

When the volume of fluid is increased, the joint capsule stretches and intra-articular pressure gradually builds. The raised pressure is effective in reducing bleeding into the joint cavity. Because of their muscular walls, small arterioles collapse at an intra-articular pressure 20 to 30 mm Hg less than blood pressure inside the vessel. Little fluid is needed to maintain clear vision when this effect of raised pressure is combined with the use of a thigh tourniquet. For a 45-minute meniscectomy with incisions along the cartilage peripherally in the vascular area, one needs an average flow of under 3 L. To benefit fully from pressure and flow variation, however, an arthroscopy pump (such as Gambro-Crafon AB, Sweden) with a speed-regulating footpedal for direct control by the surgeon himself is needed.

HANDLING OF PATIENTS

Almost all patients under 50 years of age are treated as ambulatory cases. General anesthesia is strongly preferred. Local anesthesia can be also used for total meniscectomies, but is practical only for resection of flaps or other minor repairs. Ambulatory patients are given simple instructions to follow postoperatively. When fully awake, they are instructed to stand and actively hyperextend their knees by quadriceps muscle contraction. Second, they should practice standing on each leg separately with the other knee flexed to a right angle, then actively hyperextending again, and finally trying to walk as normally as possible. Few ask for crutches. Patients are checked in 6 days and instructions added or changed.

SURGICAL TECHNIQUES

Partial Meniscectomy

The surgical technique for partial meniscectomies using a midline telescope differs little from techniques already described by others. Basket forceps are preferred only for the inner half of the cartilage, whereas the combined use of a protected arthroscopy knife (such as that manufactured by Stille-Werner AB, Sweden) and lockable grasping forceps is appropriate for the tough, outer half.[7] Motorized tools are not used initially. but are better for trimming than basket forceps. Trimming is seldom needed after clean knife cuts.

Long flaps are treated by resection of the flap only. Short flaps posteriorly in the medial meniscus usually follow the radial collagen fibers out to the periphery and necessitate more radical treatment.

Repair of Bucket-Handle Tears

The principles for treatment are simple. The protected knife with a horizontal, round-cutting blade on the carrier handle cuts from the high contralateral portal tangentially and divides the anterior segment leaving no tags behind. The mobile end of the meniscus is caught from the ipsilateral portal, is lifted high, and is stretched around the femoral condyle by the grasping forceps so that the surgeon can excise the posterior end of the lifted meniscus with the knife just superior to the tibial spine. These cuts are made with a vertical blade. For this operation, the instruments are inserted only once.

Total-Subtotal Meniscectomy

Radical removal of the meniscus still remains the treatment of choice for patients with multiple ruptures, meniscal tears secondary to previous injury, and radial and flap tears extending to the meniscal periphery. The principle is to cut tangentially around the tear leaving, when possible, a 2- to 3-mm tissue rim peripherally. The excision is routinely performed through the 2 anterior portals described; an accessory posterior portal is seldom needed. Even in many tight joints, the posterior dissection can accurately be performed anteriorly with a vertical, preferably curved blade. If, however, sharp knives are used between the condyles without a protective sheath, extensive articular damage may follow. Such injury may be too high a price to pay for the removal of a torn meniscus. On the other hand, if the instrument is equipped with an atraumatic protective sheath, it can be squeezed between the condyles without any damage to the articular cartilage or the instrument itself.

The anterior segmental surgical procedure is performed with the surgeon directing the knife from the contralateral, superior portal as is the final division posteriorly. In cases of a lateral, almost circular meniscus, a cut is also needed through the ipsilateral portal for the division close to the anterior cruciate ligament.

The patient's lower leg is hanging. The surgeon sits at the end of the operating table while he excises the anterior half of the meniscus. The joint capsule should be adequately distended at 100 to 120 mm Hg until the anterior segment has been fully mobilized; otherwise, a remnant without function may be left.

Medial segmental excision and posterior dissection can only be performed from the ipsilateral, inferior portal. The instrument must work almost parallel to the tibial condylar plane and thus must enter close to the superoanterior meniscal segment. For this stage of the operation, a straight-end cutting blade is preferred. To facilitate excision of this segment, the intra-articular pressure should be lowered to 60 to 80 mm Hg to relax the joint capsule. This maneuver allows the meniscus again to glide in over the tibia for support from inferiorly while being cut. The position of the meniscus is further stabilized by the grasping forceps through the contralateral portal for greater precision when sequential incisions are made along the attachment. When the surgeon reaches the midpoint of the meniscal periphery, the patient's leg position has to be 20° of flexion and valgus. One of the surgeon's hands opens the axilla of the incision by pulling the grasping forceps while the other cuts; the arthroscope is kept in position by the assistant or nurse. For dissection from the posteromedial or posterolateral corner toward the midline, a curved, vertical blade is used with a pro-

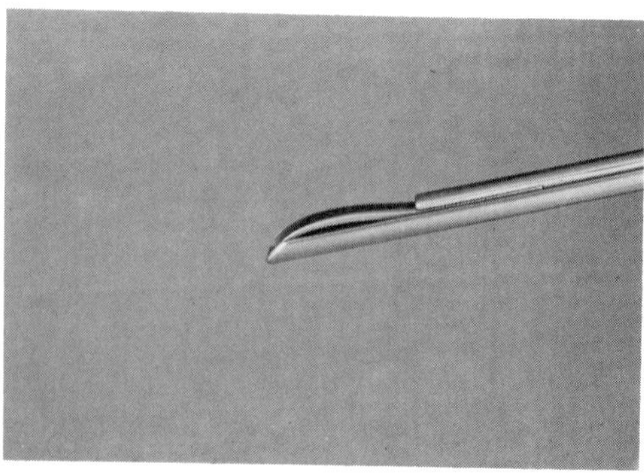

Fig. 18–3. A curved-end cutting blade with its protective sheath covering the knife edge in the noncutting position. The instrument is used for posterior dissections from an anterior entry point.

tective, retractable carrier (Fig. 18–3) through the ipsilateral portal until less than 1 cm remains posteriorly. The cartilage then slips into the intercondylar notch by the constant pull from the contralateral portal. The final cut is then made as described for repair of a bucket-handle tear.

The intra-articular pressure during the posterior dissection should not be higher than needed to occlude the vessels for control of bleeding. A high pressure distends the posterior joint capsule, overstretches the attachments, and counteracts the anterior mobilization by the grasping forceps. The dissection posteriorly is performed with the lowest possible fluid flow, just enough to keep the operating area clear. Whenever needed, the operative field is flushed temporarily by pressing the irrigation apparatus' footpedal to increase the pump speed for a few seconds.

In a tight joint showing a posteromedial radial tear extending all the way to the periphery, it may not be possible to grasp the central posterior segment of tissue anteriorly. In such cases, an accessory portal posterior to the collateral ligament is sometimes needed for operating instruments (Fig. 18–4). Visual control over the operation is then provided by the telescope, at an optical angle of 30 or 70°, placed with its tip in the narrow triangle between the posterior cruciate ligament, the tibial spine, and the femoral condylar wall.[8] Sometimes, a posterior remnant may even be excised bimanually using the posteromedial and contralateral superior portal.

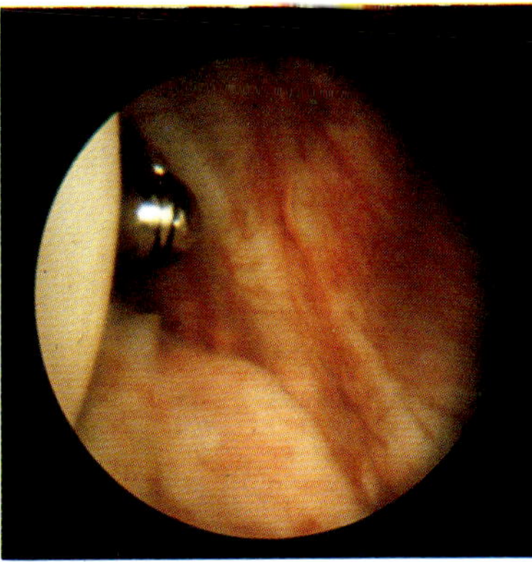

Fig. 18–4. The telescopic view is around the femoral condyle from beneath the posterior cruciate ligament to control instrument insertion and the posterior operations. At insertion, the knife blade is retracted.

RESULTS

During the past 6 years, no deep infections have occurred with this technique, and superficial drainage is unusual. Tenderness at insertion sites is not unusual the first weeks, but granulomas are seldom seen. Granulomas in the patellar tendon are not more common than at any other insertion site.

Operating times are of interest, at least for the practicing orthopedic surgeon. They vary, however, considerably with the type of tear, the surgeon's arthroscopic experience, his goal for the surgical procedure, and his endurance and patience. A bucket-handle tear can be operated on in few minutes, but the result is technically more satisfactory when 10 to 20 minutes are allowed for the procedure. A total or a subtotal meniscectomy sometimes takes less than 20 minutes, but my average time is now 45 minutes by this technique.

Official reports on sick leave in my country (Sweden) are of interest. The Social Insurance Office reported in 1981 that 28% of the patients treated at our hospital were back to work after closed meniscectomy with no sick leave at all. Mean postoperative sick leave was 9 days, as compared with 53 days after meniscectomy by traditional arthrotomy techniques. Figures on sick leave also varied with the types of meniscal tears and their treatment. Patients who underwent excision of flap tears and other minor partial resections showed a mean sick leave of only 5 days, whereas patients treated for a bucket-handle tear were working after 12 days. Total meniscectomy was followed by a shorter sick leave, 8 days, as compared with 14 days after a subtotal meniscectomy leaving a rim. This comparison may seem surprising, but total meniscectomy performed in this manner is technically less difficult than a subtotal excision of the cartilage while preserving stability in the meniscal rim. The increased surgical trauma due to such technical difficulties may explain the difference in recovery time. Whether preservation of a meniscal rim will, in the long run, compensate for and justify damage to articular cartilage during the surgical procedure is questionable. Patients with residual symptoms after treatment have been urged to undergo a check-up arthroscopy to rule out an inadequate surgical procedure as the cause of these symptoms. My rate of such "second looks" is 5% in 1 year postoperatively, but in only 2% have I found cause for further surgical correction.

Whether the long-term results of arthroscopic meniscectomy by any technique will differ from those of traditional arthrotomy remains unproved. Even if the many advantages of arthroscopic meniscectomy are no longer questioned,[9] it can be expected that overall long-term results will depend mainly on concomitant injuries to the knee as well as on proper indications for treatment.

REFERENCES

1. Oretorp, N., and Gillquist, J.: Atraumatic partial or total meniscectomy under arthroscopic control. Presented at the First Congress of the International Society of the Knee, Lyon, 1979.
2. Bullough, P., Munuera, L., Murphy, J., and Weinstein, A.: The strength of the menisci as it is related to their fine structure. J. Bone Joint Surg. (Br.), *52*:564, 1970.
3. Oretorp, N., and Risberg, B.: Studies on the fine structure of the menisci and their capsular and ligamentous connections. In press.
4. Gillquist, J., and Hagberg, G.: A new modification of the technique of arthroscopy of the knee joint. Acta Chir. Scand., *142*:123, 1976.
5. Jackson, R., and Dandy, D.: Arthroscopy of the Knee. New York, Grune and Stratton, 1976.
6. Johnson, L.: Diagnostic and Surgical Arthroscopy. St. Louis, C.V. Mosby, 1981.
7. Oretorp, N., and Gillquist, J.: Transcutaneous meniscectomy under arthroscopic control. Int. Orthop., *3*:19, 1979.
8. Gillquist, J., Hagberg, G., and Oretorp, N.: Arthroscopic examination of the posteromedial compartment of the knee joint. Int. Orthop., *3*:13, 1979.
9. Northmore-Ball, M., Dandy, D., and Jackson, R.: A comparative study of the results of arthroscopic and open partial meniscectomy. Presented at the Fourth Congress of the International Arthroscopy Association, Rio de Janeiro, 1981.

Chapter 19

PROXIMAL APPROACH TO ARTHROSCOPIC MENISCECTOMY

Dinesh Patel

Arthroscopic surgical correction of various disorders of the knee is now a well-recognized phenomenon. Improvement in optics, newer instrumentation, video cameras, and our better understanding of the anatomic structures of the knee have made this technique widely accepted. Triangulation, using single or multiple portals with or without the operating arthroscope, has made this advance possible.

In 1933, Iino studied several approaches to cadaver knees and recommended a number of different portals for insertion of the arthroscope.[1] One of these portals, the anterolateral, has been considered the standard portal for most arthroscopic diagnostic and surgical procedures. Watanabe and associates,[2] Jackson and Dandy,[3,4] O'Connor,[5] Johnson,[6] Guhl,[7] Metcalf,[8] and many other orthopedic surgeons have used this portal for much of their arthroscopic operations. Johnson[6] and Whipple and Bassett[9] popularized the polypuncture technique, whereas Gillquist and Hagberg[10] and Oretorp[11] have used the central approach (Fig. 19–1).

The existing approaches using either a single or double portal have certain disadvantages, including inadequate visualization of (1) the anterior horns of both menisci, (2) the meniscocapsular ligaments in the anterior compartment, (3) when present, the anterior intrameniscal ligament, (4) the tibial insertion of the anterior cruciate ligament, and (5) the popliteal tunnel and its contents. These drawbacks are more noticeable during a surgical procedure when the close proximity of the anterolateral, anteromedial, and central portals results in crowding and collision of the arthroscope and instruments inside the knee. This crowding causes problems in triangulation. The additional stress to the knee or instruments also increases the potential for breakage of instruments or scuffing of the articular cartilage. These problems are intensified when synovitis and enlarged fat pads also exist (Fig. 19–2).

The blind insertion of needles or instruments from the anterolateral and anteromedial approaches can damage the anterior horns of both menisci. Fat pads and the ligamentum mucosum add to the problems of triangulation, especially when these structures are inflamed and enlarged. The problems of spherical aberration, distor-

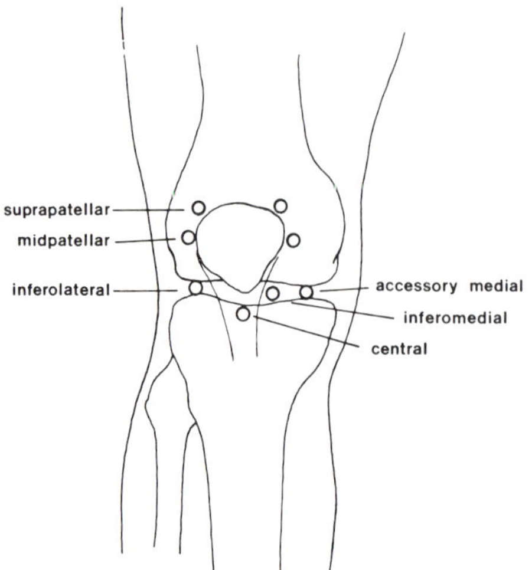

Fig. 19–1. Various approaches to the anterior portion of the knee through which the arthroscope and other instruments may be inserted.

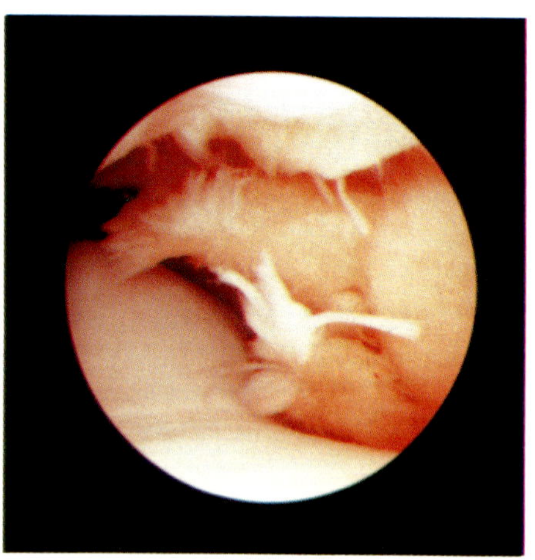

Fig. 19–2. An enlarged fat pad often makes it difficult to visualize the anterior horns of both menisci.

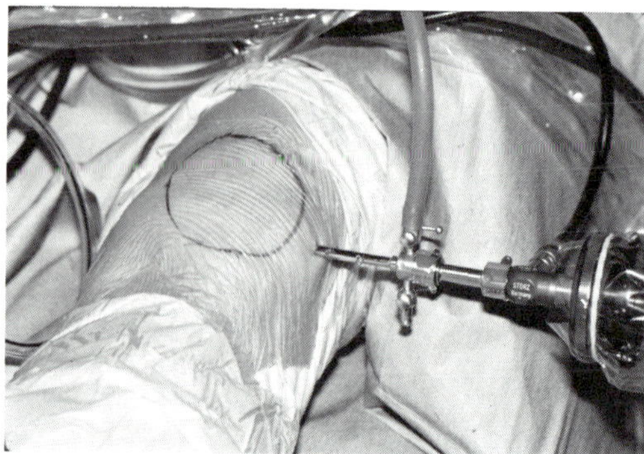

Fig. 19–3. The midpatellar lateral approach is used most often.

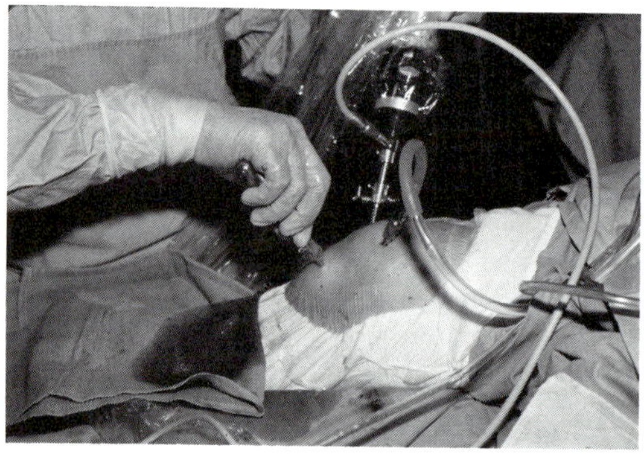

Fig. 19–4. Pressing the arthroscope through the midpatellar or suprapatellar portals eliminates crowding both inside and outside the joint.

tion, and magnification of objects arise with the conventional portal as the arthroscope is brought closer to the object. These disadvantages also apply to the central portal used by Gillquist and Hagberg.[10]

After analyzing all these problems and having experienced most of them, I have used superior or midpatellar medial and midpatellar lateral approaches (Fig. 19–3) for the introduction of the arthroscope, and I use the anterolateral and anteromedial incisions for introduction of instruments. Because the oblique tip of the arthroscope is inserted superiorly and the instruments are inserted inferiorly, crowding and collision outside as well as inside the knee are minimized (Fig. 19–4). With the arthroscope inserted superiorly, proper placement of the instruments is possible, thus facilitating operation and minimizing complications.

SURGICAL PRINCIPLES

The surgical technique, as described in detail elsewhere,[12] requires that the patient be given general or local anesthesia. The foot end of the operating table is not broken, and the patient's knee and leg are kept straight. The surgeon sits beside the knee to be operated on. I do not usually use a leg holder, but I find it no interference to the arthroscope or video camera. I perform most of the surgical procedure with the patient's knee flexed at about 15°, and I place the joint in a valgus or varus strain as necessary.

The incision for the introduction of the arthroscope is made at the broadest portion of the patella, either midpatella laterally or medially. Because the popliteal tunnel cannot be visualized by the midpatella medial approach, I prefer the midpatella lateral approach (see Fig. 19–3) and use other portals as necessary. A small incision is made close to the outer border of the patella. A standard technique for scope insertion is then used. I prefer a 30° oblique tip, although at times I have used a 70° angle.

In patella alta, the incision is naturally not made at the broadest portion of the patella, but inferior to it. When only the anterior compartment needs to be visualized, the incision may be made anywhere from the superior pole to the midpatellar position. When the patellofemoral joint is tight, one may have to make the incision inferior to the broadest portion of the patella.

The knee is systematically examined as with any other portal. The main difference with this approach is that the knee cannot be placed in the figure-4 position, which is often helpful in visualizing the lateral compartment. With the aid of a needle, seen entering the joint, the instruments can be properly inserted.

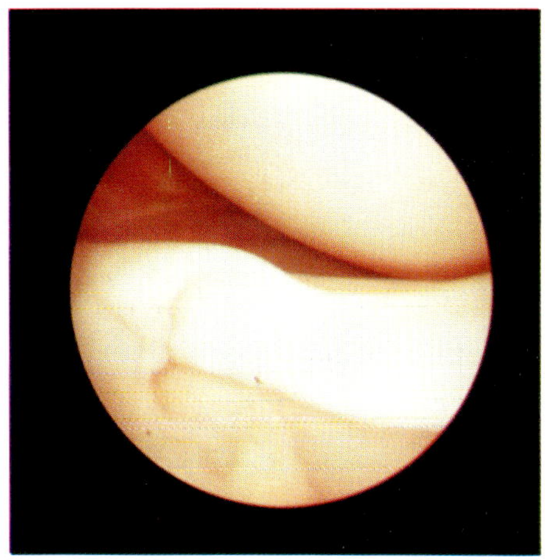

Fig. 19–6. Displaced medial meniscus seen with the scope in the midlateral position.

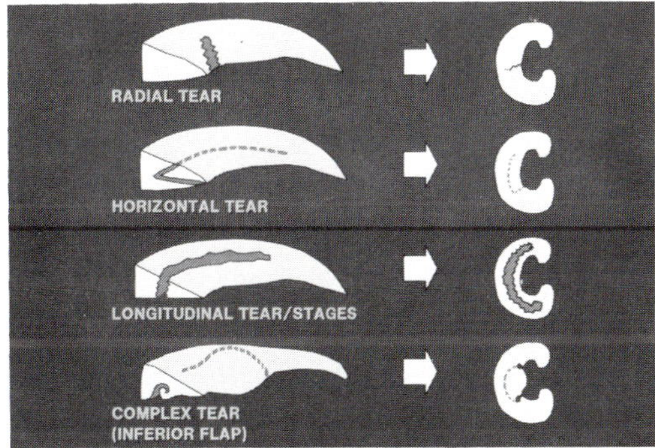

Fig. 19–7. A diagram illustrating the various types of tears that can be seen and treated with the scope in the midpatellar medial or lateral position.

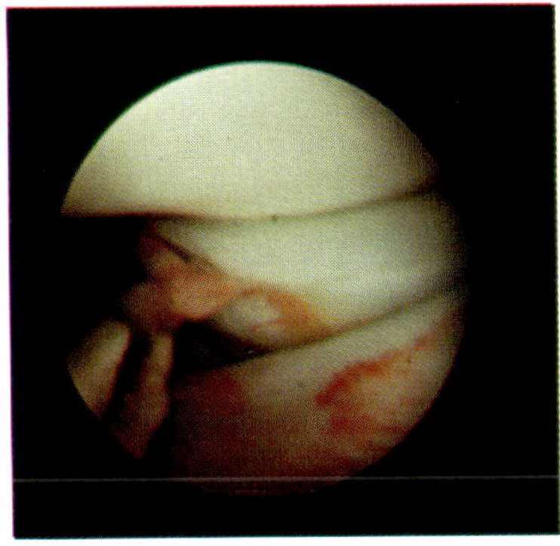

Fig. 19–5. An excellent view of the displaced lateral meniscus can be obtained with the scope in the midpatellar medial or lateral position.

Visualization of the posterolateral portion of the lateral meniscus and the posteromedial portion of the medial meniscus may be difficult. In such a case, I change portals, placing the arthroscope through another portal to complete visualization of the remaining portion of the knee (Figs. 19–5 and 19–6).

SURGICAL TECHNIQUES FOR MENISCAL LESIONS

All common tears such as radial, horizontal, longitudinal, and complex tears can be seen by this approach (Fig. 19–7). The

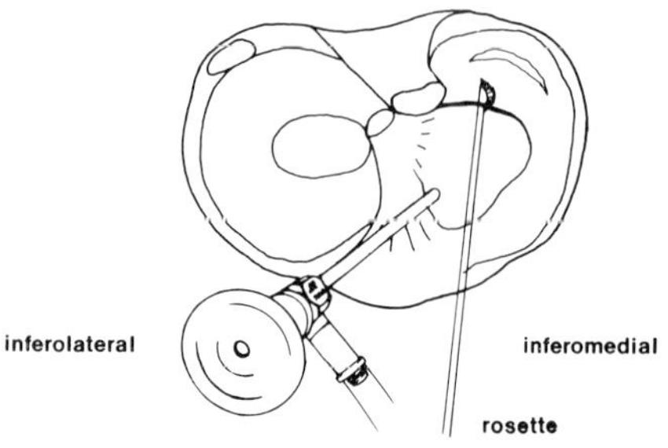

Fig. 19–8. The short longitudinal tear of the medial meniscus with a rosette knife inserted from an anterolateral approach. The posterior horn is partially divided.

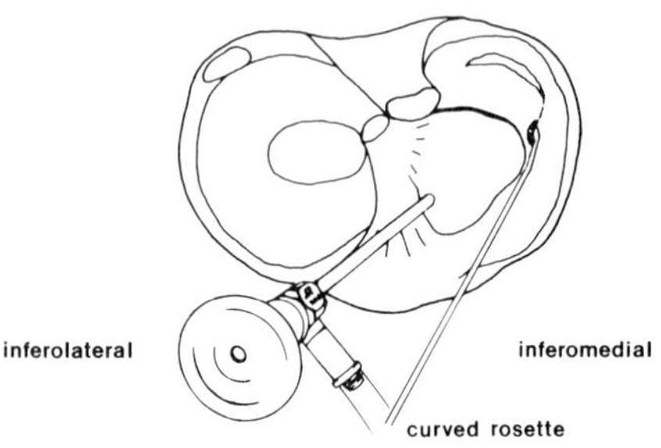

Fig. 19–9. Anterior margin of the tear is divided next.

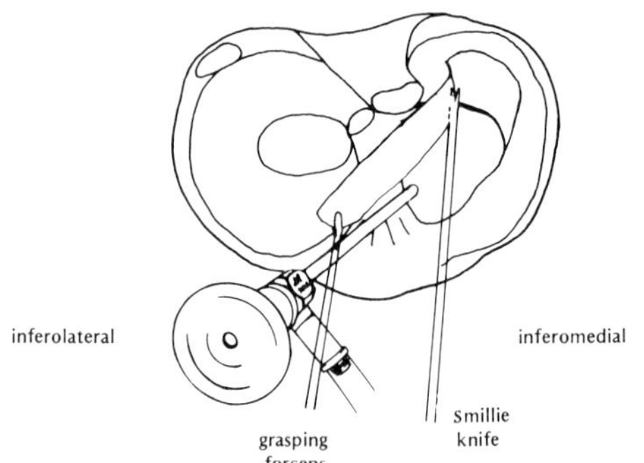

Fig. 19–10. The free anterior portion of the torn meniscus is grasped, the remaining attachment of the posterior horn is divided with a small, Smillie-type knife, and the fragment is pulled from the knee joint.

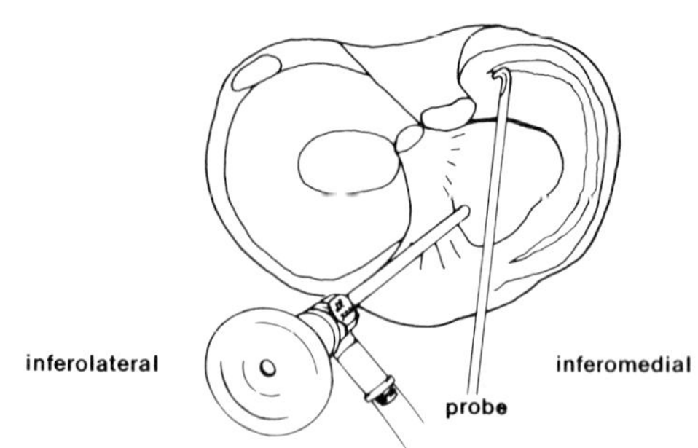

Fig. 19–11. A long vertical tear of the medial meniscus is probed to determine its mobility.

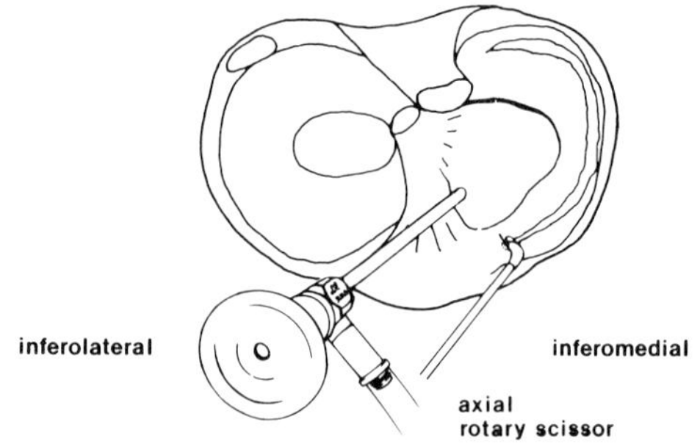

Fig. 19–12. Anterior horn of a tear is divided first, using a knife or axial rotary scissors.

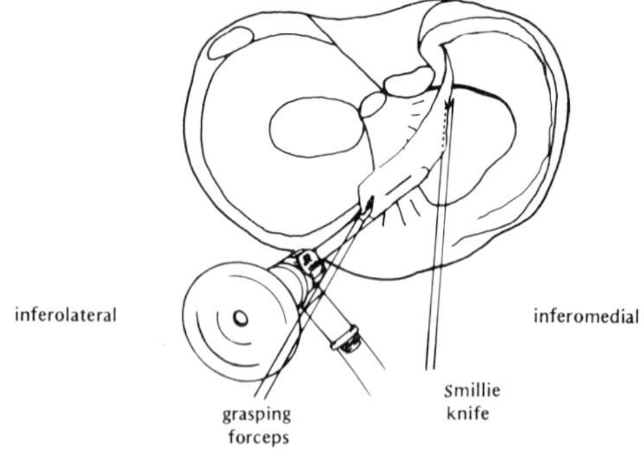

Fig. 19–13. Anterior horn is grasped, and traction is applied. The posterior horn is divided with a slightly curved Smillie knife.

short longitudinal tear is approached by placing the arthroscope at the midpatella laterally. The second incision is made close to the medial border of the patellar tendon, to permit division of the posterior horn of the medial meniscus. This short longitudinal tear of the posterior horn is partly divided to make sure that this flap does not become lodged in the posterior popliteal area (Fig. 19–8). Only three-fourths of the posterior portion of the medial meniscus are divided. A third incision an inch away from the medial border of the patella is made, and the anterior attachment of the meniscus is divided (Fig. 19–9). The displaced medial meniscus is then held taut with grasping forceps while the remaining attachment of the meniscus is divided using a rosette blade, axial scissors, or a Smillie knife (Fig. 19–10). The next step is to remove the major fragment as well as any displaced menisci and trim the rim with basket forceps; one should check the rim with a probe.

Long Longitudinal Tears of the Medial Meniscus

The technical problems of removing the displaced portion of the bucket-handle tear depend on the length of the meniscal fragment, its mobility, and the displacement of the handle of the meniscus. If the meniscal fragment is long, but is less mobile both anteriorly and posteriorly, then either the anterior or posterior horn can be detached first without the need for grasping or pulling on the fragment (Fig. 19–11).

I prefer to remove the anterior meniscal horn first because it is simpler. I use 30 or 60° axial scissors or a rosette blade to divide the anterior horn flush with the remaining rim (Fig. 19–12). The incision is made either adjacent or posterior to the patellar tendon, an accessory medial incision. This incision should be made just superior to the axilla of the anterior horn of the bucket-handle tear.

When the handle of the medial meniscus is small, short, or unusually mobile, then technically it is better to grasp the handle first, to apply traction, and then to divide its attachment anteriorly and posteriorly (Fig. 19–13). It is essential to check the mobility of the remaining rim of the meniscus. A second bucket-handle tear or displacement is often noted. A small tag of the meniscal tissue in the anterior or posterior can be troublesome in the future if both ends are not cut flush. Flap tears are approached in a similar manner. If the meniscal fragment is large and becomes lodged near the ligamentum mucosum during extraction, direct visualization of the portal will minimize this problem.

Lateral Meniscal Lesions

Lateral meniscal operations are complex and difficult for a number of reasons. One problem is the evaluation of meniscocapsular complexes in the popliteal hiatus. As we know, the lateral meniscus has an attachment on the lateral capsular ligament in the popliteal hiatus with superior and inferior meniscocollagenous fascicles. This area needs to be evaluated to ensure the integrity of the periphery of the lateral meniscus. If the complexes, commonly called superior or inferior fascicles, are torn, then the lateral meniscus will be unstable in this popliteal hiatus. The inferior fascicle has been noted to be frequently torn with a torn anterior cruciate ligament.

Another difficult problem in lateral meniscal operations is the anterolateral portion of the lateral meniscus. This anterior meniscal horn, which attaches at the base of the anterior cruciate ligament, is often difficult to visualize, and tears in this area are difficult to treat. Fortunately, such tears are less apt to produce clinical symptoms than those in the posterior portion of the meniscus. Generally, this area can best be viewed with the arthroscope introduced some distance away.

One of the most common lesions of the lateral meniscus is a radial tear in which one may see a horizontal cleavage component if the tear is of long standing. Such tears can be treated using ordinary basket forceps inserted from an anteromedial portal or right-angled rotary basket forceps inserted from the anterolateral portal.

Longitudinal Tears. Longitudinal tears are short or long. The short intrameniscal tear of the posterior horn is often associated with an anterior cruciate ligament tear. Sometimes, the longitudinal tear extends all the way to the anterior entrance of the popliteal hiatus, but usually not beyond this point. If it does, it can result in a large

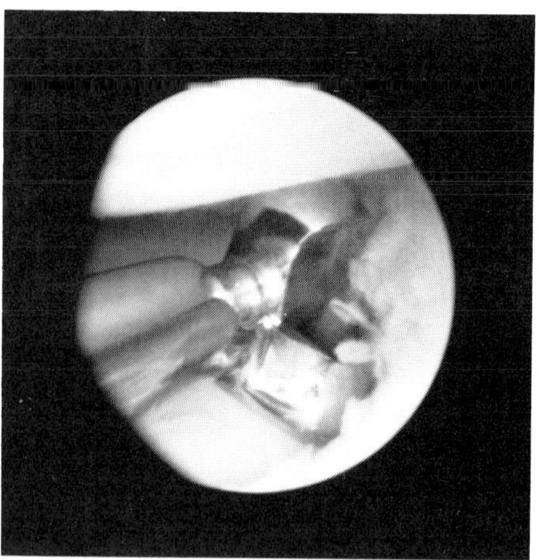

Fig. 19–14. Rotary basket forceps are used to trim the meniscal rim. This instrument is especially useful for short radial tears of the lateral meniscus and when trimming forceps must be placed in the joint from the ipsilateral side.

bucket-handle tear. This tear is removed in a manner identical to that for removal of a medial tear, with the arthroscope in the midpatellar lateral position. The second incision is made anteromedially next to the patellar tendon, which can be used to divide the anterior meniscal horn and an anterolateral incision to remove the posterior attachment. One should remember that no one position of the arthroscope or the operating instruments is always best, and changes of insertion of the arthroscope and instruments are often required. Occasionally two instruments, grasping forceps and a Smillie knife, can be placed in the same incision to detach the posterior meniscal horn. This procedure is possible if one uses rotary basket forceps that give one enough room to avoid crowding and collision inside the joint (Fig. 19–14).

In a short longitudinal tear, the inner portion of the displaced lateral meniscus is removed using either a basket punch or a hook knife to divide the anterior portion first and then the posterior portion, so the rim is well trimmed.

Complex and flap tears of the lateral meniscus are removed in an identical manner, and again, the rotary basket punch facilitates this procedure.

Whatever approach is used for the arthroscope, an enlarged fat pad can be troublesome and may render the operation impossible. In such a circumstance, it is necessary to remove the fat pad with the motorized patellar shaver. Even this procedure can be a problem because it is sometimes difficult to see the end of the shaver, and severe damage to the end of the arthroscope has resulted when the shaver operates on the end of the instrument instead of on the fat pad. One should not forget that the meniscus does not have to be removed arthroscopically. Arthrotomy is still a viable alternative.

RESULTS

The superior or proximal midpatellar lateral or medial approach is useful for arthroscopic surgical correction of all kinds of meniscal disorders, except the posterolateral portion, which is often difficult to visualize. This approach eliminates crowding and collision and thereby excessive stress to the knee or the instruments. It is also helpful in avoiding specific technical problems of the anterior compartment, such as those caused by an enlarged fat pad and ligamentum mucosum, and in evaluating the popliteal hiatus.

Dividing the anterior extent of a bucket-handle tear of the medial meniscus and handling anterior compartment problems caused by a flap tear or a swollen fat pad are facilitated with this approach. I recommend it as a primary or adjunctive approach for arthroscopic meniscal surgical procedures.

One must remember specific localization of the incision, orientation, and use of oblique arthroscopes. At the present time, I use the superior or proximal midpatellar portal for diagnosis and surgical procedures. I use the anterolateral and anteromedial portals for insertion of instruments. If difficulty is encountered, I am prepared to use other portals, both for the arthroscope and for the other instruments.

REFERENCES

1. Iino, S.: Normal arthroscopic findings of the knee joint in adults. J. Jpn. Orthop. Assoc., *14*:467, 1939.
2. Watanabe, M., Takeda, S., and Ikeuchi, H.: Atlas of Arthroscopy. Tokyo, Igaku-Shoin, 1957.
3. Jackson, R.W., and Dandy, D.J.: Arthroscopy of the Knee. St. Louis, C.V. Mosby, 1977.
4. Dandy, D.J.: Arthroscopic Surgery of the Knee. Edinburgh, Churchill Livingstone, 1981.
5. O'Connor, R.: Arthroscopy. Philadelphia, J.B. Lippincott, 1977.
6. Johnson, L.: Comprehensive Arthroscopic Examination of the Knee. St. Louis, C.V. Mosby, 1977.
7. Guhl, J.F.: Third International Seminar on Operative Arthroscopy, UCLA Extension, Maui, Hawaii, 1981.
8. Metcalf, R.W.: Third International Seminar on Operative Arthroscopy, UCLA Extension, Maui, Hawaii, 1981.
9. Whipple, T.L., and Bassett, F.H.: Arthroscopic examination of the knee. Polypuncture technique with percutaneous intraarticular manipulation. J. Bone Joint Surg. (Am), *60*:444, 1978.
10. Gillquist, J., and Hagberg, G.: A new modification of the technique of arthroscopy of the knee joint. Acta Chir. Scand., *142*:123, 1976.
11. Oretorp, N.: On the Diagnosis and Treatment of Meniscus and Ligament Injuries in the Knee, Especially on the Medial Side. Stockholm, Linkopings Tryckeri, 1978.
12. Patel, D.: Proximal approaches to arthroscopic surgery of the knee. Am. J. Sports Med., *9*:296, 1981.

Chapter 20

ARTHROSCOPIC TOTAL MENISCECTOMY

Robert W. Carson

Total meniscectomy is a radical operation, analogous to amputation or patellectomy. Arthroscopic observations and biopsies belie the claim that the meniscus regenerates if totally excised at the synovial border.[1] The additional contention that total meniscectomy leads to less articular cartilage degeneration than total meniscectomy is not supported statistically by any published study.[1] To the contrary, Tapper and Hoover's long-term study (10- to 30-year follow-up), showed almost double the percentage of excellent results (67% to 34%) from leaving an intact peripheral rim versus removing the entire meniscus.[2]

Experimental studies also favor a conservative approach to the meniscus. In 1936, King's dog experiments led him to conclude that only the mobile portion of a torn meniscus should be removed if articular cartilage degeneration was to be minimized.[3] This work was basic to O'Connor's rationale for "partial" meniscectomy under arthroscopic control.[4] Accumulating research on microanatomy,[5] physiology,[6,7] and biomechanics of the meniscus[8–11] substantiates King's conclusions and provides strong arguments for preserving meniscal tissue. This mounting evidence supports not only the minimal meniscectomy, but also the concept of meniscal repair.

All the conservative arguments notwithstanding, situations exist in which total (synovial border) resections are unavoidable. Of my first 400 arthroscopic meniscectomies, 28 (7%) were total.[12] Semantic differences account for a number of these cases; nevertheless, to consistently manage excisions arthroscopically, the ability to perform a total meniscectomy is essential.

HISTORY

Dr. Hiroshi Ikeuchi of Tokyo performed the first total meniscectomy in July of 1968 and reported a series of 13 cases in September of 1978.[13] O'Connor, in 1977, published a case report of a total meniscectomy.[4] I presented my technique of posteromedial instrumentation for subtotal meniscectomies in 1978.[14] Oretorp and Gillquist, of Sweden, described their transpatellar tendon technique in 1978[15] and later expanded this method to include total meniscectomies.

NEW DEFINITIONS

A new era of endoscopic meniscal surgery demands a re-examination of the classic definitions of the types of meniscectomies. If we are to learn from our long-term results, more specific terminology is required for the selective meniscal excisions that are now being performed. The phrase "partial meniscectomy" is meaningless. It is used indiscriminately by some as a synonym for arthroscopic meniscectomy. A meniscus can be totally avulsed from its synovial border, but if it is delivered through a puncture wound, it is usually referred to as a partial meniscectomy.

To test the hypothesis that the least meniscectomy is the best meniscectomy, I have established 3 arbitrary categories of meniscal excision, according to the amount of tissue removed. The term *partial* meniscectomy is reserved for those excisions of less than 50% of the meniscal mass. *Subtotal* is used for those of greater than 50% of the mass with a peripheral rim at least 2 mm wide. *Total* meniscectomy describes a meniscus excised at the synovial border or interrupted at the border, destabilizing the ligamentous attachments and losing the effectiveness of the circumferential fibers (Fig. 20–1). Allegedly, meniscectomies that invade the popliteal sulcus lead to rapid lateral compartmental degeneration. Therefore, the sulcus is chosen as the dividing line for the lateral meniscus, and all such excisions are placed in the total category.

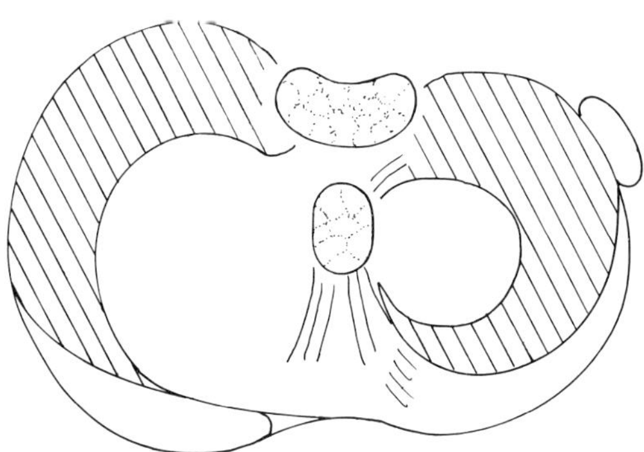

Fig. 20–1. My definition of total meniscectomy includes excision of shaded portions. If a circumferential rim of meniscus remains, then the procedure is considered subtotal. Anterior horns are not usually excised.

The anterior meniscal horns are resected only rarely. I have performed almost 600 meniscectomies over a 5-year period, and have observed no adverse effects from leaving this tissue. A prerequisite, however, is an anterior incision that makes a smooth transition through the inner meniscal rim to promote healing and to avoid the risk of a secondary tear, "a blended cut."

INDICATIONS FOR TOTAL MENISCECTOMY

The presence of a torn meniscus is not, alone, an indication for meniscectomy. Minor fibrillation, small radial tears, degenerative tears, and even stable longitudinal tears of the lateral meniscus are best left alone. Meniscectomy does not relieve the "giving way" of a pivot shift or the "locking" of a nonopaque loose body hiding in a posterior space. Only meniscal tears that are *causally related* to recurrent pain and disability or to an unacceptable interference with the patient's life style should be treated surgically.

Longitudinal Tears

Peripheral meniscal rim tears are reparable as described by DeHaven in Chapter 21. For those tears that are not repaired, completing an excision through a natural tear at the synovial margin is, by definition, a total meniscectomy.

Mixed Tears

Mixed tears infrequently extend into the peripheral meniscal rim or popliteal sulcus and require total excision of the posterior horn or a loss of integrity of its circumferential fibers. Examples are double radial tears, a combination of horizontal and radial tears, or an occasional radial tear that penetrates to the synovial border and extends longitudinally in one or both directions.

Examining Posterior Spaces

Most meniscal tears that require total excision can be fully appreciated only from the vantage point of the medial and lateral posterior spaces. Both these spaces can be examined from the anterior of the knee and indeed must be examined or serious pathologic changes will be overlooked.

Gillquist and Hagberg introduced an arthroscopic central (transpatellar tendon) approach to the knee in 1976.[16] With Oretorp, they reported a large series of posterior compartment examinations, using angled arthroscopes through the patellar tendon.[17]

The posterior knee compartments can be examined without puncturing the patellar tendon. With the standard 2-puncture technique, the lateral incision is placed adjacent to the patellar tendon and 2 cm superior to the lateral tibial crest. A 5-mm water sheath with blunt trocar is walked blindly across the medial compartment and is slipped between the cruciate ligaments and the medial femoral condyle. The knee should be in 20 to 30° of flexion, with the

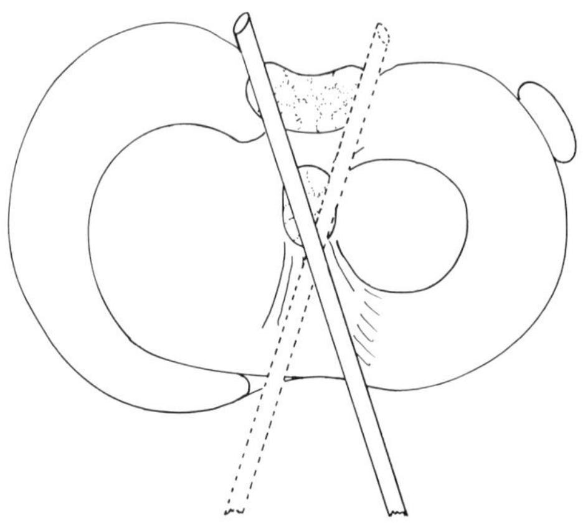

Fig. 20–2. Angled arthroscopes (5-mm outer diameter) penetrate the posterior spaces through the intercondylar notch from opposite punctures, if properly placed. This technique allows full examination of the knee without multiple accessory incisions.

tibia rotated internally. This approach may fail in a child or in an arthritic knee, leaving the posteromedial approach as described by Johnson as an alternative for viewing the posteromedial compartment.[18] The posterolateral compartment can be entered from an anteromedial puncture through the intercondylar notch, if the incision is kept near (1 cm) the patellar tendon (Fig. 20–2).

CONTRAINDICATIONS TO TOTAL MENISCECTOMY

No *absolute* contraindications are unique to total meniscectomies. Extensive mixed tears, however, should be treated conservatively if they are associated with degenerative changes of the involved compartment. The more advanced these changes are, as seen on single-leg, weight-bearing roentgenograms, the worse is the prognosis following meniscectomy. If a patient with a degenerative knee joint develops acute disabling symptoms from what appears to be a *causally related* meniscal tear, meniscectomy may be unavoidable. Removing any meniscal tissue from such a compartment may be the final insult that leads to rapid progression of degenerative disease and a medial tibial osteotomy. If a surgeon fails to warn the patient in advance of this probable outcome, the meniscectomy may receive full blame for all future symptoms in this knee.

INSTRUMENTATION

Diagnostic Arthroscopes

For surgical procedures, the primary arthroscope should have a 20- or 30°-angled lens for viewing the posterior meniscal attachments from the opposite puncture. The secondary arthroscope should have a 70° angle for examining posterior spaces from anterior punctures through the intercondylar notch. The ideal diameter for these basic instruments is 4 mm (5-mm water sheath), which is the maximum size that will penetrate the notch. This size is also a compromise between a smaller arthroscope, which passes inferior to the femoral condyle (4-mm sheath), and a larger one (6.5-mm sheath), which carries a generous optical system and a great enough flow of saline solution to maintain joint distension while using a power-driven patellar shaver.

I designed a flat diagnostic arthroscope with a thin (4 mm) vertical profile that seemed more suitable for the narrow crevices of the knee joint. Full-sized optics, fiber space, and water channel were arranged horizontally, obviating the need to compromise among small, medium, and large arthroscopes. Stryker has this instrument on the market with a 20° lens (Fig. 20–3).

Arthroscopes age, wear, and are easily damaged. The clumsy use of probes, powered shavers, and large video cameras are particular risks, as are substitute assistants and visitors. For anyone who performs arthroscopic surgery on a regular basis, backup equipment is essential. The specialty arthroscopes, such as small, large, and 120° retrograde, can serve the dual role of providing backup as well as their particular advantage.

Operating Arthroscopes

An operating arthroscope is indispensable for meniscal surgical procedures. Otherwise, extra punctures are required, instrument crowding becomes a significant problem, and the surgeon becomes dependent on an extra assistant and on video equipment. The arthroscopes, working instruments, and techniques are discussed in Chapter 3.

Instrument Sleeves

Surgical arthroscopy requires the repeated introduction and withdrawal of instruments through punctures that cut into multiple tissue planes. With any change in knee flexion or rotation, these layered punctures become unaligned. To resolve this problem, the punctures must be en-

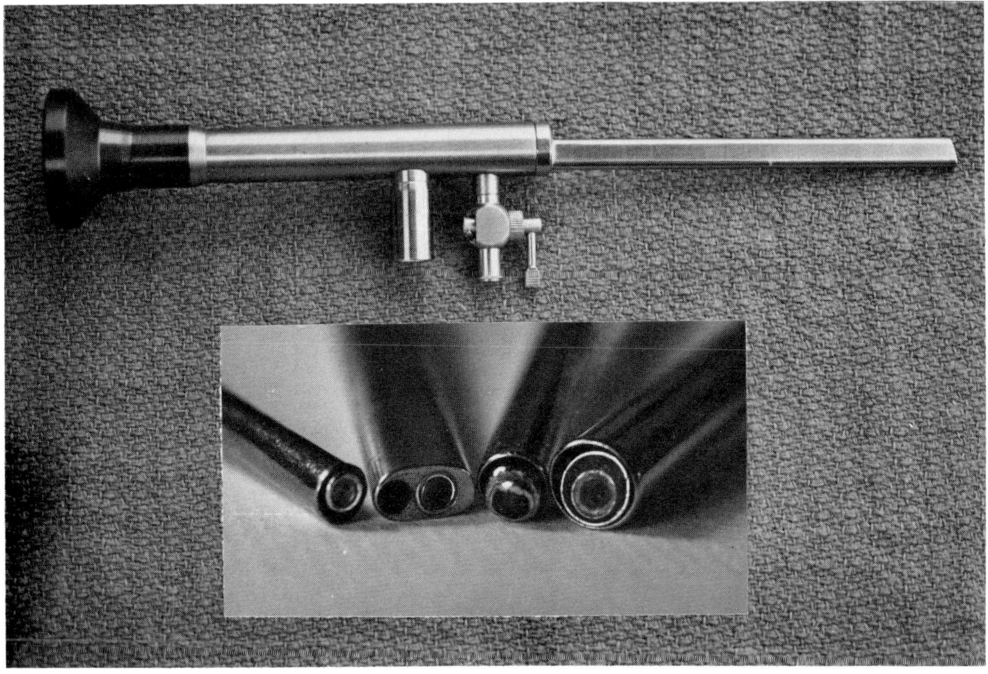

Fig. 20–3. The flat diagnostic arthroscope was designed to combine the advantages of large optics, light fibers, and (inset) the flow rate of the largest diagnostic arthroscope (6.5 mm) with the thin profile of the smallest (4 mm).

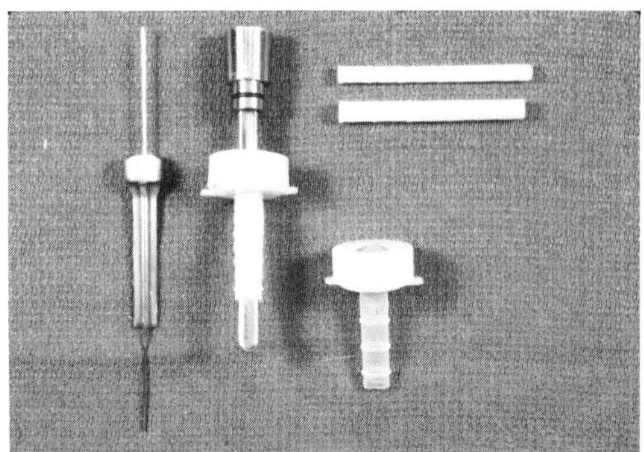

Fig. 20–4. Flexible sleeves have evolved to a commercial model that will accept flat arthroscopes, curved and angled instruments, and power-suction instruments. Specially cannulated trocars follow a guide wire through the joint capsule.

larged unnecessarily, or instrument sleeves must be used. I originally introduced flexible sleeves in 1978, to accommodate various sizes and shapes of short, curved instruments.[14] Stryker now markets a model that is disposable and has multiple self-sealing, latex diaphragms. These air-resistant, water-resistant membranes also permit the use of sunction instruments (Fig. 20–4). Several manufacturers market metal sleeves that accept straight working instruments, and Wolf markets a short-threaded metal sleeve that passes their own gently curved instruments.

Grasping Instruments

To excise a meniscus en bloc, a sturdy, self-locking clamp is essential. Kocher clamps (6- and 7-inch) can be used, but they are not ideal; to spread their jaws, the pivot point must be at or near the skin. Pituitary forceps with teeth (Schlesinger or alligator) are better, but must be locked with a towel clip. The best all-around clamp that is commercially available is a reinforced tendon passer marketed by Wolf.

Hand Cutting Instruments

Knives. Knives have many advantages as cutting instruments. They are cheap, easy to sharpen, and unlikely to break. They cut cleanly in the narrow confines near the posterior meniscal attachments, where scissors and basket forceps are likely to scuff articular cartilage. Disposable blades manufactured by Beaver have solved the problem of the dull blade. Their new arthroscopic blades are break-resistant, and their new collet has eliminated the risk of dropping a blade into the joint.

Scissors and Basket Forceps. Although short, curved, cutting instruments were suggested in 1977, the laparoscopic influence has been slow to die. Only recently, have "knee-sized" instruments (4- to 5-inch shafts) become available. At this writing, none of the curves of the commercially available instruments have a radius short enough to be useful in the knee. For triangulating instruments, a 3.4-mm diameter is a good compromise to reduce scuffing of the articular cartilage while ensuring reasonable strength.

Powered Instruments

In 1977, Leonard Bonnel of Dyonics and three others, inluding Dr. Lanny Johnson, submitted a patent for a new instrument for closed surgical procedures of the knee. This "shaver" was an important step forward for arthroscopic surgery. The instrument was designed with slow, shearing speeds and a suction to bring tissue into the shaver's mouth for cutting. Stryker, Storz, and Wolf have followed with similar devices (Fig. 20–5).

These instruments facilitate meniscectomy by improving visibility. They vacuum debris, remove synovium, and help to identify and remove tags of the meniscal rim. Once a meniscus has been fragmented by hand cutting instruments, the newer cutting heads are able to perform limited excisions of meniscal tissue.

TOTAL MEDIAL MENISCECTOMY

The natural tear line determines the ease or difficulty of any arthroscopic meniscectomy. If a tear is longitudinal and in the posteromedial corner, the most inaccessible part of the excision line is made by the

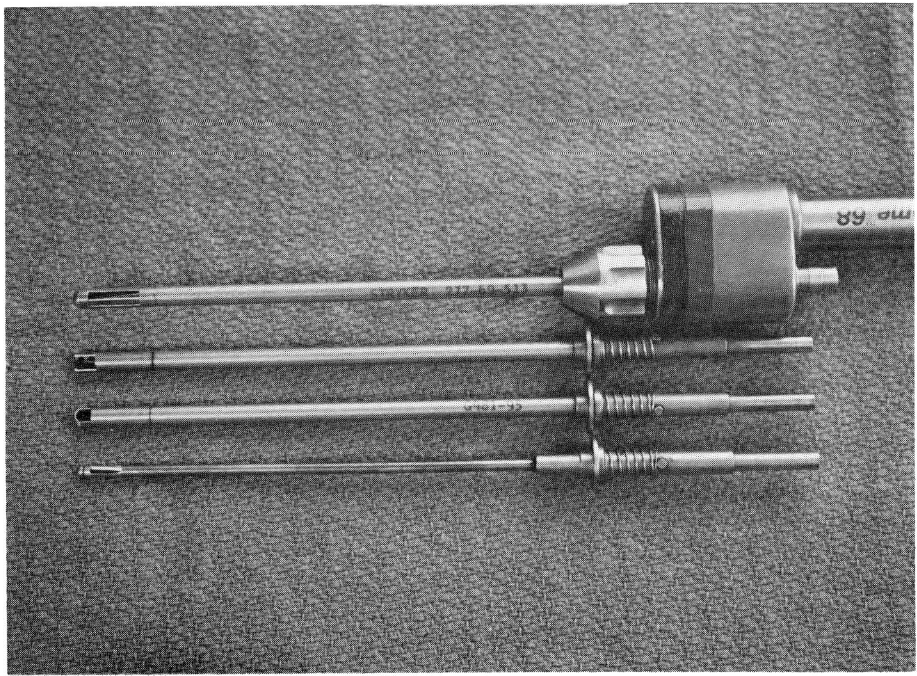

Fig. 20–5. Stryker's power-suction chondrotome system is nitrogen powered and fully autoclavable. Each manufacturer's system has unique features.

injury. The longer the tear, the less cutting remains to be done by the surgeon. The solitary, long, displaced or displaceable peripheral rim tear is the easiest total meniscectomy of all. On the other hand, the most difficult meniscectomy has no natural tear in the line of excision and must be removed either piecemeal or by en bloc resection.

Posteromedial Puncture

A posteromedial puncture can be used for instrumentation while the surgeon views with angled arthroscopes through the intercondylar notch. The puncture must be well superior and posterior to the meniscal border for instruments to have a proper cutting angle inferiorly into the meniscus and around to the midline attachment of the posterior horn.

First, a quarter-inch skin incision is made about 2 cm superior to the joint line and just anterior to the hamstring tendons, while the patient's knee hangs off the end of the operating table at 80 or 90° of flexion. Then, a fine Kirschner wire or hypodermic needle is inserted through the capsule under the direct vision of a 70 or 120° arthroscope in the intercondylar notch.

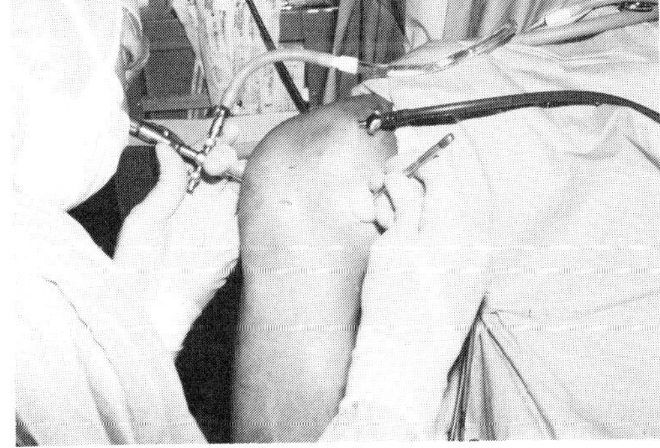

Fig. 20–6. Usually, the posteromedial puncture is used for instrumentation while viewing through the notch, but sometimes this procedure is reversed. Even the flat operating arthroscope fits this sleeve.

The wire or needle is followed by sharp then blunt trocars, preferably cannulated. These trocars are also inserted under direct vision as an assistant simultaneously pumps a 60-ml syringe full of saline solution through the arthroscope as a counter force against the joint capsule.

Finally, a flexible sleeve is inserted and is sutured to the skin to prevent its inadvertent withdrawal during manipulation of the leg or instruments. This approach can then be used to extend short longitudinal tears in either direction, or more importantly, to create a longitudinal excision line for en bloc resections of shattered menisci that would otherwise have to be removed piecemeal (Fig. 20–6).

LONGITUDINAL TEARS OF THE PERIPHERAL RIM

Whether short or long, these tears are usually associated with anterior cruciate ligament injuries. The trend is toward repair. If one elects to excise rather than to repair, the longer the tear, the easier the excision. The entire meniscus can be avulsed from the meniscal rim with only the anterior and posterior attachments remaining intact. This procedure is the simplest of meniscectomies. If a short tear is to be excised, the posteromedial puncture is used to convert it to a longer tear, which can then be managed from anteriorly with a two-puncture technique.

A short longitudinal tear can be extended centrally to the posterior attach-

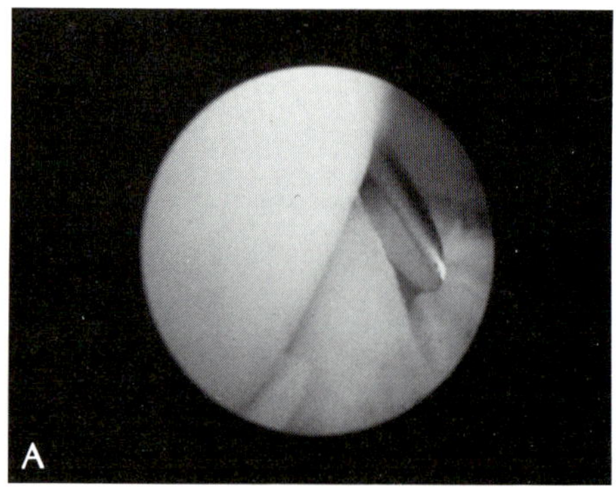

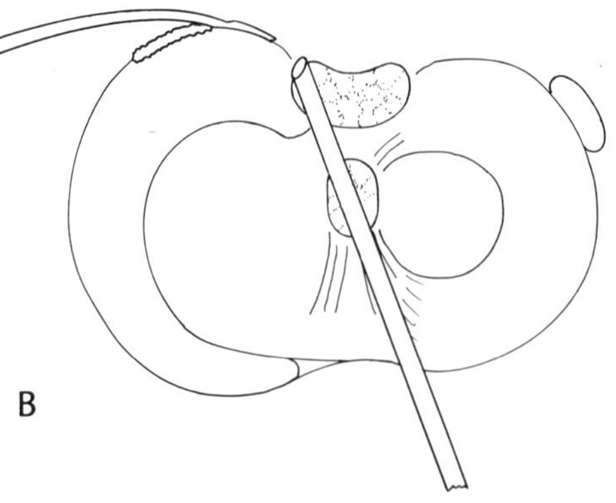

Fig. 20–7. *A* **and** *B,* **Either a curved knife or curved scissors will extend a short tear or an incision line centrally toward the medial posterior attachment.**

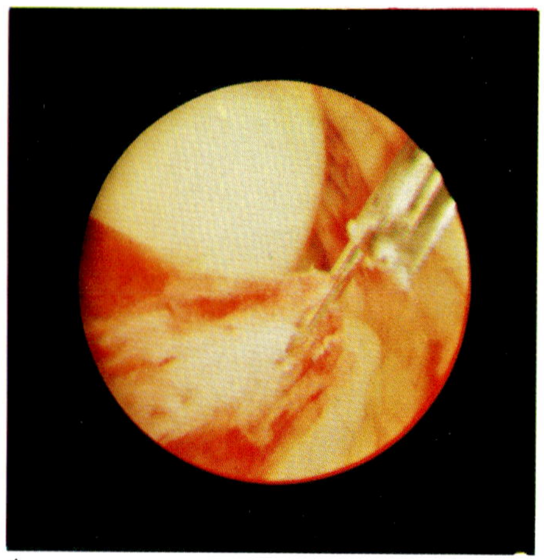

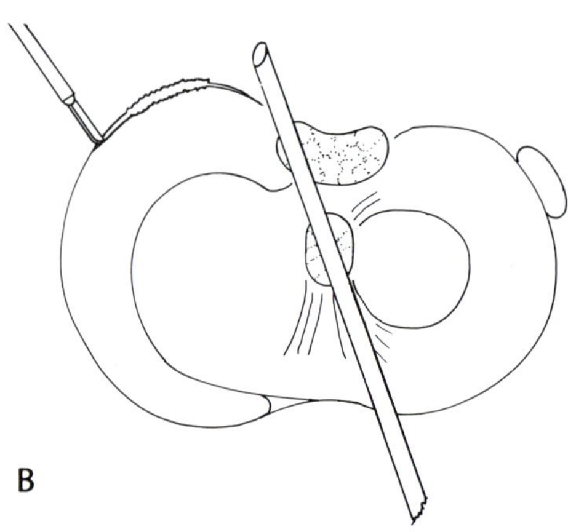

Fig. 20–8. *A* **and** *B,* **Gently curved end and side cutting knives, such as the Beaver No. 64 series, extend a short tear or an incision line around the posteromedial "corner" toward the medial collateral ligament. The puncture must be** ***superior to*** **the joint line.**

ment with a curved Smillie-type knife or with curved scissors through the instrument sleeve (Fig. 20–7). To extend a peripheral tear toward the medial collateral ligament, a side-cutting knife such as a Beaver No. 6490 blade is used. The blade is inserted into the tear and is swept medially around the meniscal rim; one should stay as close as possible to the femoral condyle to preserve the circumferential meniscal fibers. The incision is brought anteriorly as far as possible. With a 120° retrograde arthroscope, one can see anteriorly to the fibers of the medial collateral ligament, and triangulation is actually easier than with a 70° arthroscope (Fig. 20–8).

Anterior and Posterior Completion

Once a longitudinal tear has been extended, it can be managed as any other longitudinal tear, simply by releasing it anteriorly and posteriorly in a "blended" fashion. I would normally choose the operating arthroscope for completing both the anterior and posterior attachments (see Chap. 17), but alternatives are available. A retrograde knife, such as the Beaver No. 6006, can be used to both detach the posterior meniscal horn and to make the anterior cut through the inner rim. A retrograde knife is difficult to control if slightly dull and makes unaesthetic cuts in the anterior compartment (Fig. 20–9).

A side-cutting knife, such as the Beaver No. 6490, can also be used to cut anteriorly from the axilla of the longitudinal excision of the posterior meniscal horn. As it reaches the anterior third of the meniscus, however, this blade skives into a horizontal plane and leaves a poorly blended cut, unless it is switched to the lateral portal. This blade must also be handled with special care to avoid damaging the articular cartilage of the tibia (Fig. 20–10).

A posterior detachment may be partially made with scissors or a retrograde knife from the anteromedial puncture, prior to displacing the meniscus and grasping it from the lateral puncture. This maneuver reduces wear and tear and the risk of damage to the small scissors of the operating arthroscope, which are used to release the final threads.

Mixed Tears (Shattered Meniscus)

If a medial meniscus is hopelessly disintegrated with a mixture of tears, but with no significant longitudinal component, a total meniscectomy is the most tedious of all arthroscopic procedures. The alternatives are either a piecemeal resection by a two-puncture technique or an en bloc resection using a third portal posteromedi-

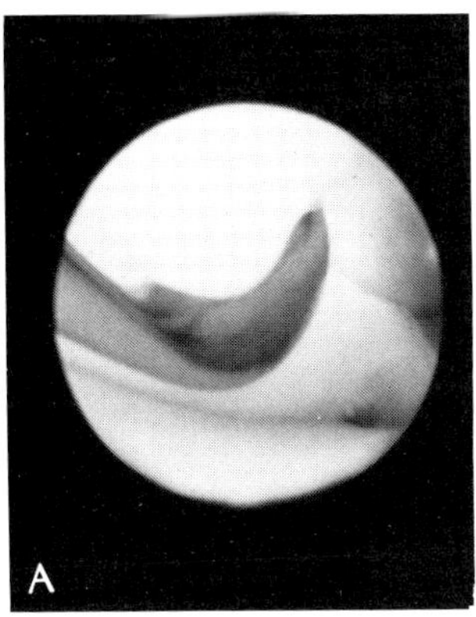

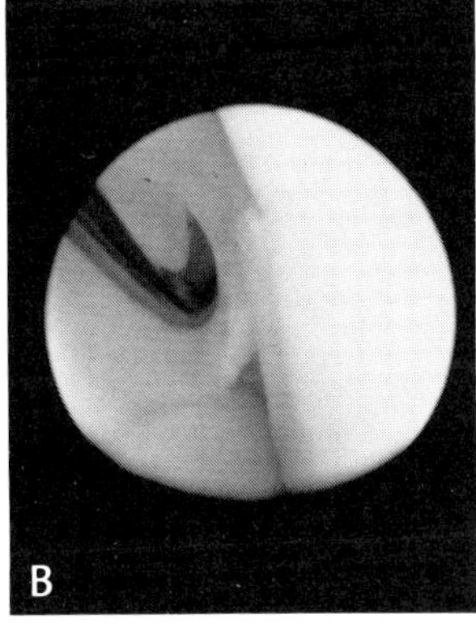

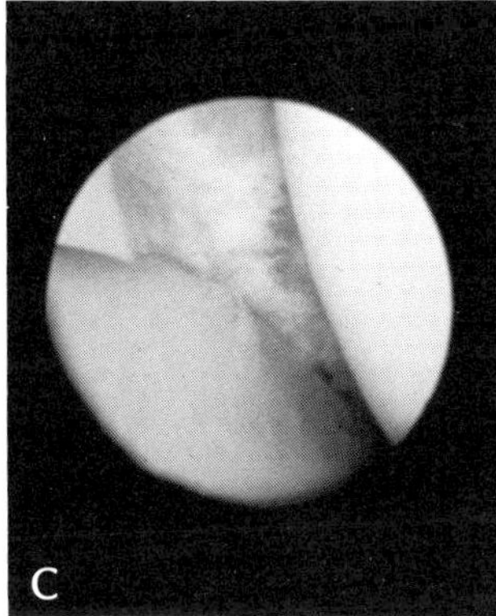

Fig. 20–9. *A,* **A retrograde knife releases posterior attachments. It must be sharp and meticulously controlled to avoid damaging the articular cartilage and the anterior cruciate ligament.** *B,* **A retrograde-knife can also be used for anterior releases.** *C,* **Retrograde knives allow less fixation anteriorly and less control. Skiving cuts such as this one may result.**

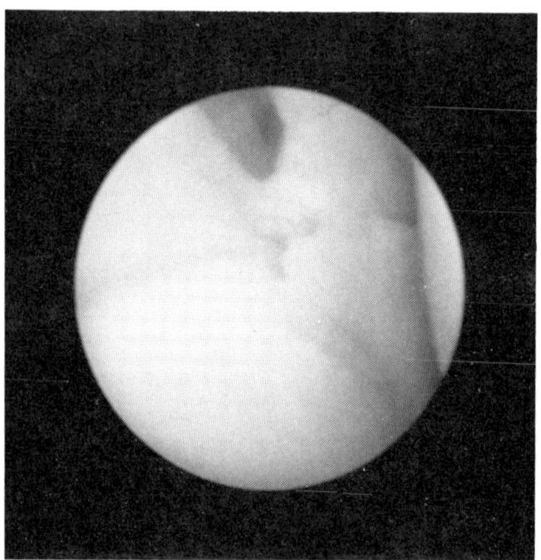

Fig. 20–10. A side-cutting blade makes an acceptable "exit" in the rim of the middle third of the meniscus. Further anteriorly, it also skives.

ally. Mixed tears are frequently associated with degenerative joint disease, may not be causally related to the patient's symptoms, and rarely deserve such radical treatment as a total excision.

Piecemeal Resection. With a 30°-angled arthroscope in an anterolateral puncture, the inner rim of a medial meniscus can be seen from its anterior to its posterior attachment. The posterior half of the meniscus can be removed piecemeal with basket forceps through a medial puncture. This technique requires patience and an extra assistant to help spread the tight medial compartment. Some surgeons use a mechanical thigh holder for this purpose.[18]

To "blend" this saucerization smoothly into the inner rim of the anterior of the meniscus, the basket forceps must be inserted through the lateral puncture, either through an operating arthroscope or with the diagnostic arthroscope transferred to the medial puncture (Fig. 20–11).

The largest basket forceps that pass inferior to the femoral condyle are those 3.4 mm in diameter. Saucerizing the posterior meniscal horn causes considerable wear and tear on these small instruments. The strongest objection to piecemeal resection, however, is the risk of scuffing the articular cartilage of the medial compartment.

Powered meniscal cutters are also helpful for piecemeal resections, in conjunction with scissors and basket forceps. The hand instruments are used to create flaps of tissue, which can then be handled by the end-cutting "keyhole" of a powered meniscal cutter.

En Bloc Resection. In a tight knee, en bloc resection is preferable to scuffing the articular cartilage of the medial compartment. This procedure can be accomplished by converting a mixed tear to a longitudinal tear through a posterior approach.

A plastic sleeve is inserted posterome-

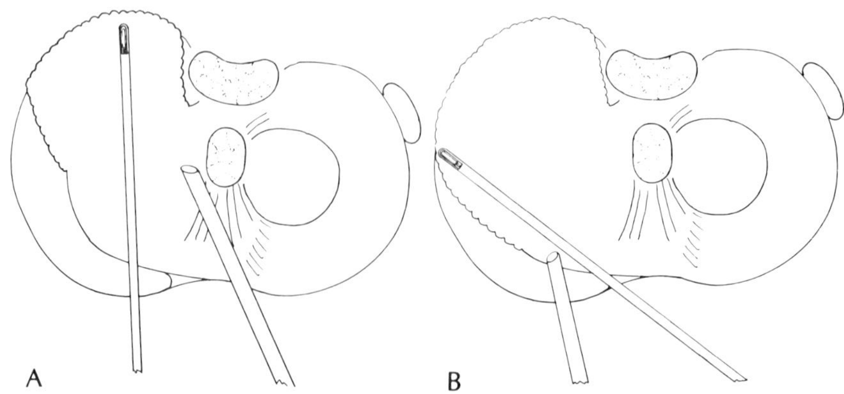

Fig. 20–11. To saucerize a medial meniscus is tedious work. Basket forceps 3.4 mm in diameter are the largest instruments that pass under a femoral condyle, and even these instruments scuff the articular cartilage. *A,* From the medial puncture, the posterior horn can be removed. *B,* To "blend" a cut safely through the junction of the medial and anterior thirds, the basket forceps must be inserted through the lateral puncture.

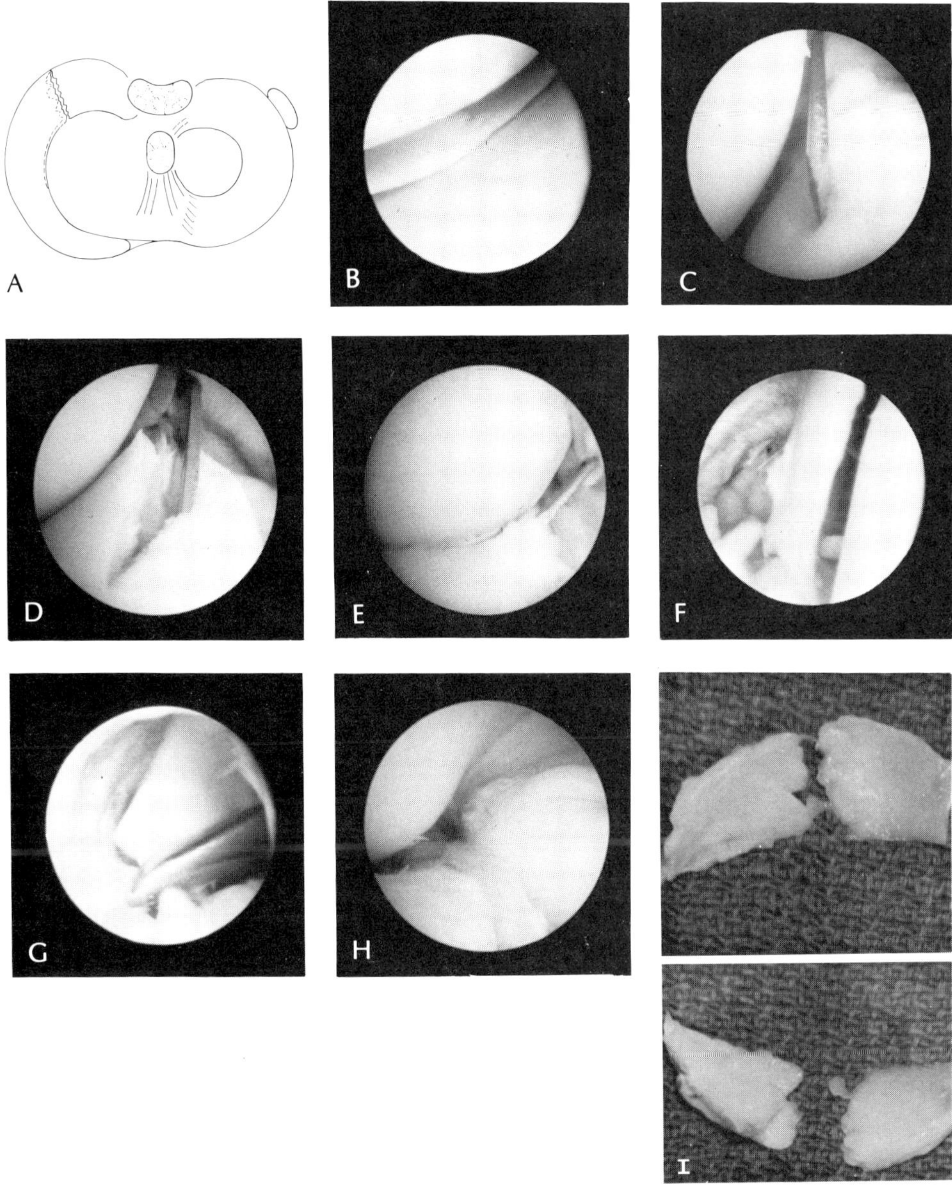

Fig. 20–12. A 56-year-old waitress caught her foot on a step at work, twisted her knee, and fell. An arthrogram showed "multiple irregularities of the medial meniscus." Arthroscopy showed (*A* and *B*) a radial tear extending to the synovial border of the posterior horn with a horizontal component in the middle third of the meniscus. *C* and *D*, Through a posteromedial puncture, a Beaver No. 64 blade was used to create a circumferential excision near the synovial border to include the axilla of the radial tear. A 70° arthroscope through the notch permits one to view toward the medial side of the knee. *E*, As seen with the 120° arthroscope, the incision was extended forward to the medial collateral ligament. *F*, Once the posterior horn was detached, it floated freely in the posterior compartment. *G*, While the operator viewed with a 30° arthroscope through the posteromedial sleeve, the meniscus was removed through the notch with down-biting pituitary forceps. *H*, At the conclusion of the procedure, a small rim remained. *I*, The anterior excision was completed from the front, and the mixed lesion can best be seen on the undersurface of the specimen (bottom).

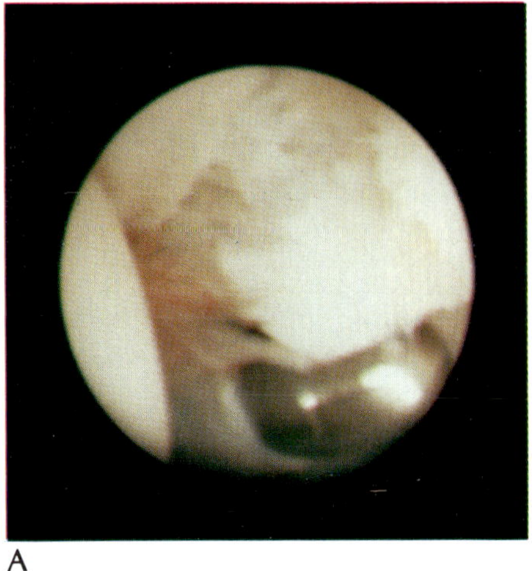

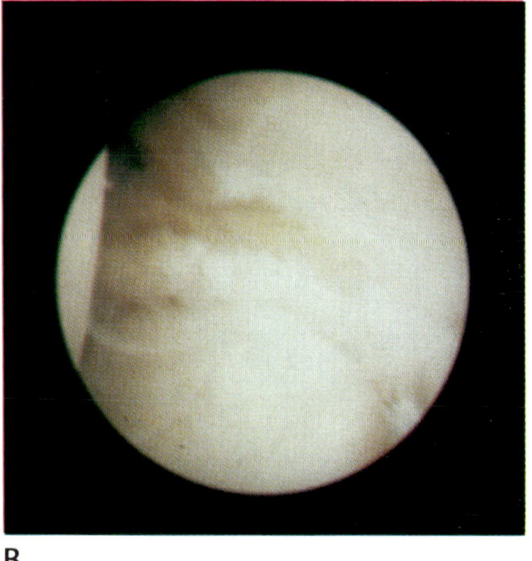

Fig. 20–13. *A,* **Shaver heads range from 3 to 5 mm in diameter. For clearing tags from the posterior horn, the posteromedial puncture is sometimes preferred.** *B,* **A notch view of a final result, showing the bare tibial surface after a total meniscectomy.**

dially as previously described. A side-cutting knife, such as the Beaver No. 6490, cuts into the top of the meniscus as far centrally as possible and as close to the femoral condyle as possible. A circumferential incision is made toward the medial collateral ligament, carrying the incision as far anteriorly as possible, staying close to the condyle. At this point, one is dealing with a longitudinal tear. The incision can be extended toward the posterior attachment with curved instruments, such as a Smillie knife or scissors, and the remainder of the excision can be managed as any other longitudinal tear of identical length (Fig. 20–12). If a stable peripheral rim (2 mm) has been preserved, this meniscectomy is *subtotal*.

Mixed tears may break under traction and may deliver in several large pieces. In this event, the posteromedial sleeve can be used for piecemeal resection by basket forceps and a power cutter and may still prevent scuffing in the tight medial compartment (Figs. 20–13).

TOTAL LATERAL MENISCECTOMY

Anatomic Features

The anatomy of the lateral compartment is so different from that of the medial that it has a significant influence on the diagnosis, natural history, and surgical management of tears of the lateral meniscus. First, the lateral meniscus is loosely attached posteriorly, and this attachment should not be mistaken for a pathologic condition.

Regarding meniscectomy, it is the *anterior* horn that is hard to manage on the lateral side. This area is broad, sweeps posteriorly toward the tibial spine, and thereby makes it difficult to effect an entry into the thin edge. The posterior compartment, on the other hand, spreads easily and allows 5-mm instruments to pass inferior to the femoral condyle without scuffing.

The lateral compartment is small and circular. That the "O"-shaped lateral meniscus rests on a convex, dome-shaped tibia may account for the so-called "silent lesions," that is, tears that do not catch, lock, or cause significant pain. It is not rare to find asymptomatic, healed, or stable tears of the lateral meniscus; these findings suggest that one should avoid overdiagnosing and overtreating this structure.

Longitudinal Tears

By definition, only excisions that include the popliteal sulcus are considered to be

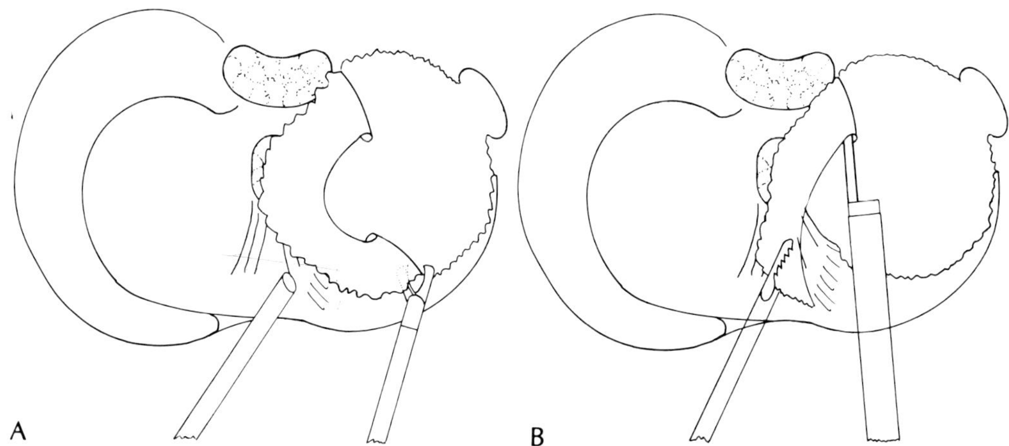

Fig. 20–14. ***A,*** **Anterior release of a displaced lateral meniscus involves so much tissue in such a small space that 5-mm scissors are usually preferred; 30 or 70° arthroscopes permit a variety of perspectives.** ***B,*** **Preliminary posterior attachment cuts are helpful, but final release with control and traction prevents loss of the fragment. The lateral meniscus is broad and thick, and it requires a generous puncture for en bloc removal.**

total meniscectomies. Lesions so treated are usually long, displaceable (bucket-handle) tears. A *displaced* (locked) tear is excised in the same manner as a locked medial bucket-handle tear. The anterior attachment is easy to resect if it is displaced, by using 5-mm scissors from the lateral puncture. The fragment is then retracted medially, and the posterior attachment is released with the operating arthroscope in the lateral compartment (Fig. 20–14).

If the anterior cruciate ligament is torn (67%), the instruments can be reversed, and the operating arthroscope inserted medially, a more comfortable position for the surgeon if the patient's leg is in a figure-4 position. A *displaceable* tear should be deliberately *displaced* to facilitate the anterior release. Conversely, it is helpful to *reduce* a displaced meniscus, in order to release the posterior attachment with 5-mm scissors, and to save the operating arthroscope for the last few threads.

To excise a *nondisplaceable* tear, the most

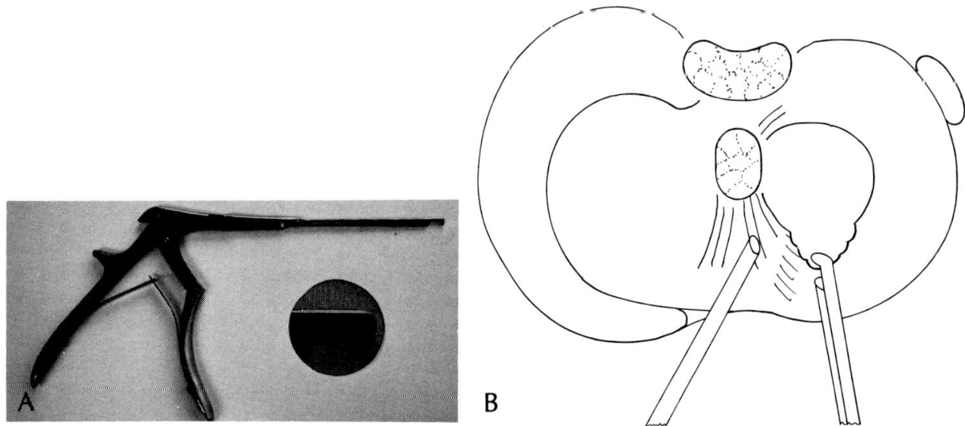

Fig. 20–15. ***A*** **and** ***B,*** **3- or 4-mm down-biting Kerrison forceps are useful for this single purpose, although the instrument also removes osteophytes, for example.**

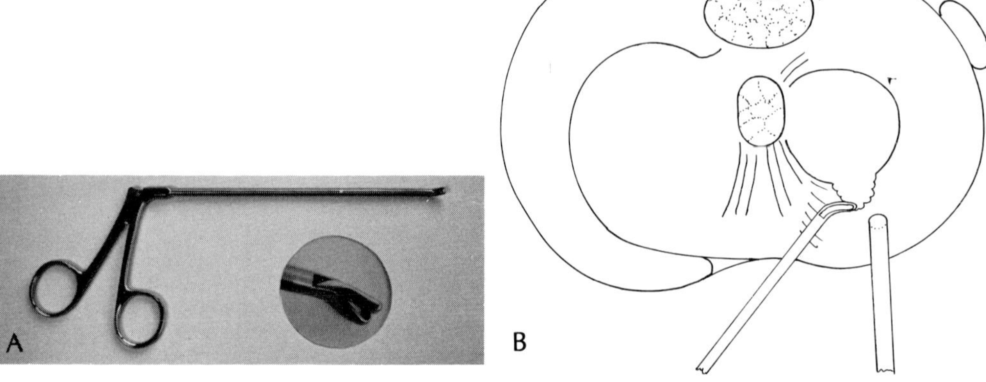

Fig. 20–16. *A* **and** *B,* **Stryker markets these versatile, angled basket forceps with right and left curves, useful in both compartments.**

difficult problem is to make a smooth entry into the thin edge of the anterior horn of the meniscus. Two instruments make this difficult cut. Stronger and more reliable are neurosurgical down-biting Kerrison forceps with a 3- or 4-mm mouth (Fig. 20–15). The advantage of this instrument, in addition to its indestructibility, is that it can be inserted into the lateral puncture, giving the arthroscopist a better perspective from the medial side. The commercial instrument has sharp edges, which should be buffed away to avoid abrading articular cartilage. The other instrument is 45°-angled basket forceps marketed by Stryker, which must be inserted through a medial puncture while the operator views from the lateral puncture. The function of these instruments is the same, to saucerize the inner rim toward the periphery for 5 to 6 mm in order to manage it as a medial meniscus (Fig. 20–16). The anterior axilla of the short tear is then connected to the saucerized entry, either by a side-cutting knife used in a retrograde manner from a lateral portal, or by scissors, preferably through an operating arthroscope, from the medial portal. The meniscus can now be displaced into the intercondylar notch, and the posterior meniscal horn can be released as described.

Although the lateral compartment spreads more easily than the medial, it is small, and the meniscus occupies most of its space. It is not always easy to execute these surgical techniques because of crowding of tissue and instruments. If this crowding becomes frustrating for the surgeon, the entire lateral meniscus can be saucerized with 5-mm basket forceps in piecemeal fashion. At times, this method is a last resort, but with each small excision, visibility improves and the procedure becomes easier.

Mixed Tears

Only rarely do horizontal, radial, or mixed tears extend into the popliteal sulcus and require a total meniscectomy. In these instances, the meniscus is saucerized with 5-mm basket forceps until the remaining anterior and posterior rims are stable and well blended; one should save as much tissue as possible in both anterior and posterior meniscal horns (Fig. 20–17).

Cystic Degeneration

In the course of almost 600 arthroscopic meniscectomies, only 1 knee was opened, and this was for total excision of a meniscus. This was the knee of a 66-year-old housewife who had cystic degeneration of the lateral meniscus. While exposing a 3-cm cyst at the joint line, we found that

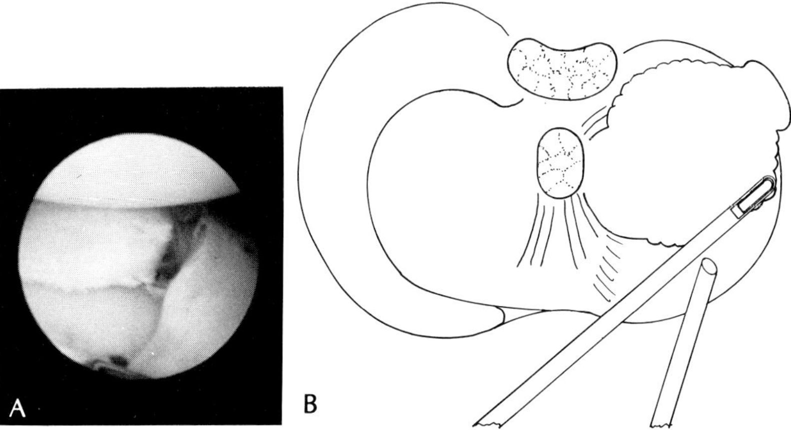

Fig. 20–17. ***A,*** **This is a rare example of a single radial tear extending into the popliteal sulcus.** ***B,*** **For total, subtotal, or partial meniscectomy, 5-mm basket forceps saucerize everything in the lateral compartment except the anterior horn.**

almost the entire meniscus was involved with mixed tears. An en bloc resection was made of the cyst and the complete meniscus. The original plan had been to excise the cyst, repair the peripheral meniscal rim, and remove any unstable fragments from the inner rim. Three medial cysts have been treated in this manner, and as yet no tears have recurred. Interestingly, this patient refused hospital admission, crutches, or a walker. Her postoperative management was the same as for all closed meniscectomies, and no significant difference was seen in morbidity.

POSTOPERATIVE CARE

Almost all arthroscopic surgical patients are treated at the short-stay facility of a general hospital. For total meniscectomies, a single suction (Hemovac) tube is inserted through a puncture during wound closure. This tube is removed an hour later in the recovery room, prior to ambulation of the patient. Ice is applied to the knee for the first 24 hours. The short-stay nurses instruct the patient in straight leg raising, quadriceps muscle setting, and antiphlebitic exercises before and after the surgical procedure. Most patients walk unassisted as soon as they have recovered from general anesthesia and are discharged usually within 2 hours.

The dressing is changed on the first postoperative day, and the knee is aspirated if an effusion of 40 ml or more is suspected (about 35%). Knee flexion to 90° begins on the first postoperative day, and gentle resistance exercises follow a day or so later. Salicylates are started on the first postoperative day and are maintained for 2 or 3 weeks for their anti-inflammatory and anticoagulant effects. Printed instructions supplement verbal orders for progressive ranging and strengthening exercises. Most patients (78%) are referred to a physical therapist for muscle evaluation and supervised exercises until the knee joint's range and strength equal that of the normal extremity.

COMPLICATIONS

In reviewing 400 arthroscopic meniscectomies, 3 synovial sinuses were found, all in posteromedial punctures.[3] This approach is not restricted to total meniscectomies, but is more likely to be used for these operations. The sinuses disappeared without treatment other than sterile dressings and elastic bandaging. Other complications were minor and rare, and the incidence was no different from that in patients undergoing partial and subtotal meniscectomies.

REFERENCES

1. Smillie, I.S.: Injuries of the Knee Joint. 5th Ed. Edinburgh, Churchill Livingstone, 1978.
2. Tapper, E.H., and Hoover, N.W.: The later results of meniscectomy. J. Bone Joint Surg. (Am.), *51*:517, 1969.
3. King, D.: The function of semilunar cartilages. J. Bone Joint Surg., *18*:333, 1936.
4. O'Connor, R.: Arthroscopy. Philadelphia, J.B. Lippincott, 1977.
5. Oretorp, N., and Risberg, N.: Studies on the fine structure of the medial meniscus and ligaments and their anatomical relations in the human knee. Linkoping University Medical Dissertation No. 63, 1978.
6. Bullough, P.G., et al.: The strength of the meniscus as it relates to their fine structure. J. Bone Joint Surg. (Br.), *52*:564, 1970.
7. MacConaill, M.A.: The movements of bones and joints: 3. The synovial fluid and its assistants. J. Bone Joint Surg. (Br.), *32*:244, 1950.
8. Hsieh, H., and Walker, P.S.: Stabilizing mechanisms of the loaded and unloaded knee joint. J. Bone Joint Surg. (Am.), *58*:87, 1976.
9. Seedhom, B.B., and Hargreaves, D.J.: Transmission of the load to the knee joint with special reference to the role of the menisci. Part II. Eng. Med., *8*:220, 1979.
10. Walker, P.S., and Erkman, M.J.: The role of the meniscus in force transmission across the knee. Clin. Orthop., *109*:184, 1975.
11. Wang, C.J., and Walker, P.S.: Rotatory laxity of the human knee. J. Bone Joint Surg. (Am.), *56*:161, 1974.
12. Carson, R.W.: Arthroscopic meniscectomy: a four year follow up. Presented at the Fourth Congress of the International Arthroscopy Association, Rio de Janeiro, 1981.
13. Ikeuchi, H.: Meniscectomy surgery using the Watanabe arthroscope. Orthop. Clin. North Am., *10*:629, 1979.
14. Carson, R.W.: Arthroscopic meniscectomy. Orthop. Clin. North Am., *10*:619, 1979.
15. Oretorp, N., and Gillquist, J.: Transcutaneous meniscectomy under arthroscopic control. Int. Orthop., *3*:19, 1979.
16. Gillquist, J., and Hagberg, G.: A new modification of the technique of arthroscopy of the knee joint. Acta Chir. Scand., *142*:123, 1976.
17. Gillquist, J., Hagberg, G., and Oretorp, N.: Arthroscopic visualization of the posteromedial compartment of the knee joint. Orthop. Clin. North Am., *10*:545, 1979.
18. Johnson, L.L.: Diagnostic and Surgical Arthroscopy. St. Louis, C.V. Mosby, 1981.

Chapter 21

PERIPHERAL MENISCUS REPAIR

Kenneth E. DeHaven

With the increasing knowledge of the functional significance of normal menisci and of the disappointing, late degenerative changes seen following meniscectomy, the rationale for attempting to treat meniscal lesions without resorting to meniscectomy, even partial meniscectomy, is obvious. A long-standing precedent exists for the concept of meniscal repair. The Scottish surgeon Annandale reported repairing the anterior horn of the medial meniscus in the mid-1800s. Repair of peripheral meniscal tears in conjunction with repairs of acute medial or lateral collateral ligament tears has long been advocated by Hughston and Eilers[1] and Allman,[2] and favorable results have been reported by Price and Allen.[3]

Menisci have long been considered avascular structures and therefore incapable of healing. King demonstrated the healing response to experimental meniscal lesions in dogs in the 1930s,[4] and these findings have been confirmed by more recent studies by Arnoczky,[5] myself and my colleagues,[6] and Cabaud and associates[7] in primates. Although clinical experience makes it apparent that spontaneous healing does not readily occur in humans, Arnoczky and Warren have demonstrated a consistent vascularity in the peripheral 10 to 20% of human menisci that indicates the potential for healing of lesions occurring in this vascular zone.[8]

In addition to peripheral meniscal repair, discussed in this chapter, anterocentral detachments of the menisci, particularly of the medial meniscus, have also been found to be reparable, sometimes arthroscopically. Stone[9] and Goletz and Clancy[10] have reported techniques and results of repair of these lesions, which are rare in my experience.

Although the repair techniques described here are open procedures, interest remains high in the concept of arthroscopic meniscal repair. Ikeuchi has reported a few peripheral tears in the medial third of the meniscus that have been repaired under arthroscopic control,[11] and it is certainly conceivable that peripheral or near peripheral tears in the posterior third may be amenable to arthroscopic repair in the future. Additionally, repair of tears within the substance of the meniscus may be feasible if a source of vascular response is present or can be created, and it is a distinct possibility that arthroscopic meniscal repair may become routine in the future.

SELECTION CRITERIA

Menisci selected for repair must have a vertical tear at or near the periphery of the

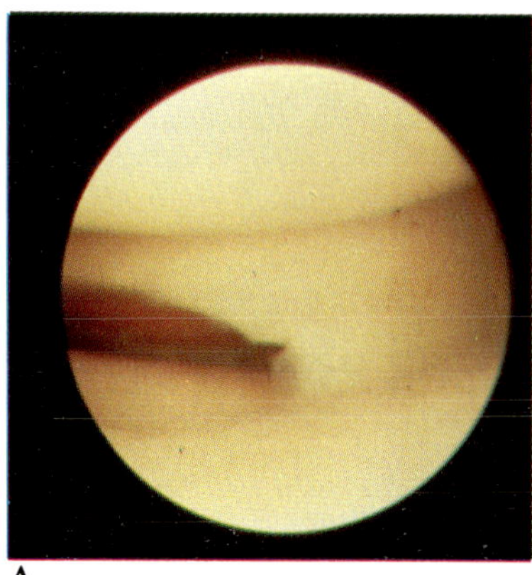

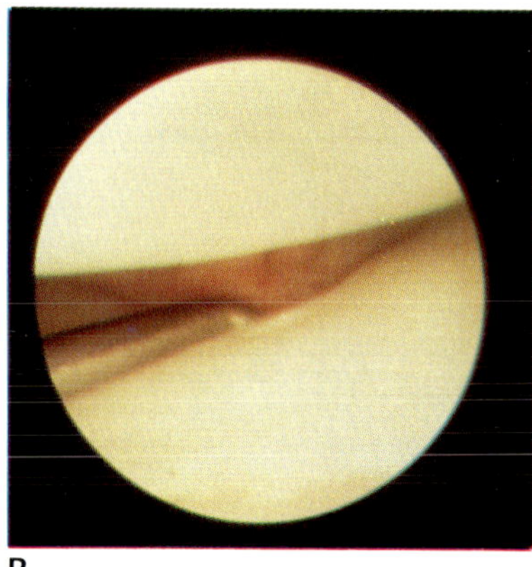

Fig. 21–1. Careful arthroscopic examination is frequently necessary to demonstrate a peripheral tear. This arthroscopic photograph of a lateral meniscus *(A)* looks normal, until examination with a probe *(B)* clearly demonstrates the posterior peripheral detachment.

meniscus, with the body of the meniscus intact. Arthrography is a useful adjunct in preselection of reparable lesions, especially chronic cases. A vertical peripheral tear with no staining of the body of the meniscus should be a good candidate for repair, whereas a similar peripheral vertical tear with significant staining into the meniscal body is not suitable.

Direct visualization of the meniscus arthroscopically is essential to confirm the peripheral or near peripheral location of the tear and to confirm that the body of the meniscus is intact. The use of a probe is frequently required to demonstrate the lesion (Fig. 21–1), and often the posterior horn of the meniscus can be subluxed inferior to the femoral condyle with the probe. It is also important to determine the length or extent of the lesion. Short tears under 5 mm in length are usually not symptomatic and rarely require treatment, but tears over 5 mm in length, particularly over 1 cm, are sufficiently unstable to be symptomatic and should be treated. If the body of the meniscus is significantly damaged, conventional repair will have little or no chance of success, and arthroscopic resection should be performed.

The period of time following injury within which successful repair is still possible remains in doubt, but if the basic criteria for selection can be satisfied, the time factor may be ignored. Some lesions present for more than a year have been successfully repaired.

SURGICAL TECHNIQUE

Following arthroscopic confirmation of a reparable lesion, the patient's leg is reprepared and draped in the usual sterile fashion before proceeding to arthrotomy for repair. The exposure is made through a direct posteromedial or posterolateral approach; one must avoid the major stabilizing structures.[12] The tear is seldom exactly at the meniscocapsular junction, and frequently, a small portion of the meniscal rim remains attached to the joint capsule. This rim is excised as required to create a well-vascularized capsular bed, which is sutured back to the rim of the meniscus using vertically oriented sutures of fine absorbable material (Fig. 21–2). The sutures are placed 2 to 3 mm apart, and one uses as many as necessary to repair the lesion. The individual sutures are tagged with hemostats until all sutures have been placed, and then are tied inside the joint sequentially, starting with the most distantly placed suture.

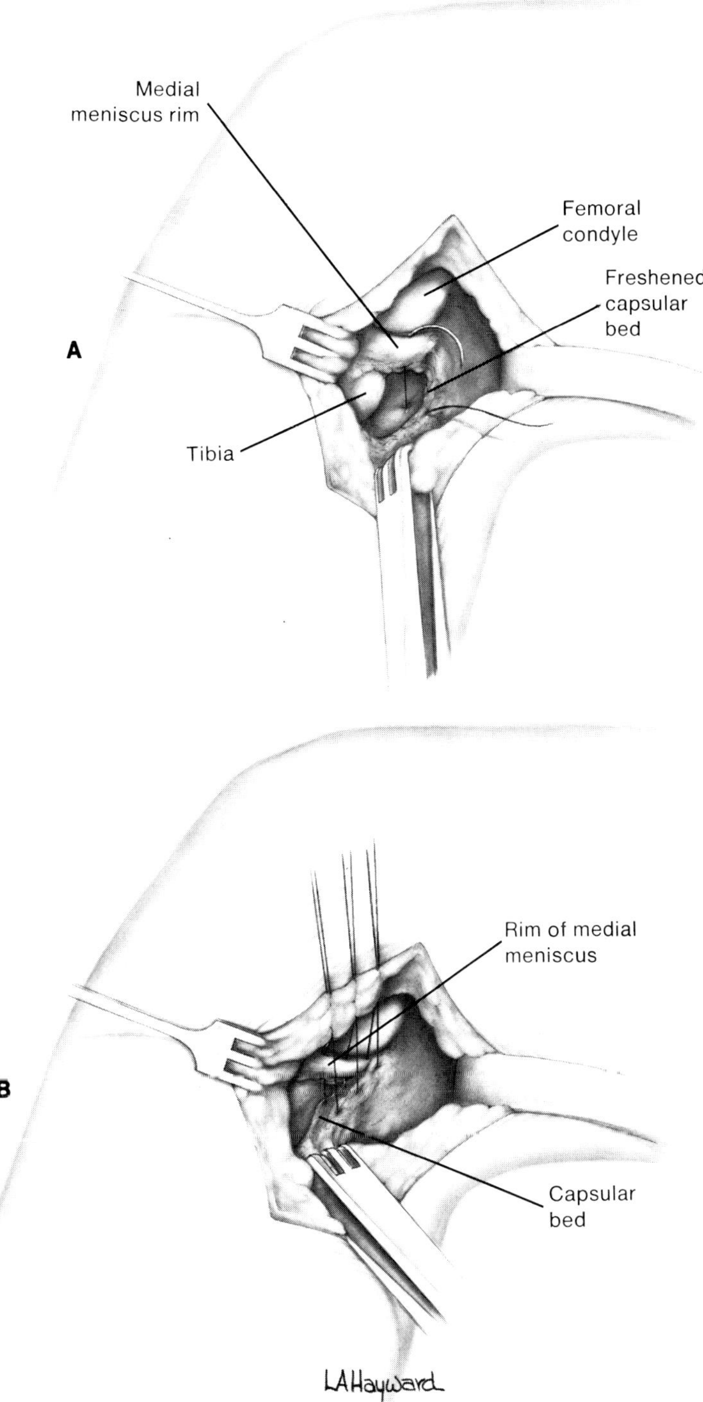

Fig. 21–2. Technique of peripheral repair of the medial meniscus through a posteromedial approach. *A,* A repair suture is placed vertically through the freshened capsular bed and then vertically through the rim of the meniscus. *B,* The repair sutures (2 to 3 mm apart) are tied after all have been placed, to reapproximate the capsular bed to the rim of the meniscus. (From Goldstein, L.A., and Dickerson, R.C. (eds.): Atlas of Orthopaedic Surgery. 2nd Ed. St. Louis, C.V. Mosby, 1981.)

Cassidy and Shaffer[13] have reported a slightly different technique for repair of the medial meniscus in which the medial head of the gastrocnemius muscle is separated from the posteromedial joint capsule, and the vertically oriented sutures are passed through the capsule and are tied outside it. The capsular incision is then closed in a plicating fashion, and the knee is immobilized at approximately 45° of flexion.

POSTOPERATIVE CARE

The knee is immobilized in flexion for 4 weeks, followed by active range of motion and isometric quadriceps muscle exercises for 2 additional weeks while the patient remains on crutches. Six weeks following the surgical procedure, progressive resistance exercises are initiated, and crutches are used until the patient is able to lift 15 pounds with the quadriceps muscles. If the patient is athletic and wishes to return to running sports, straight-ahead jogging and half-speed running are permitted when the range of motion has returned and the quadriceps muscle exercises are performed with the patient lifting 30 pounds. Full-speed running and agility maneuvers such as hard starts and stops, cuts, or jumps are not permitted for at least 6 months following the procedure, to allow time for maturation of the healing collagen. If any ligamentous repair or reconstruction was done at the same time (anterior cruciate ligament surgical procedures are frequently also performed), the protocol for the ligamentous procedure dictates the postoperative care program.

RESULTS

Between 1976 and 1981, I repaired 104 menisci using this technique. It was a young, athletic group of patients, ranging in age from 11 to 40 years, with the average being 18. The male-to-female ratio was 3:1, with 2 medial menisci repaired for every lateral meniscus. Slightly more than half the repairs were acute, within 2 weeks of the injury, and virtually all patients also had acute anterior cruciate ligament tears. The remainder (47%) were late repairs, at least 5 weeks following the injury (usually 4 to 6 months), and half the patients with late repairs also had old tears of the anterior cruciate ligament. Some of these patients underwent anterior cruciate ligament reconstruction at the time of the meniscal repair. Between 1978 and 1981, repaired menisci constituted 20% of all meniscal tears treated.

This group of patients was athletic and all returned to at least a recreational level of athletics, placing strenuous running, cutting, and jumping stresses upon the knee. With the exception of the patients sustaining retears, and a few patients who continued to have functional anterior cruciate ligament instability requiring subsequent reconstruction, patients who underwent meniscal repair procedures were surprisingly free of symptoms such as pain, swelling, or giving way.

To date, 7 menisci have retorn (7%). All were late repairs, and to date, no acute repair has retorn. Three retore through a different portion of the meniscus, which could be treated by arthroscopic partial meniscectomy leaving behind a significant peripheral rim well attached to the joint capsule (Fig. 21–3). Follow-up arthroscopic examination of 6 repaired menisci that had not retorn demonstrated satisfactory healing in each (Fig. 21–4).

In summary, selected peripheral meniscal tears can be successfully repaired, and the early results (up to 5.5 years follow-up) are encouraging, even with a return to high-demand athletic function of the knee. Long-term studies will be necessary to prove that these repaired menisci hold up, continue to function, and avoid the degenerative changes seen following meniscectomy. One hopes that repair techniques will become applicable to other types of tears, to increase the numbers of torn menisci that can potentially be salvaged, and it is likely that these procedures will be performed arthroscopically in the future.

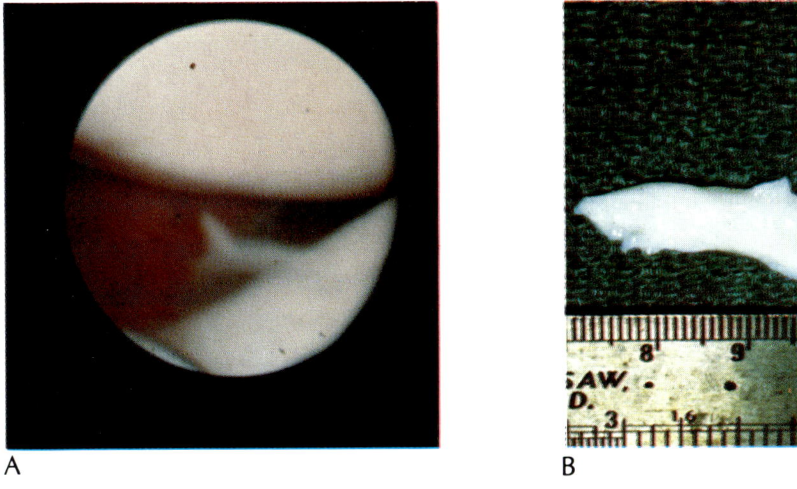

A B

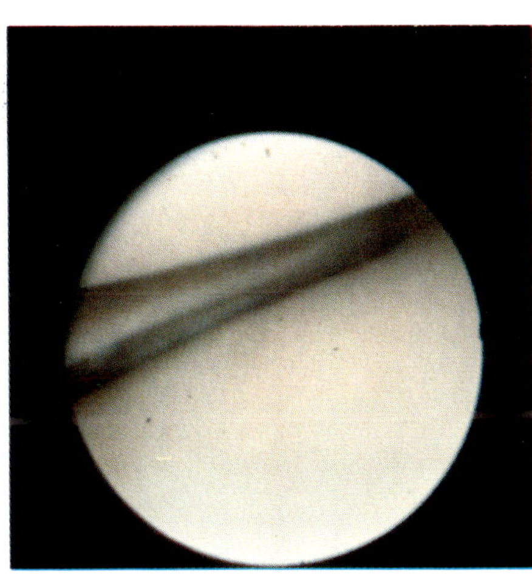

C

Fig. 21–3. Retear of a previously repaired medial meniscus. *A,* The arthroscopic picture of a medial meniscus repaired 14 months previously that retore as a displaced bucket-handle tear. The medial femoral condyle is seen superiorly, and the displaced fragment of medial meniscus inferiorly. *B,* This photograph shows the displaced portion of the meniscus that was excised arthroscopically. *C,* The arthroscopic appearance of the remaining posterior peripheral rim following resection of the retorn and displaced fragment. The femoral condyle is seen superiorly, the tibial plateau is seen inferiorly, and in between is a substantial posterior rim, which was well attached to the capsule in the area of the previous repair.

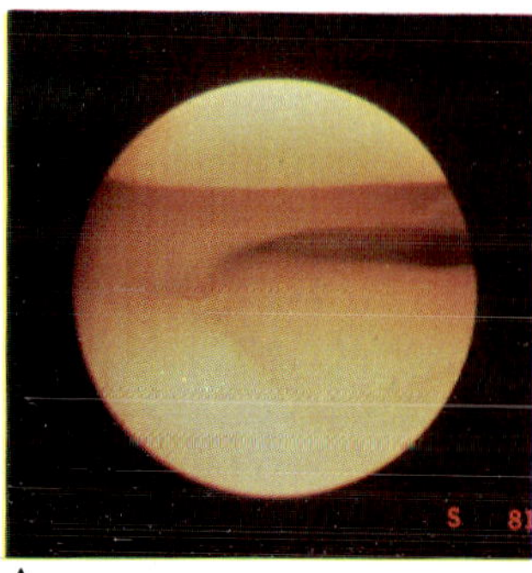
A

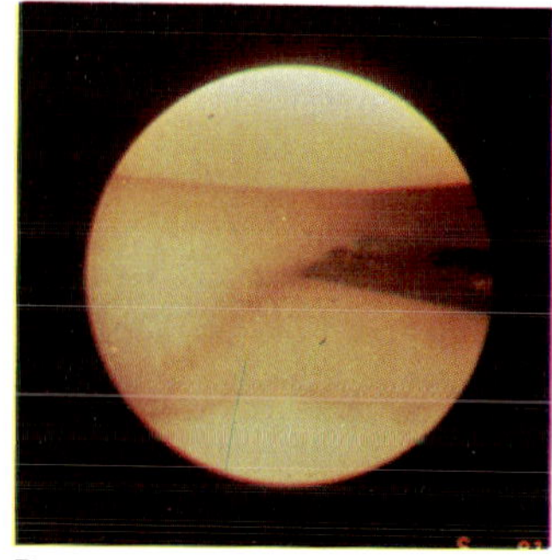
B

Fig. 21–4. ***A,*** **A previously repaired lateral meniscus is examined arthroscopically 14 months following repair at the time of subsequent anterior cruciate ligament reconstruction; this photograph demonstrates a normal appearance of the meniscus and articular cartilage of the lateral femoral and tibial condyles.** ***B,*** **A probe introduced to evaluate the posterior horn demonstrates the normal stability provided by the previous repair.**

REFERENCES

1. Hughston, J.C., and Eilers, A.F.: The role of the posterior oblique ligament in repairs of acute medial (collateral) ligament tears of the knee. J. Bone Joint Surg. (Am.), *55*:923, 1973.
2. Allman, F.L.: Personal communication.
3. Price, C.T., and Allen, W.C.: Ligament repair in the knee with preservation of the meniscus. J. Bone Joint Surg. (Am.), *60*:61, 1978.
4. King, D.: The healing of semilunar cartilages. J. Bone Joint Surg., *18*:333–342, April, 1936.
5. Arnoczky, S.P.: Experimental studies of meniscus healing. Presented at the Orthopaedic Research Society, Las Vegas, 1981.
6. DeHaven, K.E., Thorpe, W.P., and Brodell, J.D.: Unpublished data.
7. Cabaud, H.E., Rodkey, W.G., and Fitzwater. J.E.: Medial meniscus repairs. An experimental and morphologic study. Am. J. Sports Med., *9*:129, 1981.
8. Arnoczky, S.P., and Warren, R.F.: Microvasculature of the human meniscus. Am. J. Sports Med., *10*:90, 1982.
9. Stone, R.G.: Anterior central meniscus tears. Presented at the Third Congress of the International Arthrosocpy Association, Kyoto, 1978.
10. Goletz, T., and Clancy, W.G.: Symptomatic dislocation of the anterior horn of the medial meniscus. Presented at the American Orthopaedic Society for Sports Medicine Annual Meeting, Big Sky, Montana, 1980.
11. Ikeuchi, H.: Paper presented at the Second Congress of the International Arthroscopy Association, Copenhagen, 1975.
12. DeHaven, K.E.: *In* Atlas of Orthopaedic Surgery, 2nd Ed. Edited by L.A. Goldstein and R.C. Dickerson. St Louis, C.V. Mosby, 1981.
13. Cassidy, R.E., and Shaffer, A.J.: Repair of peripheral meniscus tears. A preliminary report. Am. J. Sports Med., *9*:209, 1981.

Chapter 22

USE OF THE LASER BEAM IN ARTHROSCOPIC SURGERY*

James M. Glick

Laser, an acronym for Light Amplification by Stimulated Emission of Radiation, has been used to perform many types of surgical procedures, including those to repair a detached retina, to control gastrointestinal hemorrhage, and to remove tattoos. A potential also appears to exist for laser in arthroscopic surgery, but thus far it has been used only on an experimental basis.

In a laser, the active material, whether solid, liquid, or gas, is placed in an optical cavity and energy (light, electric, or other forms) is pumped from the side to excite the molecules to a high energy level (Fig. 22–1). The light emitted by the laser material reflects back and forth in the optical cavity, multiplies, and emerges from one end of the cavity. Using this phenomenon, a highly intense, columnated, and monochromatic beam of light is produced. By focusing down the beam with a lens system, a high energy density and peak power can be achieved in a small spot.[1] Laser cuts by burning or vaporizing.

The consideration of laser in arthroscopic meniscectomy stems from the difficulties with the present equipment, which must often be used in limited spaces. Knives do not cut easily in loose or floppy tissue, and they may damage the joint surfaces. Often, it is difficult to insert the cutting instrument into the joint at the proper angle to divide certain meniscal tears. When small instruments are used, much time is required to perform the surgical procedure. A laser might circumvent these difficulties and would be most effective if it could be directed through the same optics used for viewing. It would then cut cleanly through one incision and would simplify the procedure by eliminating multiple puncture sites and by reducing the need for manipulation of various instruments.

LASER TYPES

The available lasers are CO_2, argon, hydrogen fluoride (HF), and neodym-

*Editorial note:
This chapter on the possible application of the use of the laser in performing meniscectomies was written to give the reader a glimpse of one of the advances that may have application in the rapidly expanding field of arthroscopic surgery. As yet, little has appeared in the literature on this subject, and the information given here is culled from several papers written in the past year. It is a good summary of knowledge available as of March, 1983.

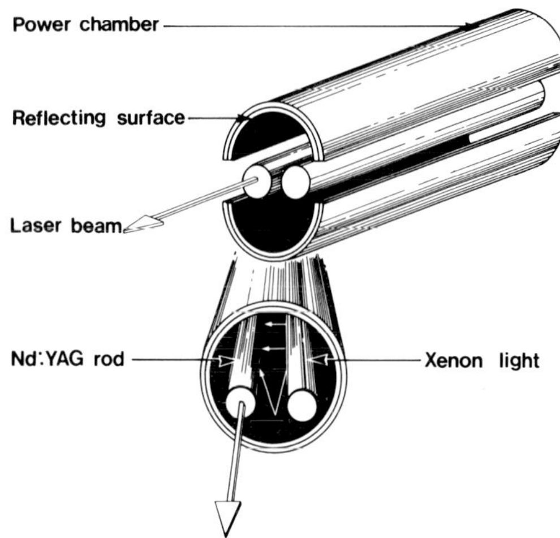

Fig. 22–1. Laser Source. See text for details.

ium:yttrium-aluminum-garnet (Nd:YAG). CO_2 laser, which emits at 10.6 μ, has been used in performing meniscectomies in humans.[2] Two disadvantages exist, however. First, lenses capable of transmitting visible radiation do not transmit CO_2 laser at 10.6 μ radiation. Therefore, another instrument or wand through a separate portal is necessary for cutting. Second, the 10.6 μ radiation cannot be transmitted through water or saline solution, and thus one needs a gas medium for distension of the joint. Argon laser, which emits in the blue-green region of the spectrum, has been used extensively for retinal detachment procedures because of its ability to coagulate vessels. Argon laser transmits through saline solution and would be ideal for arthroscopic application. Unfortunately, argon laser with adequate power for cutting a meniscus is not available. In the case of Nd:YAG laser, the input energy source is a xenon gas lamp encased in a gold-coated coupling cavity (Fig. 22–1). In the same cavity is also placed an Nd:YAG rod of optical quality that transmits the light from the xenon source into a columnated beam of 10.6 μ radiation. This beam can be coupled through the normal arthroscopic optics, it can be transmitted through saline solution, and it is capable of producing enough power to cut a meniscus.

Glick and Kapany have used Nd:YAG laser for cutting a bovine meniscus in vitro.[3] In their experiments, the bovine meniscus was suspended from hooks in a closed plastic model that was filled with either fluid or gas. Although the Nd:YAG laser could be transmitted through fluid, it did not cut the meniscus. It appeared that the heat necessary for cutting was dissipated in the fluid. A constant wave (CW) Nd:YAG laser was directed through a 600-μ glass fiber onto a bovine meniscus in an air-filled model. A bucket-handle tear of the meniscus was fashioned. The width and depth of cutting was 1 cm by 8 mm, respectively (Fig. 22–2). The cuts on each side took about 4 minutes and 45 seconds.

HF laser uses toxic materials and consequently is not used for medical purposes.

CLINICAL CONSIDERATIONS

At this stage of development, it appears that gas is necessary for joint distension, no matter which laser is used. Arthroscopic surgery in a gas medium does have advantages. For example, the distension of the joint by gas is superior to that by saline solution, and the field of vision is wide because the scope does not need to be placed so far into the joint to avoid the soft tissues that frequently block vision. Instrumentation is therefore easier because of less crowding. Cut pieces do not float away; thus, they are easier to retrieve. The dis-

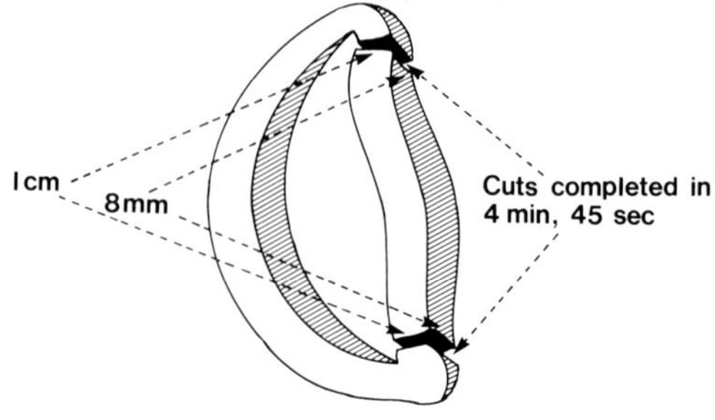

Fig. 22–2. Experimental cuts of bovine meniscus. See text for details.

advantages of a gas medium include smoke production during cutting and formation of black carbon deposits on the remaining tissue.

The type of gas used determines the amount of smoking and the deposition of carbon to some degree. CO_2 is most commonly used for distension of other organs in the body and can be used safely in joints. Smith[2] and Whipple and coauthors[4] have used nitrogen gas to minimize the problems of smoking and carbon formation. An important consideration in laser applications is its effect on surrounding tissues. To have a harmful effect, the laser beam must accidentally touch tissue such as the articular cartilage of the femoral condyle. Whipple has shown experimentally that the damage to the remaining tissues from the laser beam is minimal.[5] The beam penetrates mainly where it strikes. He also notes that healing occurs in cartilage penetrated by laser.

Using instrumentation for other surgical procedures, Smith performed meniscectomies by laser in 34 patients.[2] The procedures were difficult and slow, most likely because the instrument was not adapted for the joint. Smith inserted a 5-mm cannula in the popliteal space as an exhaust portal to clear the smoke. Once the laser instrument was in place, the cutting was precise.

The high cost of a laser system appears to be its main limitation. To be practical for arthroscopy a laser must offer the practitioner a simpler way of performing a surgical procedure. Despite the cost of a laser system, however, its possible advantages make it attractive for use in arthroscopic surgical procedures.

REFERENCES

1. Muncheryan, H.M.: Laser Technology. 2nd Edition. Indianapolis, Howard W. Sams, 1980.
2. Smith, J.B.: CO_2 laser energy for arthroscopic meniscus surgery: a preliminary report. Presented at the Annual Meeting of the Arthroscopic Association of America, January 28, 1983, Coronado, CA.
3. Glick, J.M., and Kapany, N.S.: Laser for potential use in arthroscopic surgery. Presented at the International Arthroscopy Association Meeting, August 29, 1981, Rio de Janeiro.
4. Whipple, T.L., Caspari, R.B., and Meyers, J.F.: Meniscectomy by CO_2 laser vaporization. Part I. Arthroscopic surgery in a gas medium. Presented at the International Arthroscopy Association Meeting, August 29, 1981, Rio de Janeiro.
5. Whipple, T.L.: Personal communication.

Index

Numbers in *italics* indicate figures; "t" following a page number indicates a table.

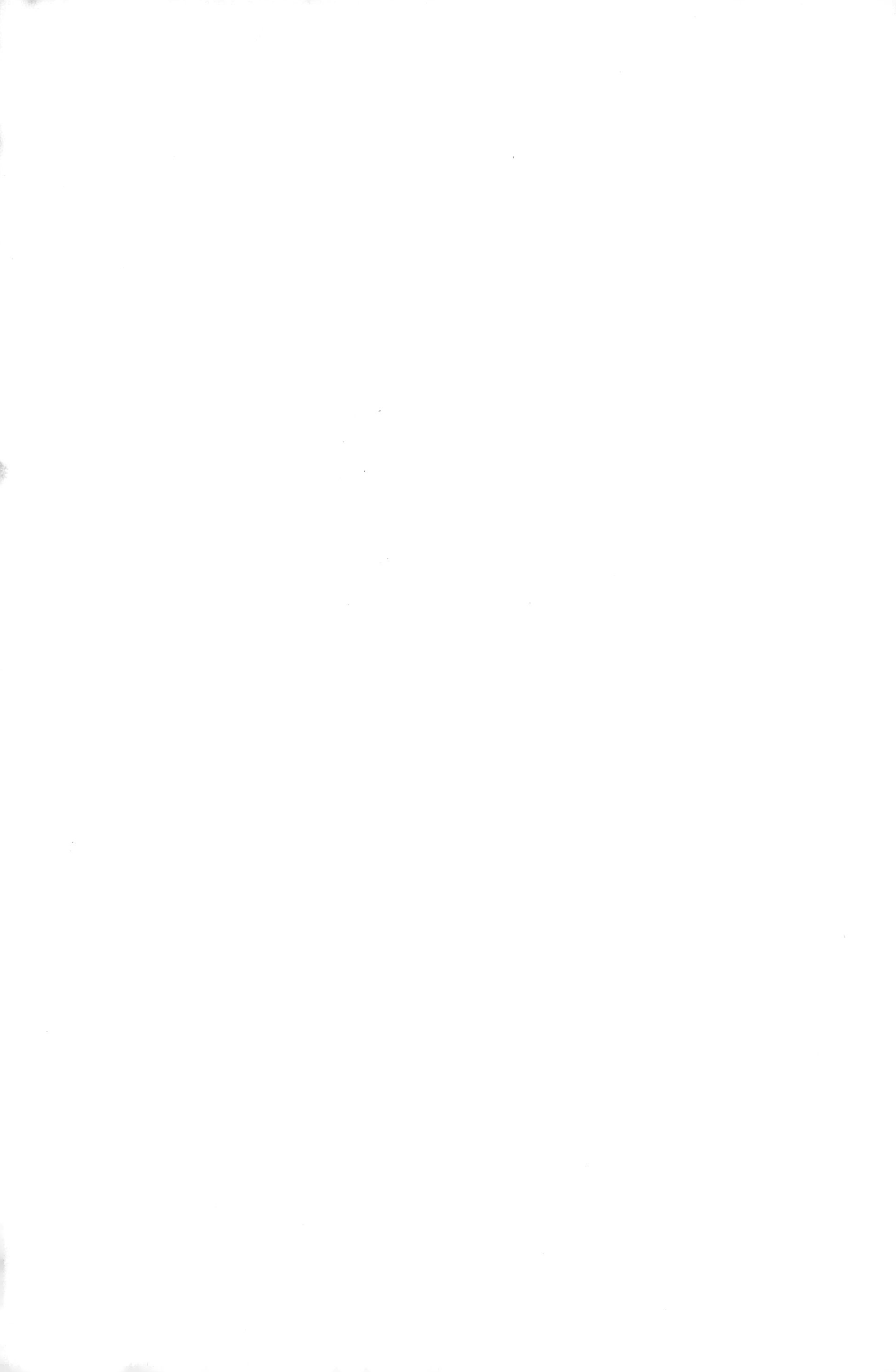